THE FAMILY GUIDE TO
SYMPTOMS &
SOLUTIONS

THE FAMILY GUIDE TO
SYMPTOMS &
SOLUTIONS

Gramercy Books
New York • Avenel

This 1997 edition is published by Gramercy Books,
a division of Random House Value Publishing, Inc.,
40 Engelhard Avenue, Avenel, New Jersey 07001,
by arrangement with Random House Reference &
Electronic Publishing Division.

Published previously as
The Lenox Hill Hospital Book of Symptoms and Solutions

Gramercy Books and colophon are trademarks of
Random House Value Publishing, Inc.

Random House
New York • Toronto • London • Sydney • Auckland
http://www.randomhouse.com/

Printed and bound in the United States

A CIP catalog record for this book is available from the Library of Congress

The Family Guide to Symptoms and Solutions
ISBN:0-517-18386-2
8 7 6 5 4 3 2 1

Contents

Acknowledgments

Many physicians, managers, trustees, auxilians, volunteers, and others at Lenox Hill Hospital have made significant contributions to the hospital's health education and community outreach programs over the years and participated in the development of various "House Call" brochures. We extend a special note of appreciation to a number of individuals who provided invaluable assistance in the preparation of this book. Many thanks to C. A. Wimpfheimer, Lenox Hill Hospital trustee, for his long and generous support of the Health Education Center and for his insights and guidance in connection with this project. Thanks to Michael F. Michelis, M.D., chairman of the Community Outreach Committee of the Medical Board, for a decade of leadership and for his steadfast commitment to public health education. Our sincere appreciation to Antony E. Pfaffle, M.D., in particular, and Roshni S. Samuel, M.D., chief medical residents, whose tireless research helped to ensure that the information in this book is as current as possible.

C.D.G.

Foreword

Progressive hospitals are no longer merely sites where people with acute illnesses come for inpatient treatment. Ambulatory care has grown dramatically, with many surgical procedures now being performed on an outpatient basis. Even when major surgery is required, presurgical testing is usually done prior to admission to help shorten the hospital stay. During hospitalization for both medical and surgical care, patient and family education in self-care can mean an earlier return home to an environment in which the patient can recuperate more comfortably and with less anxiety.

One of the most significant changes in hospitals has been their increasing commitment to public health education. This has resulted from the recognition that health care personnel must extend their reach beyond the hospital door in order to help people take better care of themselves—to reduce their risks and prevent disease, and to assure earlier diagnosis when illness occurs, so that it may be treated more effectively and at lower cost.

Lenox Hill Hospital was one of the first hospitals in the nation to take on this role of public health education when, in 1969, it launched its Community Outreach Program. At that time, the focus of the program was on the distribution of free brochures about illness prevention and self-care.

Since then, Lenox Hill Hospital has become a national leader in the provision of health information through one of the most comprehensive public health education programs offered to the public at no charge. Through its storefront Health Education Center, which celebrated its 20th anniversary in 1994, the program has impacted millions of people who live, work, or attend school in the greater New York area. The Lenox Hill Hospital Health Education Center has become the premier public health education facility in New York City, winning local and national recognition for excellence, and serving as a model for other health care institutions across the country.

The Health Education Center provides free health screenings and health information through counseling, lectures, literature, audiovisual programming, exhibits (at the Hospital and at various sites around New York City), and via the telephone. Of particular value for busy people has been the Hospital's unique array of telephone health information services. Tel-Med, the HealthLine, has received nearly two million calls since its inception in 1976. Callers select from more than 250 different subjects and listen to five- to ten-minute recordings on such topics as breast cancer, heart disease, smoking cessation, AIDS, relaxation techniques, and how to fall asleep without drugs.

This book reflects our quarter-century of experience as pioneers in helping Americans become more effective providers of their own preventive health care, as well as wiser consumers of professional health care services. We hope that *The Lenox Hill Hospital Book of Symptoms and Solutions* will bring this expertise to an ever wider audience and enhance the health of our nation.

Michael S. Bruno, M.D.
Director of Medicine
Past President of the Medical Board
Lenox Hill Hospital

Introduction

Lenox Hill Hospital is a nonprofit community and specialty care hospital in New York City. Founded in 1857, the 652-bed institution provides a wide range of inpatient medical, surgical, obstetric, pediatric, and psychiatric services. It also operates more than 60 outpatient clinics, a paramedic ambulance service and emergency department, a certified home health agency, and a number of ambulatory care programs. Special services include interventional cardiology and cardiovascular surgery, an exceptionally active obstetrics service, a high-risk neonatal care service, an AIDS center, a state-of-the-art ambulatory surgery center, and renal dialysis.

Lenox Hill Hospital is a major teaching institution. It has programs for undergraduate and graduate students in medical education and provides continuing education for its staff. The hospital is perhaps best known nationally for its innovative program of community health education. Its first efforts in this area began more than 25 years ago, leading the way for many other hospital outreach projects. In fact, over the years, Lenox Hill Hospital has won many awards as a national leader in health education.

Lenox Hill's health education program receives more than 175,000 queries annually, through telephone information service, a "storefront" walk-in health education center, workshops and lectures, and health fairs. To increase the availability of important health information, Lenox Hill Hospital developed its highly regarded "House Call" brochures, a unique series of easy-to-understand and scientifically reliable pamphlets that provide the information people need to make sensible decisions about their health.

This book was developed out of the pamphlets, the individual education services, and the input of staff physicians in each of the pertinent hospital departments. Thus the information provided is up to date and authoritative. It also simply and clearly answers the questions that people have most often put to us over the years about their bodies, their illnesses, and their health care.

Focusing on the conditions you are most likely to develop and worry about, *The Lenox Hill Hospital Book of Symptoms and Solutions*, first of all, tells you when you need a doctor's opinion and when you need emergency medical care. Then it provides the language you need to understand and explain your problem, information on the tests and treatment you are likely to require, and guidelines for self-care that may help in many circumstances, whether or not consulting a physician is necessary.

How to Use
This Book

Although some disorders can have wide impact throughout the body, most generate symptoms in just one body system. So disorders in this book are grouped by body system, such as "Heart, Blood Vessels, and Blood Disorders" and "Brain and Nerve Disorders."

In each of the 11 chapters, you will find three sections:

HOW THE SYSTEM WORKS
: A diagram of the body system, such as the cardiovascular or digestive system, and an explanation of its normal function, open each chapter. Such background is important, because when you know what normal function is you are in a better position to spot abnormal function.

SYMPTOMS AND SOLUTIONS
: When you develop a symptom of any kind, your immediate concern is often "Is this a crisis?" In the Symptoms and Solutions section, you will find a description of the most common symptoms afflicting that system, what disorders they might suggest, and clear guidelines on how to evaluate whether your situation

is an emergency and what to do right away. Boxes throughout this section highlight urgent problems and whether you should head for a hospital or just call your doctor for an appointment. You will also find tips on when to try self-care and, if so, what to do. All disorders mentioned in this section set in boldface and with page numbers given direct you to fuller discussions of the problem.

COMMON DISORDERS OF THE SYSTEM

For each of the most common disorders affecting the body system, you will find alphabetically listed entries with easy-to-understand answers to the following questions: What are the symptoms? How did I get it? How is it diagnosed? How is it treated? The self-care tips help you feel better or may help prevent the occurrence or worsening of the disorder.

THE FAMILY GUIDE TO
SYMPTOMS &
SOLUTIONS

1

Heart, Blood Vessel, and Blood Disorders

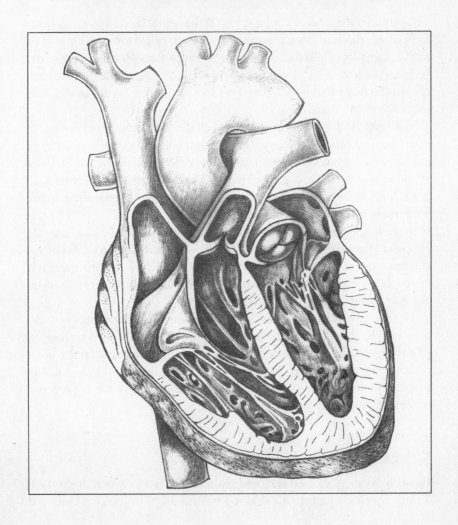

HOW THE CARDIOVASCULAR SYSTEM WORKS

The cardiovascular system—the heart and blood vessels—circulates blood through the body. We need this blood flow to supply cells with oxygen and nutrients, to remove waste from body tissues, and to maintain blood pressure and a steady body temperature. As only one example of how the system works, in warm weather, more blood is moved close to the skin to help keep us cool. In cold weather, more blood is moved into the core of the body to keep our vital organs warm.

THE HEART

The center of the cardiovascular system is the **heart.** Blood leaves the heart in large **arteries** that branch into smaller vessels called **arterioles** and then into still smaller **capillaries.** As the blood moves through these vessels, the body uses the oxygen and nutrients it contains. The blood then moves back toward the heart for reprocessing, flowing through the small **venules** that join to form the **veins.**

The heart is basically a blood pump, a cluster of muscles about the size of your fist. The pump has four chambers that are connected by a series of valves. Blood from the veins enters the **right atrium,** an upper heart chamber, and passes through the **tricuspid valve** into the **right ventricle,** a lower heart chamber. It is then pumped through the **pulmonic valve** to the **pulmonary artery** and on to the **lungs.**

In the lungs, the blood is revitalized; oxygen is added and carbon dioxide removed. After this process is complete, the blood returns to the heart via the **left atrium.** It passes through the **mitral valve** down into the **left ventricle.** Finally, blood is pumped through the **aortic valve** into the **aorta,** the main artery leading to the body.

The adult heart beats about 60 to 80 times a minute, pumping about five quarts of blood through the body. If any of the valves do not work properly, or if the heart muscle is weak, heart function may be impaired. If the heart does not pump adequately, or if the blood vessel network is blocked at any point along its path, the body may not receive enough of the oxygen and other nutrients it needs.

THE BLOOD

Blood is made up of blood cells and **plasma,** the fluid in which they travel. Taking up nearly half the total **blood volume** are three types of cells: **red**

blood cells, or **erythrocytes; white blood cells,** or **leukocytes; and plate-lets,** the smallest of the blood cells. One drop of blood contains more than 250 million blood cells.

The red blood cells carry oxygen and give blood its red color. The white blood cells are actually colorless and come in five forms: lymphocytes, neutrophils, eosinophils, basophils, and monocytes. These cells help protect the body from foreign substances and from infection. The platelets play an important role in normal blood clotting.

Blood cells are constantly being manufactured, primarily in the bone marrow, although white blood cells also are produced in the lymph nodes, spleen, thymus, and tonsils. The cells live from one week to several months. As they age, they are destroyed in the spleen or liver and are then disposed of through normal body waste. Any imbalance in the normal manufacture and destruction of blood components or any abnormality in the shape or function of blood cells may signal a blood disorder.

SYMPTOMS AND SOLUTIONS

CHEST PAIN

Chest pain is the symptom people most often associate with a heart attack. It can sometimes be an unmistakable signal but, unfortunately, **heart attack** (page 20) discomfort comes in several different forms and in several different locations.

Causes and Treatment of Chest Pain

Unfortunately, most people find it hard to believe they are having a heart attack. They take antacids, telling themselves the pain is indigestion. Or they decide to rest, thinking this is only muscle strain. Denial of this kind can lead to death. About half of all Americans who die of a heart attack each year do so before they get to the hospital, where prompt treatment may have saved their lives. Thrombolytic, or clot-busting, drugs given intrave-nously can dissolve the blood clots that cause most heart attacks, minimizing heart muscle damage.

Here's how to spot the pain of a heart attack:

Severity: It can vary from a mild ache to severe pain. People describe the sensation as pressure, tightness, burning, or crushing.

Location: Commonly at the center of the chest, the pain also may be felt

If there is even the suspicion that you may be having a heart attack, get emergency care immediately. This is especially urgent if you are over 35 years of age and experience a chest pain that lasts for more than two minutes.

• Call your doctor for instructions. Make it clear to whoever answers the doctor's phone that **this is an emergency**.
• If you can't reach your doctor immediately, call an ambulance. Again, make it clear that this is an emergency.
• If someone can get you to a hospital faster by car or taxi, get going. Don't try to go by yourself. You may collapse on the way.
• While waiting for help, remain quiet.
• Sit up rather than lie down.
• Take nothing to eat or drink.
• Take no medication unless it was previously prescribed and is urgently important or you are told to do so by your physician or emergency medical personnel.

higher up, under the breastbone, or lower, in the abdomen. It can be localized in one area, or it may spread to the neck, jaw, or the arms. Sometimes the pain is felt only in the back, shoulder, or neck.

Duration: The pain may last for hours, or it may go away in five minutes and then return minutes or even hours later.

Related Symptoms: Along with chest pain, any of the following may occur: sweating, shortness of breath, dizziness, faintness, weakness, pallor, nausea, vomiting, palpitations, an irregular heartbeat, a fluttering sensation in the chest, a feeling of impending doom.

Heart attack is not the only potentially life-threatening cause of chest pain. Chest pain in conjunction with sudden difficulty in breathing or a cough, or that worsens when you inhale, may signal a respiratory problem (see Chapter 3).

Other causes of chest pain may not be life threatening.

Chest pain may signal **angina** (page 14), another indicator that the heart is not getting enough oxygen and that severe **atherosclerosis** (page 17) puts you at risk for a heart attack.

Chest pain that worsens when you bend over or lie down, especially shortly after a meal, may be caused by stomach acid that has backed up into your esophagus—a condition known as heartburn or **reflux** (page 178). Taking an antacid eases the discomfort quickly.

Chest pain also may be caused by severe stress or anxiety, such as that provoked by panic attacks.

EDEMA

Fluid retention in body tissue causes the abnormal swelling that is called **edema.** This condition is not a disease itself but rather a signal that something is amiss. Though swelling of the lower legs and ankles is commonly associated with heart disease, edema can occur anywhere in the body as a result of an injury, illness, or other causes.

> If you have repeated episodes of leg or ankle swelling, or if you can't explain even a single episode of swelling by any of the lifestyle causes discussed in this section, call your physician. This is especially important if you are also short of breath. Describe what is happening so that the doctor can decide whether you should be seen immediately.

Causes and Treatment of Edema

Heart, kidney, liver, and other problems can cause edema. In **heart failure** (page 21), where the heart fails to pump adequately, water is retained by the body, most commonly in the lower legs or ankles. This sometimes leads to a weight gain of 10 to 15 pounds or more.

Not all edema is caused by serious illness.

Swollen feet and ankles are quite common in salespersons, mail carriers, cashiers, and others who are on their feet a lot. The problem usually can be controlled by changing your daily habits. Take hourly breaks. Sit down if you can, and raise your feet for a few minutes before going back to work.

Ankles sometimes swell because of something constricting the upper legs. Tight garters, rolled stockings, or tight underwear may cause the condition. Simply don't wear them anymore, and you will probably get rid of the edema.

The hormonal changes accompanying menstruation, pregnancy, and the use of oral contraceptives can be responsible for edema. The premenstrual swelling of the breasts and other parts of the body that women experience almost always disappears with the onset of menstruation. Some women find that cutting down on salt during this time is a help. If the problem is severe, your physician may prescribe diuretics.

Some swelling of the feet and ankles is common during pregnancy. However, always tell your doctor about any swelling because excessive fluid retention may be a signal that other problems are developing.

Birth control pills are another source of troublesome edema. Sometimes a change of brand can alleviate the problem.

Eating too much salt may cause edema in both normal people and those with special health problems. Because salt tends to hold water in the body, restricting salt intake is frequently advised and is sometimes vital for people with edema. To cut back on salt, reduce your use of prepared foods containing salt and don't use salt in cooking. You get more salty taste from less salt when you add it at the table.

PALPITATIONS

The perception of a rapid or irregular heartbeat is called **palpitation.** Episodes of palpitation can feel like a fluttering or a pounding of the heart. Palpitations are only one of many different types of **arrhythmias** (page 16) that can signal heart problems.

If palpitations continue for more than a few minutes, recur frequently, or are associated with chest pain, dizziness, or shortness of breath, call your physician. Even if there are no other associated symptoms, call your physician if palpitations cannot be explained by the lifestyle causes discussed in this section. Describe what is happening so that the doctor can decide whether you should be seen immediately.

Causes and Treatment of Palpitations

Palpitations can be a sign of heart disease or of **hyperthyroidism** (page 248). But not all palpitations are caused by serious illness.

Excessive intake of caffeine can cause palpitations in some people. If this happens to you, cut down on coffee, tea, chocolate, and cola beverages.

Use of alcohol can suddenly cause palpitations. If this happens to you, cut down or eliminate your use of alcoholic beverages.

Anxiety can also trigger palpitations. Some people notice abnormal heartbeats when they get into bed at night and review the day's events or worry about what tomorrow will bring. Meditation, a regular exercise program, and other stress-relieving techniques may help you learn how to control stress.

GENERAL FATIGUE AND WEAKNESS; PALE SKIN AND GUMS; SHORTNESS OF BREATH, ESPECIALLY AFTER EXERTION; SWOLLEN LYMPH NODES

General fatigue and weakness, pale skin and gums, and so on are called constitutional symptoms because they cause problems throughout the whole body, rather than in just one organ. For example, skin and gums may be pale because of a shortage of red blood cells. Although the problem affects blood throughout the body, its effects are more easily seen in the skin and gums.

> If these symptoms cannot be explained by lifestyle causes discussed in this section, call your physician. Describe what is happening so that the doctor can decide whether you should be seen immediately.

Causes and Treatment of Constitutional Symptoms

General fatigue and weakness, pale skin and gums, and shortness of breath may be signs of **heart failure** (page 21), **heart valve disease** (page 22), **cardiomyopathy** (page 19), or **anemia** (page 10).

When constitutional symptoms occur with swollen lymph nodes—most noticeable when you have uncomfortable swellings below the jaw, under the arms, or in the groin—they may be a sign of **leukemia** (page 31) or **Hodgkin's disease** (page 25).

Simple problems in your lifestyle may cause one or two of these symptoms, but are not likely to cause the whole cluster at once. For example, a lack of sunshine will cause pale skin but not pale gums. Overwork may cause general fatigue. Overweight may cause fatigue, weakness, and even intermittent shortness of breath, signaling that your heart has to work too hard to carry your weight around. Anxiety may cause shortness of breath, especially during a panic attack. An infection may cause fatigue and swollen lymph glands.

Even if you think you know why the symptoms are occurring, you shouldn't live with them. Take steps to change your life, and get your doctor's help in eliminating the problem.

LEG PAIN

Few people associate leg pain with heart or blood problems, but, indeed, they can be linked.

> If leg pain cannot be explained by muscle strain or an injury, call your physician. Describe what is happening so that the doctor can decide whether you should be seen immediately.

Causes and Treatment of Leg Pain

Aching legs may be expected if you have just started a new exercise program and have gone too fast or have not stretched beforehand in order to avoid "charley horse."

However, if you have pain during exercise but it disappears within a few minutes of standing still, it may be **intermittent claudication** (page 30), a warning sign of **atherosclerosis** (page 17) that warrants medical attention.

In the absence of exercise, deep pain, swelling, and tenderness in the legs may indicate **phlebitis** (page 33), an inflammation of a vein that requires an immediate call to your physician.

Varicose veins (page 36) also may cause leg pain that should not be ignored. If not treated, varicose veins can lead to serious infections and ulcers.

"SYMPTOMLESS" PROBLEMS

Some of the most serious heart and blood vessel problems may develop without warning. You may have no symptoms until a crisis occurs. For example, **hypertension** (page 27) and **hyperlipidemia** (page 26) may cause no problems until a **heart attack** (page 20) or **stroke** (page 71) occurs. For this reason, all adults should have their blood pressure and cholesterol levels evaluated at least once every two years—more often if your personal or family history indicates that this is advisable.

COMMON DISORDERS OF THE CARDIOVASCULAR SYSTEM

ANEMIA is a term that describes a variety of disorders characterized by a reduction in blood cells, especially the red blood cells. These cells are important because they contain hemoglobin, a protein that carries oxygen through the body. Normally, the body constantly produces new blood cells and destroys old ones in the spleen. Anything interfering with that process

THE HEART-HEALTHY LIFESTYLE

Your heredity, gender, race, and age may put you at risk for heart disease. Such factors cannot be changed, but many risk factors are related to your lifestyle and can be modified. Not only can a healthy lifestyle help prevent heart disease, recent studies have shown that it may be able to halt or even reverse atherosclerosis, the deposit of plaque on artery walls that leads to heart attacks. Here's how to take action for a healthier heart.

If you smoke, quit. The risk of heart disease may be as much as 300 percent greater for the heavy cigarette smoker. Within a few years after giving up the habit, the ex-smoker appears to be at no greater risk than the nonsmoker.

Eat a diet low in cholesterol and total fat, especially saturated fat. Cholesterol is found in animal foods, and your body also makes cholesterol from fat. Too much cholesterol in the blood increases risk of atherosclerosis. Have your serum cholesterol checked annually. If it is 200 or over, reduce your intake of meat, whole milk and cheese, butter, and eggs. Eat more fish, poultry, and monounsaturated vegetable oils, such as olive oil.

If you are overweight, reduce. Too much weight makes your heart work harder and increases your risk of hypertension and diabetes. Even if you can't get down to your ideal weight, losing 10 or 15 pounds can improve your health.

Exercise regularly to strengthen your heart muscle, help maintain ideal weight, prevent or control high blood pressure and diabetes, and improve the balance of good versus bad cholesterol in your blood. Gradually build up to a regimen of 30 minutes to an hour, three to four times a week, of such aerobic exercises as walking or jogging.

Reduce stress. Slow down and learn to take life a little easier. Make time every day for quiet recreation—gardening, handicrafts, reading, or playing with a pet. Learn how to relax. If stress is a special problem, take 20 minutes a day to practice a relaxation technique, such as meditation, deep breathing, or self-hypnosis.

If you have hypertension or diabetes, in addition to your doctor's recommendations, carefully follow a self-care regimen to keep your blood pressure and blood sugar levels as close to normal as possible.

can cause anemia. Some types of anemia can be fatal, especially if they are not treated promptly. However, effective treatment can cure or control most types of anemia.

What are the symptoms?
The various types of anemia have diverse specific symptoms. However, the following symptoms are common to most types: pale skin and gums; general fatigue and weakness; shortness of breath, especially after exertion; and/or rapid heartbeat.

How did I get it?
The cause depends on the type of anemia you have. Here are the most common types and their cause:

• *Iron-deficiency anemia* occurs when there is insufficient iron to manufacture hemoglobin. It may be caused by lack of iron in the diet; an inability to absorb the iron in food properly; pregnancy; some cancers; or chronic blood loss from an ulcer, heavy menstruation, or other problems.
• *Hemolytic anemia* occurs when red blood cells are destroyed more rapidly than normal. It may be hereditary or can be caused by abnormal spleen function, tumors, severe hypertension, leukemia, infectious diseases, or autoimmune disorders.
• *Sickle-cell anemia* occurs when abnormal hemoglobin produces deformed red blood cells, which are prematurely destroyed. The abnormal cells can block small blood vessels. It is an inherited disease that occurs most commonly among blacks.
• *Pernicious anemia* is caused by a deficiency in vitamin B_{12}. When seen in countries where there is not widespread famine, it is most often caused by autoimmune disorders. It also may arise from faulty metabolism, the toxic effects of certain drugs, dietary inadequacy, especially among vegetarians, or other problems.
• *Cooley's anemia* also involves defective hemoglobin and is potentially fatal. It is an inherited disorder.
• *Aplastic anemia*, a relatively rare condition, occurs when red blood cell production is lower than normal, although the cells themselves are usually normal. It may be caused by inherited problems, certain infections and viral illnesses, or exposure to chemical or radiation damage. However, the cause of about half of all cases of aplastic anemia is unknown.

How is it diagnosed?
A battery of blood tests to evaluate the quality, volume, and number of red blood cells and hemoglobin, as well as white blood cells and platelets, are performed. Additional tests, including bone marrow biopsy, may be necessary to help evaluate the cause of the anemia.

How is it treated?
If a treatable underlying cause like infection can be found, therapy to cure that problem can cure the anemia. In iron-deficiency anemia, improving the diet and taking iron supplements may be the cure. In pernicious anemia, vitamin B_{12} injections treat the condition effectively. For those cases with autoimmune disorders, hemolytic anemia may be controlled by immune suppressive drugs, for example, prednisone or azathioprine. Or removal of the spleen, where red blood cells are destroyed, may be indicated. Those with sickle-cell anemia and Cooley's anemia require frequent blood transfusions throughout life. In primary aplastic anemia, bone marrow transplantation is the only effective treatment.

Self-Care: If you are diagnosed with a type of anemia related to diet, you may find it useful to consult a registered dietitian to learn healthier eating habits.

ANEURYSM is an outward bulge in the wall of a blood vessel. Although it may occur anywhere in the body, the most worrisome site is the aorta, the major artery that carries blood from the heart. Aortic aneurysms most commonly occur either in the chest or abdomen. An aneurysm can also arise in the heart, where it can cause arrhythmias and heart failure. An aneurysm can disturb local blood flow and increase the risk of blood clot formation, leading to a heart attack or stroke. If an aneurysm ruptures, blood escapes from the circulatory system and the supply of blood to tissues beyond the aneurysm site is cut off. A major aortic rupture can cause circulatory collapse and death if not treated immediately. Of the several different types of aneurysms, those called dissecting—because the inner and outer layers of the artery split apart and blood gets between the layers—are the most prone to rupture.

What are the symptoms?
In the chest, an aneurysm may not cause any symptoms. In other cases, it may cause chest pain, hoarseness, a cough, difficulty in swallowing, or

shortness of breath. A dissecting aneurysm can cause chest pain similar to a heart attack, as well as a tearing sensation. In the abdomen, an aneurysm often can be seen just under the skin as a small throbbing lump that is tender to the touch; it may cause loss of appetite and weight. A dissecting aneurysm in the abdomen is rare but causes severe pain.

How did I get it?

The most common cause of an aortic aneurysm is atherosclerosis, the plaque deposits that weaken arterial walls. Aneurysms are also more common in people with hypertension. Left ventricular aneurysms usually develop as a result of a heart attack. However, an aneurysm may also be caused by arterial injury; an inflammatory disease, such as infectious endocarditis; or syphilis. The tendency to develop an aneurysm also may be inherited.

How is it diagnosed?

An aneurysm can be difficult to diagnose, and it may produce no symptoms until it ruptures. If you have symptoms suggestive of an aneurysm, your doctor will probably require chest X-rays, an echocardiogram, and perhaps a CAT scan.

How is it treated?

If you have hypertension, your doctor will prescribe medications to lower your blood pressure and reduce the risk of rupture. If the aneurysm is large or growing, surgery may be recommended, although some aneurysms are not amenable to surgery. Ventricular aneurysms, which cause heart failure or arrhythmias, and fail to respond to drug therapy, also may require surgical removal. A ruptured aneurysm requires emergency surgery to prevent you from bleeding to death.

> Self-Care: If you have an aneurysm, get frequent checkups to monitor the condition and carefully follow the regimen prescribed by your doctor.

ANGINA is an episode of chest pain related to an inadequate supply of oxygen to the heart. It usually is precipitated by physical exertion or some other type of stress and disappears when the exertion is stopped. Although angina may feel like a heart attack, it is not. However, the first incidence of angina or any change in a prior angina pattern must be evaluated by a doctor promptly. Although the arterial changes that cause angina also contribute to heart attacks, and some people with a history of angina eventually have heart attacks, effective treatment of angina, including lifestyle change, can lower this risk.

What are the symptoms?
Angina is described as pressure, tightness, or a burning sensation in the chest. Sometimes it radiates to the neck, jaws, arms, and upper back.

How did I get it?
Angina is caused by an inadequate supply of blood to the heart muscle, most often due to atherosclerosis, which narrows the arteries leading to the heart. When this happens, it is harder for blood—with the oxygen and other nutrients it carries—to reach the heart. When the work of the heart is increased—by exercise, emotional tension, a large meal, very cold weather, or other factors—and is not accompanied by the normal increase in blood flow, angina may occur.

How is it diagnosed?
If you experience chest pain upon exertion, you probably will be referred to a cardiologist for a complete examination, including an electrocardiogram (EKG) and an exercise stress test. If you develop chest pain during the test, you may be given a tablet of nitroglycerin to place under your tongue. Disappearance of the pain as the tablet dissolves will help confirm a diagnosis of angina. In some cases, your doctor may recommend an angiogram—a "moving-picture" X-ray taken after a dye is injected into the blood vessels—to assess blockage in the coronary arteries.

How is it treated?
The first immediate step in treating angina will probably be a prescription for nitroglycerin and directions for its use at the first sign of pain. Nitroglycerin causes the blood vessels to expand temporarily, allowing more blood to reach the heart. Nitroglycerin is safe and not habit forming. Some doctors recommend that you take it before exertion to prevent angina. Your doctor also will evaluate you for other heart risks, such as hypertension and high blood cholesterol, and will recommend a heart-healthy lifestyle. You also may be given other medications to take daily to help relax your blood vessels.

In some cases of severe angina, your doctor may recommend angioplasty, a technique that opens blocked arteries with a fluid-filled balloon. If you have more than one or two artery blockages, cardiac bypass surgery may be recommended. In such surgery, the blocked arteries around the heart are bypassed and new blood vessels, taken from elsewhere in the body, are inserted to carry blood to the heart.

Self-Care: Follow a heart-healthy lifestyle (page 11) to help halt or reverse the atherosclerosis that contributes to angina. The following steps may decrease your pain episodes:

• Avoid anything that brings on angina attacks, including more physical exertion or emotional stress than you can handle.
• Eat five light meals a day, rather than three full ones, and rest after each meal.
• If you smoke, stop. Smoking further constricts the blood vessels of your heart.
• If you are overweight, reduce to lessen the burden on your heart.
• Avoid going out in extremely cold weather.

ARRHYTHMIAS are abnormalities in the normal heart rate—about 60 to 80 beats per minute in adults. Bradycardia is a slower than normal heartbeat; severe bradycardia of fewer than 30 beats per minute can be life threatening. Tachycardia is a faster than normal heartbeat. Atrial fibrillation is a very severe form of tachycardia in which the atria, the upper chambers of the heart, beat very irregularly at 300 to 600 beats per minute, while the ventricles, the lower chambers of the heart, beat irregularly at 170 to 200 beats per minute. The heart does not fill with blood properly or pump blood effectively. This disorder tends to come and go, although the fibrillation may become chronic. The worst type of tachycardia is ventricular fibrillation. Normal beating ceases and the heart quivers. Normal rhythm must be restored within a few minutes, or cardiac arrest and death may result.

What are the symptoms?
Bradycardia often has no symptoms. However, if the heart is so slowed that it can no longer pump blood adequately, you may experience fatigue, shortness of breath, lightheadedness, or fainting. These symptoms are most likely to occur upon exertion. Tachycardia and atrial fibrillation cause palpitations that feel like a sudden, rapid, fluttering sensation in the chest. You also may feel weak, faint, nauseous, lightheaded, anxious, or short of breath.

How did I get it?
Bradycardia may be caused by atherosclerosis, congenital heart disease, a heart attack, or as a complication of thyroid problems, gastrointestinal disorders, jaundice, or drug abuse. It also may be a side effect of drug treatment for hypertension, glaucoma, or other problems. Minor tachy-

cardia may occur as a result of anxiety or excessive consumption of caffeine. More severe tachycardia may be caused by a heart attack, atherosclerosis, electrical disturbances in the heart, heart valve disease, congenital heart defects, or as a complication of thyroid or lung problems. Atrial fibrillation most commonly is caused by atherosclerosis, hypertension, or rheumatic valve disease. It also occurs in people with chronic obstructive lung disease or hyperthyroidism.

How is it diagnosed?

The presence of an abnormal heartbeat can be diagnosed by taking the pulse, listening to the heart with a stethoscope, or an electrocardiogram. However, because atrial fibrillation often comes and goes, your heartbeat may be normal when you are in the doctor's office, only to speed up the next day. Thus your doctor may prescribe use of a portable monitor to provide a continuous record of your heartbeat over a 24-hour period.

How is it treated?

Bradycardia is treated only if symptoms occur. If medications do not normalize the heartbeat sufficiently, a pacemaker may be implanted. You may be able to control minor tachycardia, caused by anxiety, simply by holding your breath for a minute or splashing your face with cold water. Chronic tachycardia often requires medication to slow the heartbeat. If you have atrial fibrillation, you also will be given anticoagulation medication to reduce risk of blood clots. When tachycardia is severe and fibrillation occurs, electroconversion—the administration of an electric shock to the heart—is essential to return the heart to a normal rate. A pacemaker may then be needed for long-term treatment.

> Self-Care: A rapid heartbeat after physical exertion is normal, and you probably know that sensation. It is not uncommon to experience mild palpitations if you drink too much coffee or when you are anxious. However, if palpitations persist or occur in the absence of environmental triggers, call your doctor right away.

ATHEROSCLEROSIS, also called hardening of the arteries, is a condition in which the walls of the arteries become thickened and lose elasticity. Arteries throughout your body may be affected, diminishing the blood supply in areas served by those vessels. Atherosclerosis of the coronary arteries, which supply the heart, can cause angina and heart attack. In the brain, the disease can cause stroke. In the kidneys, it can cause kidney failure. When the legs are affected, walking can become painful and limb loss may occur.

What are the symptoms?

Most people don't know they have this condition until they develop one of the complications of advanced atherosclerosis. These include angina, shortness of breath, heart attack, difficulty in walking, stroke, or memory loss or other signs of dementia.

How did I get it?

All blood vessels lose a certain amount of elasticity as we age. However, the serious hardening of atherosclerosis is caused by a buildup of fatty deposits, called plaque, on the inner lining of artery walls. The primary component of plaque is cholesterol. Although heredity plays a role in the development of plaque, cholesterol and fat in your diet are major contributors. Other factors that contribute to artery wall injury or plaque buildup are smoking, diabetes, hypertension, and a sedentary lifestyle.

How is it diagnosed?

Doctors can make certain presumptions about atherosclerosis based on an exercise stress test. If your doctor is concerned that your atherosclerosis may be life threatening, an angiogram may be recommended to show blockages clearly.

How is it treated?

Treatment depends on the site and degree of atherosclerosis. The first line of treatment, no matter what else is eventually done, is modification of your lifestyle. This alone may halt or reverse atherosclerosis. In addition, your doctor may prescribe medication: an aspirin daily to help prevent blood clots from forming in your clogged arteries, and drugs to help lower blood cholesterol if a strict diet fails to bring you to a healthy level. In severe cases of atherosclerosis, invasive procedures may be needed. Angioplasty to widen narrowed blood vessels or cardiac bypass surgery to open new pathways to the heart is sometimes necessary.

Self-Care: If your lifestyle is not a heart-healthy one (page 11), turn over a new leaf, especially by improving your diet. If you are over 35 years old, see your doctor for a complete checkup, including a stress test, before starting a new exercise regimen.

CARDIOMYOPATHY is a disease of the heart muscle. In primary cardiomyopathy, the muscle's structure or function changes without any known cause. In secondary cardiomyopathy, the muscle change is caused by an identifiable disease. Primary problems include congestive cardiomyopathy, in which the heart enlarges, weakens, and no longer pumps effectively, resulting in an increased risk of blood clots; hypertrophic cardiomyopathy, in which the heart muscle thickens and may impede blood flow through the heart; and restrictive cardiomyopathy, in which the heart muscle wall stiffens. Secondary problems include alcoholic cardiomyopathy, in which the muscle is believed to be damaged by thiamine deficiency; and viral cardiomyopathy. Unless a treatable cause is identified and therapy provided, cardiomyopathy may lead to heart failure, arrhythmias, blood clots, heart attack, stroke, and other problems. Sudden death is more common among younger people with hypertrophic cardiomyopathy.

What are the symptoms?
Fatigue and shortness of breath are the most common symptoms. In some cases, chest pain, dizziness, and palpitations may occur. Except when cardiomyopathy is associated with an infection, symptoms usually develop slowly.

How did I get it?
The most common underlying problem appears to be atherosclerosis. Some types of cardiomyopathy have specific causes, such as alcoholism. In most cases, though, no cause can be diagnosed.

How is it diagnosed?
Your doctor will require several tests to identify cardiomyopathy and try to determine its cause. These may include an EKG, chest X-ray, echocardiogram, angiogram, and myocardial biopsy.

How is it treated?
If you have secondary cardiomyopathy and a cause is identified and treated, further heart damage may be halted. Drugs also may be prescribed to decrease the heart's workload, regulate the heartbeat, and help prevent blood clot formation and excess fluid accumulation in the body. In congestive and dilated cardiomyopathy, the effectiveness of therapy may decrease over time. In some cases of restrictive cardiomyopathy, surgery is necessary to replace damaged valves or to thin thickened areas. If life-threatening heart failure develops, heart transplantation may be an option.

Self-Care: To help your heart function at its best, avoid excess alcohol and stress and get adequate nutrition and sleep.

HEART ATTACK occurs when the heart fails to receive an adequate blood supply and is deprived of the oxygen and other nutrients carried by blood. The particular area that has been deprived is damaged. That part of the heart muscle is called the infarct. When the infarct is small and does not interfere with the heart's electrical system, you have only a minor to moderate attack and probably will recover fully. When the infarct is large or damages the heart's electrical system, there is a greater likelihood that the attack may be fatal. This occurs in about one-third of all heart attacks. The severity of the attack depends on the cause and the duration of the impaired blood supply. A heart attack is also known as a myocardial infarction or coronary thrombosis.

What are the symptoms?
The primary symptom of a heart attack is pain in the center of the chest that lasts longer than a few minutes. The pain—described as a sense of fullness, pressure, or squeezing—may spread to the shoulders, neck, or arms. In addition to pain, you may experience dizziness, sweating, shortness of breath, pallor, nausea, or vomiting. The symptoms may arise, disappear, and then return, or they may be constant.

How did I get it?
The primary underlying cause of heart attack is atherosclerosis—arteries that have been narrowed by the buildup of fatty plaques. Then, in most cases, a blood clot becomes lodged in one of the coronary arteries, blocking the flow of blood. In some cases, no clot is present; rather, a critical artery goes into spasm and the constriction blocks the blood supply. Such spasms may occur for no known reason, although cocaine use is known to cause them. The site of the clot or spasm determines what part of the heart will be deprived of blood and oxygen.

How is it diagnosed?
Your doctor will diagnose heart attack based on your description of your symptoms and by checking your pulse and blood pressure, listening to your heartbeat with a stethoscope, and taking an electrocardiogram (EKG). The diagnosis can be confirmed six hours later by blood tests that reveal an increase in certain enzymes. However, it is likely that therapy will be started immediately without waiting for confirmation.

How is it treated?

If you arrive at the hospital early in the attack, you may be given one of the new thrombolytic drugs that dissolve blood clots and effectively halt the heart attack, thus limiting damage to the heart muscle. (In some communities, the drugs may be started in the ambulance by paramedics who are in radio contact with a physician at the hospital.) These drugs are given intravenously, and you must be carefully monitored for potential adverse effects, especially excessive bleeding. You also are given medication to alleviate pain, anticoagulants to decrease the risk of more clots, and other drugs to reduce the workload of the heart. If abnormal heart rhythms occur, drugs are administered to stabilize the heartbeat. If your heart stops, it is electrically stimulated to restart it. You will probably recuperate from the attack in the hospital's coronary care unit. In the aftermath of a heart attack, your doctor may recommend an angiogram to evaluate the extent of atherosclerosis in the coronary arteries. If only a few localized obstructions are found, angioplasty may be done to open them. Angioplasty involves the insertion and inflation of a balloon to compress the plaque and widen the artery channel. If multiple severe obstructions are found, cardiac bypass surgery may be recommended.

> Self-Care: Rehabilitation after a heart attack may require drastic changes to a heart-healthy lifestyle (page 11) in order to reduce risk of further attacks.

HEART FAILURE is a frightening term. It sounds like a condition in which the heart suddenly stops forever. That's not the case. Rather, the term refers to the heart's diminished capacity to properly do its job of pumping blood through the body. When the heart is unable to pump sufficient blood to meet the body's needs, there is a diminished blood flow to all the body's tissues. Also known as congestive heart failure (CHF), this is one of the more common illnesses of the heart. If left untreated, it can lead to death. However, if you get early treatment, normal activities may be possible for many years.

What are the symptoms?

Although heart failure can occur suddenly, it most often develops slowly, with symptoms manifested gradually. No pain occurs. The most important warning sign is edema—the retention of fluid in the body. When the heart fails to pump effectively, blood backs up in the veins. Fluids also build up in the body tissues because poor blood circulation fails to perform its cleanup role. This is the "congestive" aspect of CHF. As extra fluid collects throughout the body, you may notice puffiness of all extremities. Most noticeable, however, is swelling in the ankles after you have been standing. When you recline, fluid settles in your chest, especially the lungs. You may have difficulty in breathing, or breathing may be accompanied by a rattling sound. Or you may feel a heaviness in your chest when lying down. Coughing or shortness of breath may interrupt sleep, with temporary relief only when you sit upright. You also may experience an overall feeling of fatigue and weakness.

How did I get it?
Many different diseases can weaken the heart's ability to pump. Most common are atherosclerosis, abnormalities of the heart valves, infection of the heart, and congenital malformation of the heart. In many cases, treatment of the underlying cause provides excellent relief from CHF.

How is it diagnosed?
A complete examination and special tests are necessary. Key elements will be an EKG, a chest X-ray—possibly revealing an enlarged heart—and the doctor's listening for certain sounds in your chest as you breathe.

How is it treated?
To reduce the workload of the heart, temporary bed rest may be an important first step. Obese patients will be encouraged to lose weight. Medications like digitalis can strengthen the heart muscle's pumping action. They increase cardiac output and slow the heart rate. Water and salt balance are controlled by diet changes and, sometimes, by diuretic medications. These help the kidneys to get rid of excess salt and water. Finally, your doctor will seek to identify and treat the underlying cause of your CHF. Once the CHF is under control, you usually are able to return to normal activity, unless there are other complicating factors.

> Self-Care: Your daily activities have a critical impact on your treatment. You have to reduce the amount of salt you eat and cut back on physical exertion. If you are overweight, you must reduce. Other measures will be related to the underlying cause of the heart failure.

HEART VALVE DISEASE is any disorder in the function of the four valves that control blood flow into and around the heart. A stenosed valve is abnormally narrow, and a sufficient amount of blood cannot move through it with each beat. An incompetent valve does not close properly, and some blood moving through it regurgitates or leaks back into the prior heart chamber with each beat. In either case, the heart must work much harder to pump adequate blood. The muscular wall of one or more chambers may thicken. The resulting heart enlargement means the heart needs more oxygenated blood to do its job. One common type of incompetence is mitral valve prolapse, where one or both of the flaps that open and close to form the valve bulge into the left atrium during each heart beat. Mitral valve prolapse may cause a clicking sound that can be heard by the physician as blood regurgitates. Some heart valve problems cause vibrations in blood movement called a heart murmur. Some heart valve disorders present no problems, but others can increase your risk of abnormal heart rhythm, heart failure, heart attack, stroke, and heart infection.

What are the symptoms?
Many heart valve problems, especially mitral prolapse and most other types of incompetence, cause few if any symptoms, particularly in their early stages. More advanced cases of incompetence and mitral stenosis may cause shortness of breath, angina, fatigue, and other symptoms of heart failure. Pulmonic valve problems cause pale skin and cold hands and feet. Tricuspid problems can cause an uncomfortable fluttering sensation in the neck. Aortic stenosis may cause dizziness and even fainting, especially upon exertion.

How did I get it?
Most heart valve disorders, especially aortic stenosis and incompetence, are congenital (present at birth). Mitral stenosis is almost always caused by rheumatic fever. Mitral incompetence may also be caused by a heart attack. Tricuspid valve disorders almost invariably occur only in conjunction with other heart valve or lung problems.

How is it diagnosed?
Some signs of heart valve disorders, such as a heart murmur heard through a stethoscope, may be detectable during a physical examination. A complete evaluation is likely to include a chest X-ray, an electrocardiogram, an echocardiogram, cardiac catheterization, and coronary arteriography.

How is it treated?
Mild heart valve problems may not need treatment. Others may require only medication to help prevent blood clot formation, to slow the heart rate, to

avoid arrhythmias, or to decrease fluid buildup in the body. More severe problems may require surgery to repair or replace the valve. Some valve problems present life-threatening emergencies and require immediate surgery.

Self-Care: Most people with mitral heart valve problems are advised to take antibiotics prophylactically before surgery or certain kinds of dental work to prevent infections.

HEMOPHILIA is excessive bleeding due to abnormalities in your body's ability to form blood clots. The condition only affects males. Hemophilia is a chronic disease that cannot be cured. If not treated properly, a person with hemophilia may bleed to death from even a minor injury. Although hemophilia was once often a fatal disease, current therapies markedly reduce such risks.

What are the symptoms?
Although milder forms of hemophilia may not appear until adulthood, symptoms usually show up in infancy or childhood. For example, parents may notice that the youngster bruises very easily and bleeds for a long time from even a minor cut. A fall may lead to internal bleeding and severe swelling, which can be especially painful if the bleeding occurs in a joint.

How did I get it?
Hemophilia is a genetic disorder. Although it may occur as a result of genetic mutations, it is most commonly inherited. Women carry the genes that cause the disorder, but they do not suffer with the disease. Rather, they pass the defective genes on to their sons. As a result, the boys lack Factor VIII, a blood protein essential for normal clotting.

How is it diagnosed?
Hemophilia is diagnosed by blood tests. If hemophilia has occurred in your family, you may want to seek genetic counseling before starting a family to determine your risk of passing on the disease.

How is it treated?
Hemophiliacs are given transfusions of concentrated blood products containing the factors missing from their own blood. If you have severe hemophilia, you may need such transfusions after even minor cuts or bruises. You are certain to require transfusions before any surgical procedure. Un-

fortunately, many people with hemophilia who received transfusions in the early 1980s, before a blood test for the virus that causes AIDS was developed, may have received blood containing that virus.

Self-Care: Avoid contact sports that increase your risk of injury. Avoid aspirin and other drugs that interfere with normal blood clotting. Have regular dental care to help avoid problems that may require dental surgery. Wear identification indicating you are a hemophiliac to help ensure proper medical care if you are in an accident and are unable to communicate with medical personnel.

HODGKIN'S DISEASE is a form of cancer that involves the lymph glands. Lymph glands produce blood cells called lymphocytes that help the body fight infection. They are located throughout the body, primarily in the neck, under the arms, in both groins, and in the chest and abdomen. Hodgkin's disease starts in a single lymph node and eventually spreads to others. The disease tends to remain in the lymph nodes for a long time. Usually only in the late stages of the illness do such vital organs as the liver, spleen, lungs, and bone marrow become involved. The outlook for people with Hodgkin's disease has improved remarkably. If diagnosed in an early stage, the odds for a permanent cure are excellent. Even if you have advanced Hodgkin's disease, therapy is often successful in arresting the disease for extended periods of time.

What are the symptoms?
The most common symptom is swollen lymph glands, especially in the neck, armpits, or groin. You also may experience sweats, fever, chills, weakness, and weight loss.

How did I get it?
The cause of Hodgkin's disease is unknown. It occurs most often in young adults between 15 and 34 and in the elderly. There is some evidence that a virus may cause the condition. However, if this is the case, only a few people exposed to the virus actually develop the disease. Most likely, the disease cannot be passed from one person to another.

How is it diagnosed?
A biopsy of an involved lymph node is required. After the diagnosis has been established, your doctor must determine how far the disease has progressed before selecting the best treatment. This may require special

X-rays, including a lymphangiogram and a CAT scan, and possibly an exploratory operation to evaluate abdominal organs and to obtain further biopsies.

How is it treated?

If the disease is in a place in the body where radiation can be given safely, radiation therapy can usually cure it. Unfortunately, large doses of radiation cannot be given to the liver, lungs, or bone marrow without destroying these vital organs. In cases where vital organs are involved, chemotherapy is the preferred treatment. The new combinations of anticancer drugs are better able to treat the disease than the single medication that was previously available. The type of treatment you receive depends on many factors. Either radiation alone, chemotherapy alone, or a combination of the two may be used.

> Self-Care: If you are living with Hodgkin's disease, you may want to join a support group for cancer patients to help cope with your feelings about the disease. A registered dietitian can help you plan meals to manage problems presented by radiation and chemotherapy.

HYPERLIPIDEMIA is an excess of the fatty substances in the blood called lipids. These include cholesterol and triglycerides. The condition may also be called hyperlipoproteinemia because lipids circulate in the blood attached to proteins; the fat-protein complexes are called lipoproteins. They include low density lipoprotein (LDL), high density lipoprotein (HDL), and very low density lipoprotein (VLDL). LDL transports most of the body's cholesterol. It is known as the "bad" lipid because it tends to carry serum cholesterol from the liver to the arteries, where it is deposited on arterial walls. HDL is known as the "good" lipid because it tends to transport cholesterol away from arterial walls and back to the liver. VLDL largely contains triglycerides. In one type of hyperlipidemia, hypercholesterolemia, there is a high level of LDL relative to HDL.

What are the symptoms?

Those with familial forms of the disorder may develop pinkish-yellow deposits of fat, called xanthomas, under the skin, especially around the eyes. In most people, hyperlipidemia causes no noticeable symptoms unless it reaches a severe stage. However, inside the body, hyperlipidemia tends to accelerate atherosclerosis. Risk of coronary heart disease is likely to rise in direct correlation with increased levels of blood lipids.

How did I get it?
Familial hypercholesterolemia is hereditary. Other types may occur as a complication of diabetes, nephrosis, hypothyroidism, alcoholism, and other diseases. But hypercholesterolemia, the most common form, seems to be related to eating foods containing cholesterol and fat, especially saturated fat.

How is it diagnosed?
Lipid levels are measured by blood tests. A total serum cholesterol level of under 200 mg/dl is recommended for adults, with LDL under 130 mg/dl and HDL over 50 mg/dl. If HDL levels are particularly high, and LDL levels correspondingly low, a higher total serum cholesterol level may be acceptable. Triglyceride levels above 250 mg/dl are considered abnormal.

How is it treated?
The first step in treating hypercholesterolemia is a heart-healthy lifestyle, including a low-cholesterol and low-fat diet. A low-carbohydrate diet and avoidance of alcohol are prescribed for hypertriglyceridemia. Weight reduction and increased exercise help both conditions. If such measures do not provide sufficient benefit, drug therapy may be necessary.

> Self-Care: A heart-healthy lifestyle (page 11) can often prevent or cure hyperlipidemia.

HYPERTENSION, also known as high blood pressure, is a disease in which the force of blood against the walls of the arteries is higher than normal. This force is generated by the heart pumping blood throughout the body. When the doctor takes your blood pressure, two things are measured: the systolic pressure, which occurs when the heart muscles contract to push blood out of the heart into the body; and the diastolic pressure, which takes place when the heart rests between beats. Blood pressure is reported as the systolic over the diastolic pressure. The average normal pressure is less than or equal to 120/80. However, blood pressure is dependent on age, sex, and other factors. Although the diastolic pressure is usually considered more important in assessing hypertension, the systolic pressure cannot be ignored. A diastolic reading of 90 or over, or a systolic reading of 140 or over, requires medical attention.

What are the symptoms?
There are no outward symptoms of high blood pressure. You can have hypertension for years without knowing it, unless your blood pressure is

checked annually by your physician. If untreated, hypertension can cause immense damage in the body and lead to heart attack, kidney damage, stroke, and premature death.

How did I get it?

The cause of essential or primary hypertension is unknown. The disease is more common in those over 40 and tends to run in families. It afflicts men and women equally, but is twice as common in blacks as in whites. The far less common secondary hypertension is more likely to occur in younger people as a result of kidney disease or a hormonal disorder; when the underlying disorder is treated, the hypertension disappears. Pregnancy and the use of oral contraceptives also may precipitate high blood pressure.

How is it diagnosed?

Hypertension cannot be diagnosed based on a single abnormal blood pressure measurement. Indeed, some people experience a rise in blood pressure simply because they are anxious when in the doctor's office, a condition known as "white coat hypertension." If your doctor finds a high pressure reading, a schedule of repeated testing—in the office and possibly at home—will be recommended. Only when a pattern of higher than normal readings is found will hypertension be diagnosed.

How is it treated?

If your pressure is only borderline, your doctor may recommend lifestyle changes to help lower the pressure. These may include a low-salt diet, weight loss, quitting smoking, exercising regularly, cutting back on caffeine and alcohol, lowering the levels of stress in your life, and practicing relaxation techniques. If your hypertension does not respond adequately to these measures, or if it is much higher than borderline at the outset, medication will be prescribed. A wide range of drugs is available to help lower pressure. However, it is important to remember that hypertension is a chronic disease. Once you have it, you must pay ongoing attention to the condition for the rest of your life.

Self-Care: Monitor yourself carefully when you start taking anti-hypertensive medication. If you experience any side effects—dizziness when standing up, fatigue, or, in men, a change in the quality of your erection—tell your doctor. A change in dosage or medication may

resolve your problems while still treating your hypertension effectively.

HYPOTENSION, also known as low blood pressure, is a condition in
which the force of blood against the walls of the arteries is lower than
normal. (See HYPERTENSION for an explanation of blood pressure.) The
typical healthy blood pressure for adults is 120/80, the first number repre-
senting the systolic pressure and the second the diastolic pressure. In chronic
hypotension, healthy people may have systolic pressures as low as 90 and
diastolic pressures as low as 70. Even though such pressures are lower than
average, they are not lower than normal. Chronic low blood pressures are
not a problem when they are part of your body's normal function and cause
no symptoms. In fact, most people with chronic hypotension have a better
than normal life expectancy. In acute hypotension, there is a sudden or
gradual drop in pressure that can be life threatening if not treated. Intermittent hypotension or low blood pressure that is caused by some other disease
also warrants medical attention.

What are the symptoms?
People with chronic low blood pressure that presents no problems usually
have no symptoms. Orthostatic or postural hypotension occurs when you
change position from lying down to standing up. It may be accompanied by
weakness, pallor, lightheadedness, fainting sensations, or partial blacking
out. If hypotension causes any symptoms, the condition warrants medical
attention.

How did I get it?
Chronic hypotension is usually hereditary. Acute hypotension may be
caused by severe hemorrhaging from an artery or vein that leads to shock,
or shock caused by infections, burns, falls, or other accidents. If the pressure
drops so low that blood is not propelled to the brain adequately, fainting
may result. Intermittent low blood pressure can have many causes. The most
common type is orthostatic hypotension, which may occur after a long
illness in which you have been bedridden. Or it may occur during treatment
with medication for high blood pressure or glaucoma, indicating that your
medication dosage requires adjustment. Hypotension may result from severe
varicose veins that cause blockage of blood in your legs. Standing rigidly at
attention for long periods also may produce postural hypotension, as can
chronic anxiety and emotional tension. In some cases, persistent low

systolic pressure may be a symptom of certain diseases: the low adrenal gland function of Addison's disease, or low thyroid or pituitary gland function. Occasionally, blockage of blood flow out of the heart, as well as a chronic infection such as tuberculosis, leads to hypotension.

How is it diagnosed?

Blood pressure is measured with an inflatable cuff attached to a sphygmomanometer. Because a variety of everyday circumstances affect blood pressure at any moment, the diagnosis of hypotension is made only after repeated readings over a period of weeks or months—unless an extraordinarily low pressure develops suddenly.

How is it treated?

Chronic low blood pressure that causes no symptoms need not be treated. Acute hypotension requires emergency treatment of the shock that caused it. This may involve stopping the hemorrhaging and providing a blood transfusion. If orthostatic hypotension is caused by medication, a change in dosage usually returns pressure to normal. In organic diseases, pressure returns to its normal level when the underlying problem is treated.

> Self-Care: If you experience slight dizziness when getting out of bed, get up slowly, hang your feet over the side of the bed, and sit for a minute or two before standing.

INTERMITTENT CLAUDICATION is an impaired blood supply in a peripheral muscle, most often the leg, that occurs only when exercising. The impaired blood supply is called ischemia. If it becomes severe, the poor circulation may cause skin ulcers on the lower leg or foot and, in the worst cases, gangrene. Intermittent claudication is a sign of atherosclerosis. It also may indicate arterial disease elsewhere in the body. The incidence of coronary heart disease leading to heart attack is higher in people who have intermittent claudication.

What are the symptoms?

Symptoms include discomfort that can range from a tired feeling to a crampy ache or severe pain that occurs in the leg while you are walking or exercising your legs. The discomfort most commonly occurs in the calf but also may arise in the foot, thigh, hip, or buttocks. Your distress is likely to worsen if you try to walk rapidly or uphill. Within one to five minutes of rest, either by standing still or sitting, the discomfort disappears. As the disease worsens, the distance you can walk before pain occurs gradually decreases. Your foot may often be painful, cold, or numb, with the skin becoming dry and scaly.

How did I get it?

Intermittent claudication is caused by atherosclerosis as a result of fatty deposits, called plaque, on the inner lining of artery walls. Although heredity plays a role in the development of plaque, the amount of cholesterol and fat in your diet is a major contributor. Other factors that contribute to the problem include smoking, diabetes, hypertension, and a sedentary lifestyle.

How is it diagnosed?

The unique pattern of discomfort upon exercise and rapid relief upon rest will make your doctor suspect atherosclerotic intermittent claudication. When your doctor checks your pulse over arteries in the leg or ankle, the beat may be weak or absent. Doppler ultrasonography and a special type of X-ray called an arteriogram can identify the precise areas of blocked blood flow.

How is it treated?

A heart-healthy lifestyle (page 11) may help arrest or slow the progress of intermittent claudication. You will be urged to walk an hour a day, stopping as necessary for discomfort to abate. This exercise regimen will increase the distance you can walk before pain occurs. If you smoke, you must quit. Your doctor also may prescribe drugs to help dilate your blood vessels. However, when the disease becomes severe, treatment to open the vessels may be necessary. For one or a few isolated blockages, the vessel can be opened by angioplasty—inserting a small balloon into the obstructed artery and inflating it to compress the plaque. In other cases, surgery may be necessary to bypass the affected arteries.

Self-Care: To help prevent being awakened by the pain of severe claudication, use blocks to raise the head of your bed four to six inches. Gently wash your feet daily with lukewarm water and a mild soap. Check them for any sores or other problems. These should be promptly treated. Never self-treat corns, calluses, or any other foot problem. Avoid elastic hose or constricting garters. Wear shoes that fit well.

LEUKEMIA is a form of cancer that affects the blood-forming organs of the body: the bone marrow, lymph nodes, and spleen. These organs release blood cells into the blood vessels and lymph system. When leukemia strikes, abnormal white blood cells are released. These cells cannot fight infection properly. In advanced leukemia, the uncontrolled multiplication of abnormal cells crowds out the production of normal white cells to fight infection, of platelets to control bleeding, and of red blood cells to prevent anemia. Patients may die from raging infections or from bleeding that would normally be prevented by the platelets. However, considerable progress has been made in treating leukemia to prevent such deaths.

What are the symptoms?
In its early stages, leukemia may cause no symptoms. The symptoms that prompt most leukemia patients to see their doctors hardly seem life threatening. Depending on the type of leukemia, they may include pallor, fatigue, weakness, shortness of breath, frequent or persistent infections, fever, lip and mouth ulcers, a tendency to bruise and bleed easily, swollen lymph glands, loss of appetite, or night sweats. These symptoms may also be signs of many much simpler problems.

How did I get it?
The cause of leukemia is not fully understood. Some types may involve a hereditary disposition, and others may be triggered by a virus. People who have been exposed to unusual amounts of radiation and certain chemicals, such as benzene, are much more apt to develop leukemia. However, not everyone exposed to such agents gets the disease.

How is it diagnosed?
Blood tests and bone marrow biopsies are necessary to diagnose leukemia and determine whether it is acute or chronic and lymphocytic or myelogenous (also known as granulocytic). These terms refer to the origin and course of the disease and affect how it is treated and what your prognosis is. Most cases of leukemia strike adults and are about evenly divided between the acute and chronic types. Acute lymphocytic leukemia most commonly hits children.

How is it treated?
Chemotherapy can induce remissions and prolong life for many people with chronic lymphocytic and granulocytic leukemia, most often without hospitalization. Initial treatment for the acute leukemias usually requires hospitalization. Therapy includes blood transfusions, antibiotics to reduce the risk of infection, and chemotherapy to kill the leukemic cells. Such treat-

ment often induces a remission, although the disease may recur. However, bone marrow transplantation may provide a permanent cure for those with acute disease.

Self-Care: If you are living with leukemia, you may want to join a support group for cancer patients to help cope with your feelings about the disease. A registered dietitian can help you plan meals to manage problems presented by chemotherapy.

PHLEBITIS, a common but potentially dangerous disorder, means inflammation of a vein. It may lead to the formation of a blood clot, also called a thrombus. The clot sticks to the wall of the vein and partially or completely blocks the flow of blood. Technically, this is thrombophlebitis or venous thrombosis, but these terms often are used interchangeably with phlebitis to describe the presence of a clot in a vein. Although most cases are easily treated, phlebitis warrants prompt medical attention because its complications can be life threatening. Clots can break free and travel through the blood. If the clot lodges in the lungs, where it is called a pulmonary embolus, the result can be fatal.

What are the symptoms?
Phlebitis most often occurs in the legs. If the clot is in a vein close to the skin surface, vein swelling may appear as a cord-like bump. If the clot is in a deep vein, there usually is pain, tenderness, and swelling of the leg. The skin may become bluish in color and feel warm to the touch. You may run a fever. If the condition is acute, you may feel a severe heaviness, aching, or pain in the leg. Pain probably will be worse when your leg is hanging down and less when it is elevated.

How did I get it?
Physicians do not fully understand why phlebitis occurs. Three factors can create a predisposition to the condition: slowing of the blood flow because of bed rest or inactivity; damage to the vein wall through injury, bacteria, or certain chemicals, such as some intravenous solutions used after surgery; and coagulation changes in the blood, as may occur in some women who use oral contraceptives. For example, long sedentary periods, such as on car or plane trips, may contribute to clot formation in the elderly. Those most apt to develop phlebitis are people with varicose veins; pregnant women; those who are bedridden for long periods; those in plaster casts for fractures; and people who have recently had surgery. In rare cases, phlebitis may strike

apparently healthy, active people. Unexplained phlebitis may be associated with undiagnosed cancer somewhere in the body.

How is it diagnosed?
Sometimes the physician can make the diagnosis simply by observing the symptoms or by performing a sonogram. This is a painless test that uses sound waves to generate images. A definitive diagnosis requires a special kind of X-ray done after a dye is injected into your bloodstream. This shows where the flow of blood is stopped by the clot.

How is it treated?
Your physician will probably prescribe an anticoagulant to help reduce the likelihood of future blood clots. Frequent blood tests may be required to monitor how well the drug is doing its job and to modify your dosage. You should avoid staying in one position for long periods, whether standing, sitting, or in bed. Your physician also may recommend warm compresses to help ease vein inflammation and elastic support stockings to help reduce the swelling. If you smoke, quit promptly. With such care, phlebitis usually clears within a few weeks. However, phlebitis can recur and new symptoms should be reported to your physician promptly. Persistent severe cases may require surgery to open the blocked vein and remove the clot. If the vessels are so damaged that repair is not possible, veins made of synthetic materials can be inserted to bypass the affected area.

Self-Care: While taking anticoagulants, alert your physician to any symptoms of internal bleeding or other problems: changes in the color of your urine or stools, prolonged or profuse menstrual flow, bleeding from your gums, unexplained skin bruising, abdominal pain, severe headache, diarrhea, weakness, or dizziness. Do not take any other medication—even aspirin—while taking anticoagulants without informing your physician. Aspirin interferes with clotting, and the combination may lead to excessive blood thinning.

RHEUMATIC HEART DISEASE refers to the various heart disorders that may occur as a result of rheumatic fever. Any part of the heart may be damaged by the inflammation of rheumatic fever, but the most common problem is damage to the heart valves. Those with rheumatic heart disease also have a greater risk of developing endocarditis, an inflammation of the lining of the heart muscle. Rheumatic fever and subsequent heart disease have become fairly rare in the United States since the development of antibiotics.

What are the symptoms?
Symptoms may include shortness of breath, palpitations, arrhythmias, swollen feet, dizziness, and chest pain.

How did I get it?
Rheumatic fever is an infectious disease that usually occurs in children between the ages of 5 and 15. It develops after a sore throat caused by streptococcal bacteria. Any child with a sore throat should be seen by a physician to check for strep. A culture of the infected tissue should be done. If the sore throat is not treated promptly with antibiotics, the infection can spread to other parts of the body, including the heart. However, even if penicillin is given, about 60 percent of those already afflicted with rheumatic fever develop some degree of subsequent heart disease.

How is it diagnosed?
Sometimes a heart murmur develops right away. It can be heard with a stethoscope. In other cases, more severe problems become immediately apparent. However, in about half of all cases, symptoms of heart disease do not appear after a single attack of rheumatic fever. Rather, they develop slowly in young adulthood or middle age, as the heart must work harder. Diagnosis of the full impact of rheumatic heart disease may require a chest X-ray, electrocardiogram, echocardiogram, and coronary angiogram.

How is it treated?
Nothing can be done to reverse the heart damage. If problems are identified in youth, your doctor may recommend that antibiotics be taken daily until the age of 30 to prevent recurrence of rheumatic fever and to help avoid the development of endocarditis. Further therapy depends on the type of heart damage. Drugs may be prescribed to help slow a rapid heartbeat or prevent the development of blood clots. If heart valves have been severely damaged, surgery may be needed to replace them.

Self-Care: If you have had rheumatic fever, inform any physician and dentist who treats you. You may need antibiotics before any medical or dental surgery to help prevent infection and subsequent endocarditis.

VARICOSE VEINS are abnormally enlarged veins. They can be uncomfortable and unsightly. Varicosities also signal a breakdown of normal flow of blood. Varicose veins warrant prompt medical attention.

What are the symptoms?
Typically, they appear as knot-like, twisting blue bulges just below the skin, most commonly in the legs. In addition to, or instead of, these bulges, other symptoms may include feelings of heaviness or dull, stabbing pain in the legs, leg cramps at night, itching around the ankles, or tenderness and soreness along the veins. If varicose veins are not treated, you may develop infections and leg ulcers that are very difficult to heal.

How did I get it?
Varicose veins result from malfunction of valves found at regular intervals in veins. The valves normally control the flow of blood back to the heart, preventing a backup of blood. When a series of valves degenerate, the weight of the blood in the vein distends it. Varicose veins are most often seen in people who are on their feet for long periods. An increase in internal pressure of the blood also can strain the valves. This may be caused by heavy lifting, pregnancy, and abdominal tumors. Varicose veins also seem to run in families.

How is it diagnosed?
If your varicose veins show, no special testing may be necessary. If they don't show but are suspected, your doctor may simply wrap an elastic tourniquet around your leg to cause varicosities to stand out. In some cases, special X-rays may be necessary to determine the severity and locations of the weak valves.

How is it treated?
The choice of treatment depends on the severity and location of the varicosities. Your physician may recommend support stockings and medications to alleviate the swelling of mild varicose veins. For more severe problems, you may need surgery to remove the distended veins and close off the weak valves. Injections into the veins may be used to close them up.

Self-Care: The following steps can help prevent the development of varicose veins or ease your discomfort if you already have them:

• If your job requires you to stand for long periods, take breaks to sit down and elevate your legs, preferably above the level of your chest.

• On long trips, take breaks from sitting. Get up and stretch your legs at regular intervals.
• Get regular exercise to improve your circulation.
• If you are pregnant, discuss the use of support stockings with your physician.
• Never wear round garters or elastic girdles for long periods of time. They impair circulation.

2

Brain and Nerve Disorders

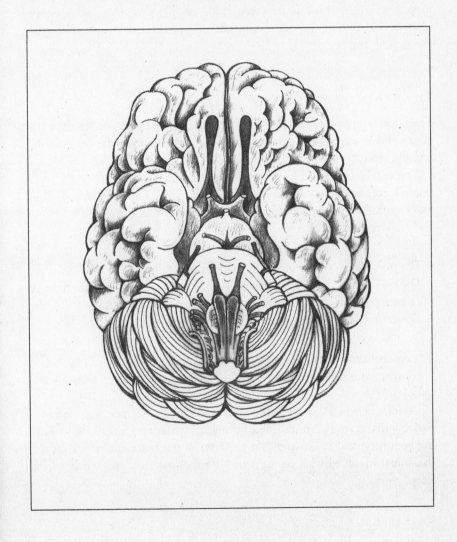

HOW THE BRAIN AND NERVOUS SYSTEM WORK

Your **brain** is the most complex organ in your body, regulating all its activities. It is the seat of consciousness, sensation, and emotion, and it directs or controls all voluntary acts and thought processes. The brain acts through the two parts of the nervous system that connect along the spinal cord: the **central nervous system** comprises the brain itself and the spinal cord; the **peripheral nervous system** encompasses a network of nerves throughout your body. The nervous system initiates and regulates all our activities—walking, talking, seeing, hearing, and eating. It accomplishes this work by acting as a communications center receiving and sending messages. These messages are conveyed as impulses traveling along nerve fibers from the brain, through the spinal cord, and through peripheral nerves throughout the body.

THE BRAIN

The brain is unusually well protected from injury, being encased in the hard bones of the skull. It has three major parts: the cerebrum, the cerebellum, and the brainstem.

The **cerebrum** looks like a large mushroom cap seated at the top of the brain. It consists of two **cerebral hemispheres,** which are largely responsible for our intellectual capabilities of thought, memory, and speech, as well as body movement. Each hemisphere is composed of four lobes:

- The *frontal lobe*, where motor function is controlled
- The *parietal lobe*, where sensations, such as hot and cold, are interpreted
- The *temporal lobe*, where hearing and memory are important
- The *occipital lobe*, which is involved with vision

The **cerebellum** is located underneath the cerebrum at the back of the head. It controls your sense of balance and coordinates movement through the muscles.

Directly beneath the cerebellum is the **brainstem,** connecting the brain to the spinal cord. It is responsible for many involuntary functions, including breathing and circulation. At the base of the brainstem is the **hypothalamus,** involved with our appetites for food and sex and our need for sleep.

THE CENTRAL NERVOUS SYSTEM

The **spinal cord** is less than a half inch in diameter and is enclosed in the bones of the spinal column.

An extension of the brain, the spinal cord essentially functions as a message relay system, carrying information from the brain to the peripheral nerves and back again.

A liquid called **cerebrospinal fluid** flows through the spinal cord and the brain. It is kept separate from the rest of the body by a membrane known as the blood-brain barrier. Although this barrier protects the central nervous system from certain infections, it also can make it difficult to deliver medicines to the brain.

THE PERIPHERAL NERVOUS SYSTEM

Peripheral nerves are divided into four main categories, based on where they connect to the spinal cord. At the top of the cord is the **cervical** region, which links to nerves in the head, throat, shoulders, and arms. Next is the largest area, the **thoracic** region, which connects to nerves in the chest and abdominal area. Toward the lower back is the **lumbar** region, which connects to nerves in the lower back and the front of the legs and feet. At the base of the back is the **sacral** region, which connects to nerves in the buttocks, the back of the legs, and the outer foot.

NERVE FUNCTION

The brain and nervous system are among the least understood parts of the body. Just as a rubber coating protects a telephone wire, a substance called **myelin** protects nerves within the spinal cord and throughout the body. This sheath is also called **white matter.** The basic units of the nervous system are nerve cells called **neurons.** The neurons of the brain and nervous system are sometimes referred to as **gray matter.**

Neurons branch into smaller offshoots called **dendrites** and **axons.** The space between neurons is called the **synapse.** Nerves have two methods of communication: they can send information along nerves using electricity, and they can send and receive messages to and from each other across synapses using chemical messengers known as **neurotransmitters.** Among the most important messages carried are those that tell muscles how and when to move.

In contrast to most other cells throughout the body, neurons do not regenerate when destroyed. Each person is born with a finite number, and they are meant to last a lifetime. However, dendrites, axons, and synapses can regrow after damage. This is how some function can be regained in areas where nerve damage has occurred.

Anything that short-circuits messages passing between the brain and the nervous system can impair function. The extent of the impairment depends on where the damage occurs. For example, damage to a nerve in the upper arm can mar function of the lower arm or hand only. Damage lower down on the spinal cord impairs lower body function. Damage higher up on the spinal cord is more apt to have widespread impact throughout the body.

SYMPTOMS AND SOLUTIONS

MEMORY LOSS AND PERSONALITY CHANGES

Dementia, any disorder that affects the brain's thinking and reasoning ability, is most common among the elderly. However, less than 3 million of the 27 million Americans now over 65 years of age have signs of mental deterioration, and only about one-third of them are severely incapacitated by those symptoms. Symptoms vary, depending on the individual and the cause of the dementia. The most common problems are memory loss, decreased intellectual function, and altered personality of sufficient severity that social and occupational functioning are impaired.

If you notice any persistent memory loss or personality changes, such as increased irritability, in yourself or a member of your family, or if you can't explain and remedy even a single episode of memory loss or unusual behavior by the lifestyle causes discussed in this section, call your physician. Describe what is happening so that the doctor can decide whether you should be seen immediately.

Causes and Treatment of Memory Loss and Personality Changes
Alzheimer's disease (page 54) causes about 50 percent of all dementia. The type of memory loss involved is not that you forget where you put the car keys but that you forget how to use them.

Multiple infarct dementia caused by **stroke** (page 71) is involved in about another 25 percent of cases of intellectual impairment in the elderly. The condition may be caused by a major stroke or by a series of minor strokes that result in the loss of brain tissue and function. Although not reversible, early diagnosis and treatment may prevent progression of multiple infarct dementia.

Potentially reversible causes lead to another 25 percent of memory loss or personality change. Most common are emotional problems, such as stress and **depression** (page 60). Even social isolation—loss of loved ones, relocation to an unfamiliar home, or fear of leaving your home because of physical inability or crime in the community—can cause treatable mental deterioration.

The side effects of some drugs, especially when several drugs are being taken simultaneously, can impair mental function. Often, merely changing dosages can solve the problem.

Other possibly treatable causes of mental impairment include alcoholism, nutritional deficiency, infections, **brain cancer** (page 56), and **brain damage** (page 57) due to trauma or other problems. In addition, several broad areas that may contribute to memory loss and personality changes include metabolic and endocrine problems (see Chapter 8) and eye and ear diseases (see Chapter 10).

Anyone with signs of intellectual impairment or personality change should have a comprehensive evaluation to determine the cause. This may include assessments by a cardiologist, neurologist, psychiatrist, and other specialists. Treatment will depend on the cause of the dementia.

SPEECH IMPAIRMENT

A problem in speaking may involve slurred speech caused by muscle problems in the throat or an inability to form the words that are in your mind, suggestive of a problem in your brain.

If you experience any episode of speech impairment, call your physician. Describe what is happening so that the doctor can decide whether you should be seen immediately.

Causes and Treatment of Speech Impairment
Speech impairment may be caused by **Alzheimer's disease** (page 54), for which no effective treatment is available.

However, it is more likely to be caused by some other problem in the brain. If you also have numbness or loss of movement on one side of the body or blurred vision, **stroke** (page 71) might be suspected. If the problem develops after an accident, **brain damage** (page 57) might be the cause. Depending on the severity of the stroke or brain damage, speech therapy may be able to return normal speech.

If slurred speech is accompanied by a drooping eyelid, double vision, or muscle weakness, especially in a woman between the ages of 20 and 40, it could be **myasthenia gravis** (page 65). If speech is expressionless, with abnormal tone and phrasing, and you also have a hand tremor, it could be **Parkinson's disease** (page 68). Although medications can alleviate the symptoms of these disorders temporarily, both are progressive diseases.

MUSCLE WEAKNESS

Muscle weakness may be experienced as a heaviness in your arms or legs, an inability to raise your arms, difficulty in walking, or arm or leg stiffness.

> If you experience any persistent muscle weakness, or even a single episode not explained by lifestyle causes discussed in this section, call your physician. Describe what is happening so that the doctor can decide whether you should be seen immediately.

Causes and Treatment of Muscle Weakness

Isolated episodes of muscle weakness are most likely to be caused by excessive use of a muscle group that is not fully fit. This may occur, for example, if you help a friend move and spend a day carrying heavy boxes. Commonly known as a "charley horse," the condition should disappear within a day or two with adequate rest. You can ease discomfort with hot baths or heating pads.

Any new episode of muscle weakness occurring after an accident that involved a bump to your head could signal **brain damage** (page 57). Immediate medical attention is necessary. The severity and location of damage will determine whether healing may restore normal muscle strength.

Persistent or recurrent muscle weakness or stiffness in an adult, especially a woman between the ages of 20 and 40, might be **myasthenia gravis** (page

65). Symptoms, including a droopy eyelid and possibly double vision, tend to come and go with exertion.

If such persistent or recurrent muscle weakness occurs in someone over 40, especially if it starts as weakness and cramps in the hands, it could by **amyotrophic lateral sclerosis** (page 55), also known as Lou Gehrig's disease.

Although medications can alleviate the symptoms of myasthenia gravis and amyotrophic lateral sclerosis temporarily, both are progressive diseases.

When muscle weakness begins in infancy or childhood, other disorders are suspected. In infants who have floppy muscles and difficulty sucking the breast or bottle, **cerebral palsy** (page 58) may be suspected. By six months of age, such youngsters demonstrate arm and leg stiffness and muscle spasms. Although drugs cannot reverse muscle weakness, physical therapy can help children maintain maximum mobility.

If in a boy, muscle weakness, stiffness, and difficulty in walking don't begin until a child is a toddler, Duchenne **muscular dystrophy** (page 117) may be suspected. This diagnosis is more likely if there is a family history. Physical therapy and the use of canes or braces can help youngsters maintain mobility as long as possible. However, Duchenne muscular dystrophy is a progressive and ultimately fatal disorder.

SEIZURES

Also known as convulsions, seizures are caused by disorganized electrical impulses in the brain. These surges cause changes in consciousness in conjunction with involuntary muscle movement.

Unless you have diagnosed epilepsy that is under treatment, call your physician if you experience any type of seizure. Even if you are under treatment for epilepsy, call your physician if you experience any change in the severity or frequency of your seizures. Describe what is happening so that the doctor can decide whether you should be seen immediately.

Causes and Treatment of Seizures

The most well-known cause of recurrent seizures is **epilepsy** (page 61). Although epilepsy may be triggered by **brain damage** (page 57) or **brain cancer** (page 56), its cause is unknown in most cases. If brain damage is the problem, seizures may abate with healing. If brain cancer is the cause, surgery or radiation therapy may ease seizures. Fortunately, antiseizure medications can reduce the frequency and severity of seizures in most people, even if the cause is not known.

People who suffer with alcoholism may experience seizures if they stop drinking abruptly. Therefore, "drying out" should always take place in a medical facility where immediate care is available at all times.

When seizures occur in a child, most often the cause is a high fever due to an infectious disease (see Chapter 9). Call your doctor for instructions on how to control fever. Never give aspirin to a child with an undiagnosed fever because it may cause a potentially life-threatening disorder known as Reye's syndrome.

In some cases, seizures in a child may be due to **cerebral palsy** (page 58). Again, antiseizure medications can usually alleviate the problem.

People with **diabetes** (page 244) who are being treated with insulin may experience a sudden and severe drop in blood sugar level called hypoglycemia. This condition may also lead to seizures. Such individuals need an immediate source of sugar to return their blood sugar levels to normal. Diabetics who know they are prone to such reactions usually carry a sugar gel with them.

If you observe someone having a seizure, do not attempt to interfere with the uncontrolled body movements. Ease the person down onto the ground, put a pillow under the head, and clear the area of objects that could cause injury. It is a myth that people having a seizure are at risk of swallowing their tongue. Never attempt to pry someone's mouth open or insert any object into the mouth during a seizure. The episode should end in a few minutes.

HEADACHES

A headache is any pain in the head. Most of us experience occasional minor headaches due to noise or tension, but some headaches are more serious and warrant medical attention.

Causes and Treatment of Headaches

Most minor headaches are due to stress or other environmental causes. Such tension headaches produce a steady, nonthrobbing, moderate pain that may feel like tightness or soreness at the back of the head or like a band around the head. Relaxation techniques may help prevent and ease these headaches, which also may be relieved by aspirin, ibuprofen, or other mild painkillers.

If you experience recurrent headaches that are not eased by a mild painkiller such as aspirin or acetaminophen and explained by factors discussed in this section, or if you have even a single extremely severe headache, as described here, call your physician. Describe what is happening so that the doctor can decide whether you should be seen immediately.

If you cannot reach your doctor, get immediate medical care at a hospital emergency room if you experience a headache that reaches a peak in seconds or a headache accompanied by any of the following symptoms:

- Fever and a stiff neck
- Confusion
- Difficulty in walking or speaking
- Pain or weakness in your arms or legs
- Visual difficulties

Prior to going to the emergency room:

- Take nothing to eat or drink.
- Take no medication unless it was previously prescribed and is urgently important or you are told to do so by your physician or emergency medical personnel.

If you have throbbing pain, particularly if it is limited to one side of the head, accompanied by nausea and vomiting, it could be migraine. If extraordinarily severe headaches center around or behind one eye, it could be cluster headaches. Such vascular **headaches** (page 62) require powerful medications and lifestyle change to decrease their frequency and severity.

Headache that occurs after an injury to the head could signal **brain damage** (page 57). This symptom warrants immediate emergency medical attention. You may be bleeding inside your skull and require surgery.

If headache is accompanied by eye pain and blurred vision, it could be **glaucoma** (page 317). Pressure is rising inside your eye and requires immediate relief with special medications or possibly surgery. If you can't reach your doctor, go immediately to a hospital emergency room.

If the headache is on your forehead or either side of your nose, you may have **sinusitis** (page 96). This is more likely if you have recently had a cold or suffer from an allergy. Warm compresses or a hot bath or shower may "clear your head." If the problem persists for more than a few days, call your doctor. You may need medical treatment for an infection.

If you regularly have a headache when you awaken in the morning, and it is not caused by excessive alcohol consumption the night before, it may only signal **sinusitis** (page 96) or it may be a sign of **hypertension** (page 27) or **brain cancer** (page 56). Make a prompt appointment with your doctor for evaluation.

Headaches may be caused by a variety of lifestyle factors: hunger, too much very bright sunlight, stuffy or smoky rooms, or consumption of too much alcohol. You can avert such headaches by avoiding the situations that cause them. They usually respond to a mild painkiller.

If you drink a lot of coffee or cola beverages and then skip one day, you may get a headache from caffeine withdrawal. The immediate solution may be a sip of coke or coffee, but this warning should alert you to lower your caffeine consumption gradually.

ABNORMAL SENSATIONS OR PARALYSIS

Sensations in your arms or legs, such as weakness, pain, numbness, or the tingling that is commonly called "pins and needles," are usually not normal. Paralysis is the inability to move an arm or leg or other body part and is never normal.

Causes and Treatment of Abnormal Sensations or Paralysis

Everyone experiences occasional pins and needles in a limb. After you have been in a cramped position for an extended period, circulation or nerve communications to the area beyond the pressure may be cut off. Some people say "my foot fell asleep." Shaking out the part and using it should return it to normal within a few minutes. Any unusual leg or arm sensations beyond this minor problem are cause for concern.

If you gradually develop pain, weakness, tingling, and numbness in just one area, usually a hand or foot, it could be **peripheral neuropathy.** This is a condition in which one or more nerves develop inflammation. Because of interference with nervous system messages, you slowly develop abnormal sensations in the affected part.

Milder forms of peripheral neuropathy may result from poor posture or activities that require cramped positions for long periods, such as squatting to garden. Learn to use your body properly, and take frequent breaks from any tasks that require a position that places any strain on you.

If the symptoms are persistent, make an appointment with your doctor. Any inflammatory problem or disorder that damages a small segment of the nervous system can cause peripheral neuropathy. Such damage may arise from an accident or surgery that injures a nerve, **diabetes** (page 244), **AIDS** (page 265), certain types of cancer, vascular disorders like **atherosclerosis** (page 17), or rheumatic disorders such as **rheumatoid arthritis** (page 121), **lupus** (page 116), **scleroderma** (page 346), or **Lyme disease** (page 282). The problem also may arise as a side effect of a drug or from nutritional deficiency, as is seen in alcoholism. Depending on the underlying cause and the extent of the nerve damage, the neuropathy may or may not disappear after the problem is treated.

If you experience any abnormal sensations in an arm or leg not explained by the lifestyle factors discussed in this section, call your physician. Describe what is happening so that the doctor can decide whether you should be seen immediately.

If you cannot reach your doctor, get immediate medical care at a hospital emergency room if you experience any paralysis or any abnormal sensations accompanied by any of the following symptoms:

• Fever and a stiff neck
• Confusion
• Difficulty in walking or speaking
• Headache
• Visual difficulties

Prior to going to the emergency room:

• Take nothing to eat or drink.
• Take no medication unless it was previously prescribed and is urgently important or you are told to do so by your physician or emergency medical personnel.

If the abnormal sensations occur in conjunction with paralysis of any part of the body, even more serious disorders may be the cause. If the symptoms come and go, it could be **multiple sclerosis** (page 64), or **MS**. MS is more likely to be suspected if you also have extreme weakness or fatigue, hand trembling, and vision or balance problems. The disorder requires treatment with anti-inflammatory medications and physical therapy to help preserve muscle function.

If abnormal sensations in conjunction with paralysis of any part of the body arise after an accident, your problems may signal **brain damage** (page 57). If they occur in an older person, it could be a **stroke** or mini-strokes, called TIAs (page 71). Inability to move any body part should never be ignored. In both these disorders, the severity of the damage will determine how much normal sensation and function will return with healing and physical therapy.

If you develop a weakness on one side of your face, the corner of your mouth droops, and you are unable to close the eye on that side, you probably have Bell's palsy, also known as facial palsy. Certain facial muscles are paralyzed because of a disorder of the nerve that controls them. It occurs when a nerve becomes swollen and is pinched at a site where it leaves the skull. Bell's palsy may be caused by an **ear infection** (page 313), **Lyme disease** (page 282), or arise for no known cause. Healing of the underlying disorder usually resolves the paralysis within a few weeks or months. Steroid medications may be prescribed to hasten a return to normal function. In some cases, surgery may be required to relieve pressure on the nerve.

CHRONIC DROWSINESS

Not everyone needs the same amount of sleep. Eight hours a night is often recommended, but this does not apply to everyone. Some people feel groggy if they sleep less than 10 hours, and others feel bright and chipper with only four. Children need more sleep, and elderly people seem to need less, perhaps because they may be less active or may nap during the day. However much you sleep, you should awake feeling refreshed and able to function in an alert manner all day.

> If you are chronically drowsy all day for more than a few weeks and cannot explain your fatigue by the lifestyle factors discussed in this section, call your physician. Describe what is happening so that the doctor can decide whether you should be seen immediately.

Causes and Treatment of Chronic Drowsiness

The most common cause of chronic drowsiness is **insomnia.** The three major types of insomnia are an inability to fall asleep within 30 to 45 minutes of getting into bed; awakening one or more times during the night but returning to sleep; or awakening much earlier in the morning than normal, before your sleep cycle is complete. Occasional insomnia that lasts only a few nights is not serious and is most often due to stress; a transient illness that causes pain or itching; or an environmental factor, such as excessive consumption of caffeine or alcohol, a large meal eaten just before bedtime, or excessive noise or light.

Longer-term insomnia is most often caused by anxiety or **depression** (page 60). When the problem causing the anxiety is solved or passes, the insomnia usually disappears. When major depression is the cause, psycho-

HOW TO FALL ASLEEP

• Exercise regularly during the day, but not before bedtime, so you don't feel full of energy when you go to bed.

• Avoid daytime naps and heavy meals late in the evening, although a glass of warm milk may help you to relax.

• Go to bed at the same time every night, and set an alarm for the same time every morning, to establish a regular pattern. Avoid staying up late—and sleeping later—on weekends, which may make it difficult or impossible to return to a regular schedule on Monday.

• Don't overstimulate yourself with exciting TV shows or family arguments before going to sleep. Instead, undertake some quiet activity in the late evening, such as reading or sewing or relaxation exercises, to prepare yourself for sleep.

• Avoid caffeine (in coffee, tea, and colas), alcohol, and cigarettes before going to bed.

• Make sure your bedroom is at a comfortable temperature, with minimal light and noise, that your night clothing is not too tight or too loose, and that bedsheets are smooth.

• Don't watch the clock as the night hours pass. This only leads to anxiety, which will, in itself, keep you awake.

• If you can't fall asleep right away, don't turn on the light to read. The light only reawakens your brain when it needs to calm down. Instead, just try to relax in the dark.

• Practice finding a comfortable position and lying perfectly still—resisting all temptation to move even a little—to let your body quiet and relax to sleep. Motionless lying is often the key to getting to sleep.

• If these techniques fail, learn progressive relaxation or self-hypnosis techniques that can help you get to sleep.

therapy and drug treatment of the illness are necessary. Physical causes of insomnia may include conditions causing pain, such as various types of arthritis (see Chapter 4), **ulcers** (page 209), or **headaches** (page 62); **prostate enlargement** (page 226), which causes frequent wakening to urinate; **asthma** (page 86); chronic **sinusitis** (page 96); or **epilepsy** (page 61).

If you don't get sufficient sleep one night, don't try to change your sleep schedule the next by going to sleep much earlier than normal. This can worsen the disruption in your normal sleep schedule. Neither should you get into a state of panic about insomnia or believe that you can't go to sleep without a sleeping pill. Just try to relax and return to your normal sleep pattern.

If you are persistently drowsy during the day and your sleeping partner says that you snore, you may suffer with sleep **apnea** (page 85). This is a respiratory disorder that merits evaluation and treatment to prevent serious complications. Therapy may include weight loss, devices to maintain an open airway at night, or even surgery.

If you are so drowsy that you have repeated sleep attacks during the day—suddenly falling asleep for periods ranging from 10 minutes to several hours—you may have **narcolepsy** (page 66). This is a neurological disorder of unknown cause that can be difficult to treat, although medications are available. If the disorder persists, you will have to avoid driving, piloting a plane, and any other activities that might be dangerous if you were to fall asleep.

TICS

Tics are any repetitive motions or sounds that you seem to be unable to control.

If you experience any persistent tics that cannot be explained by the lifestyle factors discussed in this section, call your physician. Describe what is happening so that the doctor can decide whether you should be seen immediately.

Causes and Treatment of Tics

Most tics are nervous mannerisms caused by anxiety or chronic stress. They may involve wrinkling your nose, smoothing your hair, or twitching your mouth. If you focus on the tic, you can control it. Although these tics do not indicate serious illness, they do suggest that you are on emotional overload and need to lower stress levels in your life.

Minor tics may also occur in children. If parents do not get worked up over the tic, but instead try to decrease stress on the youngster, the tic is likely to disappear.

A persistent tic that you cannot control may result from a neurological disorder. The most severe type of neurological tic disorder is **Tourette syndrome** (page 72). Symptoms may include facial tics, such as rapid eye blinking or facial twitches; body tics, such as shoulder shrugging, head jerking, arm flapping, or foot stamping; and vocal tics, such as sniffing, throat clearing, coughing, grunting, barking, shrieking, stuttering, or repeating other people's words, your own words, or inappropriate or obscene words. Although Tourette is difficult to treat, medications are available to decrease the severity and frequency of tics.

BACKACHE

Most backaches are caused by bone or muscle problems. See Chapter 4 for a full discussion of backaches.

However, pain in the lower back that shoots down the leg, especially if you are over 35, is probably **sciatica** (page 70), caused by pressure, injury, or inflammation affecting the sciatic nerve. Bed rest usually helps, but if the pain persists make an appointment with your doctor to determine the underlying cause and to get relief.

BLURRED VISION

Although blurred vision may be caused by **stroke** (page 71) or **myasthenia gravis** (page 65), it is more likely to be due to a localized problem in the eye. See Chapter 10 for a full discussion of blurred vision.

DIZZINESS

Although dizziness may be caused by **stroke** (page 71), **brain damage** (page 57), **depression** (page 60), or **multiple sclerosis** (page 64), it is more likely to be due to a vestibular disorder in the ear. See Chapter 10 for a full discussion of dizziness.

COMMON DISORDERS OF THE BRAIN AND NERVOUS SYSTEM

ALZHEIMER'S DISEASE is a disorder in which degeneration of certain brain cells impairs thinking and reasoning ability. It is the most common cause of mental breakdown in older people, accounting for about half of all cases of dementia and responsible for more than half of all nursing home admissions. Although Alzheimer's usually occurs in the elderly, it sometimes can start in the 40's or 50's.

What are the symptoms?
The first symptoms can be hard to recognize and may be blamed on emotional problems. You may be unable to concentrate as well as you used to, and disturbing patterns of memory loss occur. Although you may remember where you put the car keys, you may be unable to remember how to use them. You may ask the same questions several times or forget people you know well. Routine tasks take a great deal more time. As the disease progresses, agitation, irritability, and restlessness become noticeable. Personality and mood may be affected. As Alzheimer's progresses over a period of years, you become unable to communicate meaningfully with others and handle daily self-care. Incontinence may occur. The person with Alzheimer's may be unaware of the full extent of the disease.

How did I get it?
The underlying cause of Alzheimer's is unknown, but it is not a result of normal aging. In Alzheimer's, the brain's nerve structure changes, with nerves becoming tangled and cellular debris accumulating. Alzheimer's is not contagious. It tends to be inherited but not to the extent that every descendant of every Alzheimer's patient is afflicted.

How is it diagnosed?
Anyone suspected of having Alzheimer's disease must see a doctor as soon as possible for a comprehensive evaluation, usually by a neurologist and psychiatrist as well as an internist. Symptoms similar to those provoked by Alzheimer's may be caused by other treatable diseases, such as anemia, stroke, thyroid disorders, and arteriosclerosis. These diseases require prompt therapy to halt or reverse symptoms. Only when other causes are ruled out is the diagnosis of Alzheimer's made.

How is it treated?
Currently, there is no effective treatment to slow the course of Alzheimer's
or to cure it. It is a progressive, chronic disease that ultimately is fatal. If
problems with sleep or depression arise, medication can help alleviate them.
A careful exercise program under the guidance of a physical therapist can
aid overall good health and self-esteem.

Self-Care: The person with Alzheimer's disease should be encouraged
to continue daily routines as normally as possible. Although he or she
is unable to function as well as before, even small accomplishments
can improve mental outlook and pride. It is best to maintain an
orderly, routine environment to avoid the necessity of learning new
things. During the early phases of Alzheimer's, care can usually be
provided at home. However, the disease can cause great frustration
and emotional and physical strain for the family when constant
supervision is needed. Periodic breaks for family caregivers are essential to prevent exhaustion. Alzheimer's can be one of the most
crushing of all family burdens. When the condition becomes severe,
the family may decide that a nursing home can better provide the
proper full-time care needed.

AMYOTROPHIC LATERAL SCLEROSIS, also known as ALS, is a
degenerative disease that causes progressive muscle weakness and destruction throughout the body. It is also known as Lou Gehrig's disease, after the
famed baseball player who succumbed to the disorder. ALS most commonly
begins in people over the age of 40.

What are the symptoms?
Initial symptoms usually are cramps and weakness in the hand, although
muscle weakness in the arms or legs may come first. Leg weakness or stiffness
may cause difficulty in walking. In some people, muscles in the throat fail
first, causing slurred speech and difficulty in swallowing. Although progression of the disease varies significantly from one person to another, muscle
destruction throughout the body eventually leads to paralysis and death.

How did I get it?
The cause of ALS is unknown, although some hereditary factors may be
involved. The actual destruction of muscles starts with a problem in the
nervous system when certain nerve cells begin to die. These motor neurons

extend from the brain to muscles throughout the body and control muscle movement. As muscles lose their nerve supply, they waste away.

How is it diagnosed?

If ALS is suspected, your doctor will order X-rays, blood tests, and other evaluations to rule out other possible causes. Finally, you will be given a test known as electromyography that measures electrical activity in muscles and can confirm the diagnosis of ALS.

How is it treated?

No specific treatment to cure or halt the disease is available. Rather, therapy is designed to ease the symptoms and impact of the disease and to help you stay independent as long as possible. You may be given drugs to reduce muscle cramps and spasms. Physical therapy can help maintain muscle function. When swallowing is impaired, you may benefit from drugs to increase saliva production or surgery to establish a permanent opening from your abdomen into your stomach for liquid feeding.

> Self-Care: Because mental function is not impaired, people with ALS are fully aware of what is happening to them and may suffer depression. Counseling or participation in an ALS support group can help you cope.

BRAIN CANCER is any malignancy that occurs in the brain. Primary tumors are those that originate in the brain. Secondary tumors originate elsewhere in the body and spread to the brain by a process called metastasis. Brain cancer is relatively uncommon, accounting for only about 14,000 new cases of malignancy in the United States each year. The severity of a brain tumor depends on its size and location in the skull, as well as its rate of growth and grade of malignancy.

What are the symptoms?

No symptoms may occur until the tumor has become significant enough in size to put pressure on surrounding tissue. The symptoms of brain cancer are similar to those of many other disorders. They may include mild to severe headaches, vomiting, vision disturbances, convulsions, drowsiness, lethargy, or a variety of personality changes, ranging from mild changes in behavior and impaired thinking to psychotic episodes.

How did I get it?
As with most types of cancer, the cause of brain cancer is unknown. Although it can occur at any age, brain cancer is most common in young adults and those in their middle years. Secondary brain cancers most commonly have spread from primary sites in the breast or lungs.

How is it diagnosed?
If brain cancer is suspected, you will probably be referred to a neurologist for a complete examination. Testing will include complex vision and hearing exams, a CAT scan, which is a special X-ray of the brain, and MRI, another painless technique for imaging the brain. If a brain tumor is identified, other tests may be performed to help determine if it is a primary or secondary tumor. For example, a chest X-ray may be done to look for a primary tumor in the lungs.

How is it treated?
Surgery is almost always the first step in treating cancers of the central nervous system. Complete removal of the tumor gives the best chance for cure of an early primary brain cancer. If some cancer cells cannot be removed by surgery, radiation therapy may be successful in finishing the job. In cases where surgery might cause as much or more damage than the cancer itself, radiation or chemotherapy may be a better approach. Even if the tumor cannot be cured, treatment can often alleviate symptoms and extend life.

Self-Care: The diversity of symptoms points to the importance of reporting even mild persistent headaches to your physician. The earlier brain cancer is diagnosed, the better are the chances of effective treatment.

BRAIN DAMAGE—an injury to the brain due to illness or injury—may involve a difficult recovery. It can take months or even years for normal physical and mental activity to return.

What are the symptoms?
Symptoms depend on the part of the brain that has been damaged and the extent of the damage. You may have weakness in an arm or leg on one side of the body. You may have difficulty speaking. Hearing or vision may be impaired or lost. There may be changes in personality and behavior. Even moderate degrees of brain damage may impair your control over emotional

responses: Someone who wants to frown may instead cry, or a smile may become a laugh. As the brain begins to heal, these symptoms gradually become less severe. In time, some symptoms disappear completely.

How did I get it?

Brain damage can be caused by a fall, a car crash, a diving accident, a stroke, brain cancer or its treatment, or even a severe illness.

How is it diagnosed?

When brain damage has occurred, you will probably be referred to a neurologist for evaluation and treatment. Testing may include complex vision and hearing exams, a CAT scan, which is a special X-ray of the brain, and MRI, another painless technique for imaging the brain.

How is it treated?

Treatment involves helping the brain to relearn abilities it has lost. As soon as you are able to be moved about, therapy can begin. Depending on the nature of the brain damage, treatment may include physical therapy exercises to maintain joint and muscle mobility and promote circulation; occupational therapy to redevelop skills for daily activities; speech therapy to regain effective communications skills; and mental exercises to help redevelop thought processes. Because skills may continue to return slowly, for as long as a year or more after the damage, therapy must proceed for an extended period. If severe depression occurs, psychological counseling may be necessary.

> Self-Care: Therapists and family members can help the person with brain damage by devising techniques to work around lost skills. For example, if you are unable to say a word, you may still be able to write it, tap it out on a computer, or point to a picture of it. Similarly, if your hearing has been damaged, you may be more comfortable in a quiet environment with communication in writing. Whatever the deficit, don't give up. Thinking, talking, and hearing need to be mentally exercised just as muscles need to be physically exercised. Although the slowness of recuperation can be very discouraging, it is important to persist. Not all victims of brain damage recover completely. However, many eventually are able to return to useful, happy lives and become at least partly self-sufficient.

CEREBRAL PALSY, also known as CP, is an umbrella term used to describe a group of disorders characterized by impaired movement arising from damage to the central nervous system. Cerebral palsy causes partial or complete paralysis of one or more muscle groups as well as spastic movement.

What are the symptoms?
The type and severity of symptoms vary widely, depending on the extent of nervous system damage. In infants, you may notice the baby has difficulty sucking the breast or bottle and seems to have floppy muscles. By six months of age, stiffness of the limbs, muscle spasms, and unusual body postures may be observed. The disorder may be quadriplegic, affecting both arms and legs; hemiplegic, affecting the arm and leg on one side of the body only; or paraplegic, affecting only both legs. Normal development of walking and talking usually are delayed. Problems with hearing, vision, balance, and coordination may occur, as well as convulsions. Although some children with CP have normal or even high intelligence, many have various degrees of mental retardation.

How did I get it?
Although the exact causes of CP are unknown, these problems are believed to derive from developmental abnormalities that occur before birth or from damage to the central nervous system during or shortly after birth. CP is more common in the babies of women who used drugs or excessive alcohol or had rubella during pregnancy. Babies may be deprived of oxygen during delivery and suffer nervous system damage, although this occurs less frequently now than in the past. In less common cases, CP may arise due to head injuries, meningitis, or severe convulsions in infancy or early childhood.

How is it diagnosed?
CP can be very difficult to diagnose before the age of two, when characteristic motor impairments are more obvious. However, early evaluation can rule out other potentially treatable causes of the symptoms. A complete evaluation will include blood tests, an electroencephalogram to measure brain waves, and a CAT scan or MRI to provide images of the brain.

How is it treated?
No medical treatment is available to cure CP palsy or to alleviate the abnormal motor function. Medications can be given to ease muscle stiffness and to reduce the frequency and severity of seizures. If limbs develop permanent stiffness, surgery may be able to facilitate movement. However,

therapy is largely devoted to helping youngsters with CP to develop and maintain maximal independence within the limits of their handicaps. This may involve physical and occupational therapy, speech therapy, as well as braces, corrective eyeglasses, and hearing aids.

Self-Care: Children with mild CP are usually able to attend regular schools and have relatively normal lives. Those with more severe problems will benefit from evaluation by an educational psychologist and may require special schooling. Parents can be helped in establishing a good life for their children by family support groups.

DEPRESSION is more than just feeling sad. The condition doctors call major depression is a consistently low mood for at least two weeks, accompanied by other physical symptoms. Major depression may be triggered by real problems in your life or may start without reason, but the depression persists for months or even years. Even if there seems to be a good cause, the degree of depression may be completely out of proportion to the problem. People in every age group, from children through the elderly can develop major depression.

What are the symptoms?
Severely depressed people have feelings of great sadness, misery, pessimism, low self-esteem, and even undefined guilt. You may have a look of sadness and hopelessness that other people notice. You tend to lose interest in people and activities around you. Your feelings may interfere with your work or social life, and you may not be able to see the good side of anything. You may feel suicidal. In addition, many depressed people experience weight loss or gain, insomnia, loss of appetite, nausea, fatigue, loss of sexual desire, dizziness, or other physical symptoms. You may attribute your problems to these symptoms and not recognize that you are depressed.

How did I get it?
The cause of major depression remains unclear. It may be due to physiologic dysfunction of the brain rather than just psychological problems. A tendency toward the disorder may be inherited.

How is it diagnosed?
First, you need a complete physical examination to determine if you have any other disorder that might be causing your symptoms. When such problems are ruled out, depression may be diagnosed based on the presence of the low mood and other symptoms for more than two weeks.

How is it treated?
Although depression can be treated and cured, less than half of all those with the disorders are properly diagnosed and treated. Medication can help ease your distress and clear your thinking, so that you can look at your problems more objectively. In many cases, psychotherapy alone or in conjunction with drug therapy can help ensure long-term relief.

Self-Care: You can often self-treat minor depression by getting involved in new activities, such as a vacation or hobby, but major depression requires professional care. Medical treatment should be supplemented by a program of regular aerobic exercise, such as walking, jogging, biking, or swimming, at least three times a week. Such exercise appears to release brain chemicals that help lift your mood.

EPILEPSY is a disorder of the central nervous system usually associated with abnormal electrical rhythms in the brain. When these abnormal rhythms occur in a lengthy disturbance, they can cause an epileptic seizure, also known as a fit or convulsion. Most children with epilepsy attend regular schools and participate in all activities. Most adults are capable of working in all but the most hazardous jobs. People with epilepsy generally have normal abilities, except during a seizure or in its aftermath.

What are the symptoms?
There are many forms of seizure. Some, known as petit mal, are very minor, causing momentary blackouts or perhaps twitching of the eyelids. Some seizures cause changes in consciousness, sensation, or behavior. The most common type, known as grand mal epilepsy, causes generalized convulsive movements. During such a seizure, you lose consciousness and the body stiffens and twitches uncontrollably for several minutes. Sometimes an aura of unusual sensation precedes a grand mal attack; you may "see," hear, or smell something every time a seizure occurs.

How did I get it?
An injury or illness that caused brain damage accounts for about one-third of all cases of epilepsy. Abuse of alcohol and sedative drugs is also commonly associated with seizures. However, the cause of most cases of epilepsy remains unknown. It is neither contagious nor strongly hereditary. Although it can occur at any time, epilepsy usually begins before the age of 20. Most people with epilepsy have normal intelligence.

How is it diagnosed?
A neurologist diagnoses epilepsy based on physical examinations and multiple diagnostic tests. Most valuable is an electroencephalograph (EEG), which measures discharges from nerve cells in the brain.

How is it treated?
A small percentage of epilepsy cases is caused by curable underlying disorders, such as an infection or a brain tumor or brain abnormality amenable to surgery. When the cause is treated, the epilepsy disappears. However, in most cases, treatment involves medications such as dilantin or phenobarbital to reduce the frequency of or eliminate the seizures. Finding the right drug may require a period of trial and error.

> Self-Care: Always take your medication on schedule. Wear a tag or carry a card that says you are an epileptic and gives simple instructions on how you are to be treated. This can aid strangers assisting you if you have an unexpected attack. If your seizures are not fully controlled, avoid potentially hazardous situations: don't drive a car or fly a plane, operate machinery, ski, ride a bicycle, or climb ladders. Also avoid alcohol, fatigue, caffeine, and stimulants, which can precipitate an attack in some people.

HEADACHES are among the most common causes of pain. Virtually all of us experience an occasional headache when we are tired, tense, hungry, stressed, or have been straining our eyes excessively. However, more serious headaches plague more than 40 million Americans. The most common types of severe headaches are tension, migraine, and cluster headaches.

What are the symptoms?
Tension headaches produce a steady, nonthrobbing, moderate pain that may feel like tightness or soreness at the back of the head, in a band around the head, or at the temples. They may occur at any time of the day and generally worsen at night.

Migraines cause throbbing, severe pain usually limited to one side of the head. They are frequently preceded by warning signs called an aura; this may include such visual disturbances as seeing flashing lights or a "hole" in a page you are reading, or noticing a strange odor. Attacks may last for hours or days and are usually accompanied by nausea, vomiting, dizziness, and sensitivity to light.

Cluster headaches are extraordinarily severe headaches that come on suddenly and center around or behind one eye. They commonly last less than an hour but occur in groups or clusters—recurring as often as ten times a day for weeks or months at a time, then disappearing for a year or longer, only to return again. Cluster headaches often awake people from sleep and may cause tearing in the eye on the affected side.

How did I get it?
Tension headaches are associated with stress that may cause muscles in the head to contract and go into spasm. Migraines and clusters are vascular headaches and seem to be caused by abnormal expansion and contraction of blood vessels in the scalp, although neurological and hormonal factors also may be involved. Migraines are more common in women; they occur most often just before menstruation and often vanish after menopause. They also may be triggered by certain foods, odors, and changes in barometric pressure. Clusters occur more commonly in men; they may be seasonal in the spring and fall and may be triggered by smoking or alcohol consumption. Serious headaches also may accompany an upper respiratory or sinus infection or may be caused by head injury, glaucoma, hypertension, brain tumor, brain hemorrhage, or other serious problems.

How is it diagnosed?
Keep a record of the frequency, location, and severity of your headaches. This will be a big help in the diagnosis. Evaluation will also include a complete physical examination; blood tests; and a CAT scan, a special X-ray of the brain. Thorough testing is important to rule out underlying disorders that may be causing the headaches.

How is it treated?
If a treatable underlying cause is found, therapy will depend on the type of headache. For tension headaches, your doctor may urge you to learn relaxation techniques such as yoga or meditation and to use medication judiciously. Drugs are available to ease tension and muscle spasm. The key to therapy for migraine and cluster headaches is prevention. Your doctor may prescribe powerful drugs, including ergot derivatives or beta blockers, to be taken daily for extended periods to reduce the severity or frequency of these headaches. Other potent medications can be taken to halt these headaches, but they often require overnight hospitalization.

Self-Care: If use of mild painkillers, such as aspirin or ibuprofen, and relaxation techniques do not ease any single severe headache or even recurrent mild headaches, consult your physician. In rare cases, headaches can signal potentially life-threatening problems. Call your doctor immediately if you have a headache accompanied by fever and stiff neck; confusion, difficulty in walking or speaking, or pain or weakness in your arms or legs; visual difficulties; or any headache that reaches a peak in seconds.

MULTIPLE SCLEROSIS, commonly known as MS, is a disease of the nervous system that can affect movement, sensation, vision, balance, speech, and other functions of the body. The disease attacks myelin, the protective nerve coating. As myelin deteriorates, messages traveling to and from the brain are short-circuited. Although MS is a chronic and slowly progressive disease in some people, it can be rapidly debilitating in others. MS is often associated with dramatic exacerbations and remissions. You may have symptom-free periods lasting weeks or months between flares, especially in the early years of the disease.

What are the symptoms?
Symptoms vary widely from person to person and may come and go. They may include partial or complete paralysis of parts of the body, which can cause difficulty in walking and coordination; numbness or a prickling "pins and needles" sensation in parts of the body; noticeable dragging of one or both feet; loss of control over urinary or bowel habits; staggering or loss of balance; extreme weakness or fatigue; trembling of the hands; blurred or double vision; temporary blindness or pain in one or both eyes; dizziness; pain in one or both sides of the face; and difficulty in speaking or slurred speech. Also common are psychological changes, such as mood swings, apathy, and lack of judgment.

How did I get it?
The cause remains unknown. However, doctors believe that an immunologic abnormality, possibly triggered by a virus, may be involved. Some environmental factors may also play a role, because MS is far more common in temperate climates than in the tropics. MS usually starts between the ages of 20 and 40, but can occur at any age. Six out of every ten victims are women.

How is it diagnosed?
There is no single laboratory test for MS, but many contribute to the diagnosis. These may include brain scans and X-rays of the skull and spine.

The physician usually concludes that you have MS only after all other diseases causing similar symptoms have been ruled out. Diagnosis may be difficult because symptoms may come and go before you get to the doctor for examination.

How is it treated?
There is no cure for MS. However, certain medications that suppress inflammation or the immune system may be able to reduce the severity of attacks. Supplemental treatment is aimed at maintaining strength so that you can better withstand attacks. This may include extra rest, special exercises, and braces. Physical therapy can help preserve muscle function.

Self-Care: Try to avoid undue physical and emotional stress, which may be associated with flares. Get adequate sleep and eat a well-balanced diet. Try to maintain as normal and active a life as possible. Because MS can be a frustrating and isolating illness, consider joining a support group.

MYASTHENIA GRAVIS is a neuromuscular disorder that can cause muscle weakness throughout the body, although the problem is often limited to the eyes and mouth. It may begin at any time but most commonly starts between the ages of 20 and 40, and is more common in women than in men.

What are the symptoms?
The first sign usually is a drooping of the eyelid over one or both eyes. Sometimes there is double vision, followed by difficulty in chewing and swallowing. In many people, muscle weakness is limited to the eyes and mouth. In others, generalized myasthenia develops, leading to muscle weakness in the hands and legs and difficulty in handling objects and standing and walking. Symptoms can come and go over a period of hours or days.

How did I get it?
Myasthenia gravis appears to be an autoimmune disorder. The immune system normally forms antibodies to attack and destroy foreign invaders like bacteria. However, in myasthenia, the immune system also forms antibodies that destroy the body's acetylcholine, a chemical important in the transmission of messages along nerves. As a result, communication between nerves and muscles is interrupted, leading to the muscle weakness. Hereditary

factors may cause a predisposition to the disease because it often runs in families. However, in rare cases, it can be triggered by abnormal drug reactions.

How is it diagnosed?
A complete examination will include blood tests and electromyography to evaluate muscle responses. The pivotal diagnostic test involves an intravenous injection of a drug called edrophonium. If you have myasthenia, this drug dramatically causes all symptoms to disappear for about five minutes.

How is it treated?
To alleviate immediate symptoms, you will be given drugs to normalize the transmission of messages between nerves and muscles. To slow down the progression of the disease, you may be given steroid drugs or immunosuppressives to lessen the autoimmune attack. If generalized myasthenia develops, removal of your thymus gland may be recommended. In some cases, plasmapheresis may be performed to remove the offending antibodies from your blood. This process takes several hours but may provide a symptom-free remission for months. In the worst cases, if the muscles that affect breathing are involved, you may need a respirator.

Self-Care: Because fatigue seems to worsen the expression of myasthenia, you should get plenty of sleep and balance your day between periods of activity and rest. You may need to wear an eye patch temporarily when double vision occurs. Joining a myasthenia gravis support group can provide emotional help for dealing with the unpredictable nature of the disease.

NARCOLEPSY is a sleep disorder in which the brain is unable to maintain normal wakefulness during the day. It is more common in men than in women and seems to have no impact on general health.

What are the symptoms?
You have repeated "sleep attacks" throughout the day. Sleep episodes usually last only about 15 minutes but may extend for as long as three hours. Despite this extra sleep, you are probably drowsy all the time. In addition, your sleep at night may be interrupted by vivid dreams and you don't awake feeling refreshed. Many narcoleptics also suffer with sleep paralysis or catalepsy. They are unable to move for a few seconds either just before falling

asleep or upon wakening. Others also experience hallucinations, which are similar to dreams but occur when they are wide awake.

How did I get it?
The cause of narcolepsy is unknown, although it sometimes begins after a head injury or brain infection. It usually begins in adolescence or young adulthood and persists throughout life.

How is it diagnosed?
Although the symptoms themselves virtually define the diagnosis, you are likely to be referred to a neurologist or sleep specialist. An evaluation of your brain's electrical impulses may be performed with an electroencephalogram, and other studies may be done in a sleep laboratory.

How is it treated?
Narcolepsy is difficult to control. Stimulants such as amphetamines may be prescribed to help you stay awake during the day, although they may further interfere with sleep at night.

> Self-Care: Unless your narcolepsy is fully controlled by medication, you must avoid all situations in which suddenly falling asleep would be dangerous. For example, you should not pilot a plane, drive a car, or operate hazardous machinery. Certain athletic activities should also be avoided, including skiing, bicycling, and walking or jogging on a treadmill.

NEUROFIBROMATOSIS, also known as NF, is a genetic disorder that can cause tumors to grow on nerves anywhere in the body at any time throughout an individual's life. The tumors are not cancerous. The manifestations and severity of the disorder vary widely from one person to another. Although some people with NF may have severe medical problems, most do not and are able to lead normal lives. The severity that caused the disease to receive the nickname "Elephant Man" disease is extremely rare.

What are the symptoms?
The first indication is usually the appearance of several brown, irregularly shaped spots on the skin called café-au-lait marks. Many people have one or two café-au-lait marks, but a person with NF has six or more, each at least three-quarters of an inch in diameter in an adult and one-quarter of an inch

in a child. Café-au-lait marks are usually present at birth or soon after and may increase in size and number throughout childhood. Subsequently, benign tumors that vary in size, shape, and number occur anywhere there are nerves in the body. These tumors may affect eyesight, hearing, the bones, circulation, and physical appearance. They may or may not be painful.

How did I get it?

In about half of all cases, the disorder is inherited. Affected individuals have a 50 percent chance of passing NF to each offspring, with males and females equally affected. However, other victims have no family history of the disorder. NF is found among all races and ethnic groups and occurs once in 3,000 births. Often the tumors do not develop until puberty or until a woman is pregnant, leading researchers to believe that certain hormones may have an effect on the growth of neurofibromas.

How is it diagnosed?

No laboratory test diagnoses NF. Rather, diagnosis is based on the appearance of a cluster of characteristic symptoms—the café-au-lait marks; the tumors; small growths in the iris of the eye; and other skin, eye, and bone abnormalities.

How is it treated?

No cure is available, nor is there any general treatment that will slow down tumor growth. Tumors may be removed or reduced by surgery or radiation. However, such treatment usually is undertaken only when the tumor causes serious problems, because removal usually damages or destroys the function of the underlying nerve.

> Self-Care: Tumors easily visible to others may cause considerable psychological discomfort. You may benefit from counseling and contact with others who have the disease to help you cope with your concerns.

PARKINSON'S DISEASE, also known as shaking palsy, is a slowly progressive degenerative disorder affecting special groups of nerve cells in the brain. It may cause any combination of slowed movement, muscular rigidity, postural changes, tremors, and balance problems. Parkinson's usually begins in middle-aged or older people. Men are at slightly greater risk than women.

What are the symptoms?
Parkinson's usually begins with mild tremors of the hand that are more marked at rest than when you are alert. Progressive involvement usually extends to the muscles of the hands, face, arms, legs, and head. Without treatment, symptoms may worsen. The face may become expressionless. Because muscle rigidity makes it harder to initiate and maintain movement, walking may become difficult. Posture tends to become stooped. With the loss of postural reflexes, there is a greater risk of falling. Salivation may increase. In the latest stages of untreated disease, memory loss and dementia may occur.

How did I get it?
In most cases, the cause is unknown. In a small percentage of cases, Parkinson's may occur secondary to some other problem, such as brain infection or tumors, carbon monoxide poisoning, or use of certain drugs, such as reserpine or thorazine. Symptoms seem to derive from a part of the brain that controls movement and is involved in the manufacture of the chemical dopamine.

How is it diagnosed?
Because there is no definitive test to diagnose Parkinson's, a neurologist will perform numerous tests to rule out all other possible causes of your symptoms. These will include blood studies and a CAT scan, a special X-ray of the brain.

How is it treated?
The primary drug used to treat Parkinson's is levodopa, also known as L-dopa. A metabolic precursor of dopamine, it replaces the missing substance in the brain. This drug can completely eliminate symptoms in some people and sharply decrease them in others. However, levodopa does not halt the underlying progression of disease, and increasing doses usually are needed to prevent symptoms. Other drugs may be used to supplement or replace L-dopa, if its action alone is insufficient. Physical therapy can also help maintain function. In addition, researchers are exploring new types of surgery that may provide more effective and long-term treatment.

Self-Care: Tremors may be more severe when you are fatigued or under stress. Therefore, it's important to plan a calm lifestyle and get adequate rest. About half of all victims develop moderate to severe depression that may be a result of the symptoms rather than a symptom itself. In such cases, seek out a Parkinson's support group or a psychological counselor for assistance. Also consider home modifications, such as handrails along walls to help prevent falls.

SCIATICA is a disorder that causes pain in the lower back and leg. It derives its name from the sciatic nerve, the longest and widest nerve in the body. This nerve begins at several levels in the spinal cord, and these multiple sources join to form one nerve trunk. The trunk extends down the back, past the pelvis, and into the thigh. Just above the knee, it branches into two smaller divisions, which then travel down to the feet. Its long course and large size make the sciatic nerve particularly vulnerable to pressure and injury. Pain can be severe and diagnosis difficult, but sciatica can be successfully treated.

What are the symptoms?
The primary symptom is pain, usually in the lower back and leg. Pain is usually described as shooting down the leg. You also may have muscle weakness, which may be limited to the thigh or buttock or extend to the foot. The problems caused by sciatica can range from mildly discomforting to severely disturbing. An attack usually lasts for several days to several weeks and may recur if the cause of the problem is not corrected.

How did I get it?
Sciatic pain most commonly arises from disk problems, but also may be caused by any pressure, injury, or inflammation affecting the nerve. Pressure may derive from severe arthritis, abnormal muscle spasms, or occupations that require certain types of movement. Injury to the nerve root inside the spine may be caused by a slipped disk, fractures of the pelvis or lower spine, or hip dislocation. Inflammation may arise mysteriously or, in rare cases, be traced to diabetes.

How is it diagnosed?
A wide range of tests, including X-rays, may be required to determine the precise source and cause of your pain. In most cases, you are referred to a neurologist or orthopedist for diagnosis and treatment.

How is it treated?
Until the cause is determined, the most effective treatment is bed rest in order to avoid any further pressure on or stretching of the nerve. Your doctor also may prescribe a pain reliever and hot baths or use of a heating pad.

Unless the cause of sciatica is discovered, such symptomatic treatment is the only help and may resolve your pain within a few weeks. If an underlying cause is diagnosed, specific treatment can be instituted. For example, in severe cases, surgery to remove a slipped disk or arthritic bony prominence can remove pressure on the nerve.

Self-Care: When lying on your back, you may be more comfortable with a small pillow under your knees. Some people with sciatica get relief from lying on the side with the legs bent. After you recuperate, develop a regular exercise regimen to gain muscle strength in your stomach and back.

STROKE is an interference in blood supply to the brain that can lead to a wide variety of disorders, ranging from minor speech problems to paralysis, coma, and even death. A stroke occurs when the blood flow and, hence, oxygen supply to some part of the brain are cut off. Physicians also call strokes cerebral vascular accidents or CVAs. There are three forms:

• *Thrombotic stroke*, the most common, is caused by the blockage of an artery in the brain due to atherosclerosis.
• *Hemorrhagic stroke* occurs when the wall of a blood vessel in the brain has been under a great deal of pressure for a long time; it grows weak and eventually develops a leak, interrupting blood flow to part of the brain and causing bleeding into brain tissue.
• *Embolic stroke* occurs when small blood clots from other parts of the body are carried into the brain and block the flow of blood in a small artery.

Transient ischemic attacks, or TIAs, are what some people call mini-strokes, temporary episodes of abnormal function caused by decreased blood flow to the brain. TIAs can be vital warning signals of an impending stroke or the development of problems likely to lead to a stroke.

What are the symptoms?
You may remain conscious during a stroke and feel changes occurring in your body, or you may lose consciousness. Symptoms may include blurred vision, headache, confusion or dizziness, numbness or heaviness, or an inability to move an arm, leg, or other part of your body. Because a stroke usually affects only one side of the brain, only one side of the body is affected. But, depending on the area of the stroke, you may also experience loss of memory or speech. The most common symptoms of a TIA are much milder

and very temporary (from a few minutes to a few hours) changes in your ability to see, read, write, or speak or in limb movement or sensation. If you have any such symptoms, especially a combination of symptoms on one side of the body, contact your physician right away.

How did I get it?

A variety of factors contribute to stroke risk. Atherosclerosis is the leading cause; obesity, smoking, diabetes, high blood pressure, and high cholesterol levels all contribute to the development of atherosclerosis. High blood pressure also contributes to the development of hemorrhagic stroke. Some studies have suggested that women who use birth control pills may be at greater risk of strokes.

How is it diagnosed?

Your doctor will determine whether you are having TIAs or a stroke by a complete medical examination and multiple tests, possibly including an electrocardiogram and special X-rays (such as a CAT scan or arteriogram) of your chest, brain, and the carotid artery in your neck, which is a main supplier of blood to the brain. It is important for the doctor to try and determine what type of problem is causing your symptoms, or which type of stroke you are having, in order to plan treatment.

How is it treated?

If you have had TIAs, your physician can determine the cause of the symptoms. If atherosclerosis of the carotid artery is the source, surgical correction may be possible. In other cases, anticoagulant medication may be prescribed to help prevent clotting; just one adult aspirin every other day or a daily baby aspirin may be sufficient. If a stroke due to a blood clot has occurred, medication may be given to dissolve the clot and thus limit the severity of the stroke. If there is blockage of an artery, surgery may be recommended. In the aftermath of a stroke, long-term rehabilitation may be necessary to relearn skills impaired by damage in the brain.

Self-Care: A heart-healthy lifestyle (page 11) may help to reduce your risk of a subsequent stroke, even if you already have had TIAs or a first stroke.

TOURETTE SYNDROME, also known as TS, is a neurological movement disorder. Its primary symptoms are rapidly repeated, involuntary, multiple movements called tics. These tics are not nervous habits or a behavioral abnormality. People who have Tourette cannot control such movements and sounds, although they may be able to suppress symptoms temporarily. Most people who have minor tics do not have Tourette. But because Tourette is a serious disorder, anyone who develops a tic should be evaluated by a physician. The disorder usually begins in children and teenagers, between the ages of 2 and 16. Once Tourette syndrome begins, it generally lasts throughout life.

What are the symptoms?
The tics produced by Tourette syndrome may include facial tics, such as rapid eye blinking or facial twitches; body tics, such as shoulder shrugging, head jerking, arm flapping, or foot stamping; and vocal tics, such as sniffing, throat clearing, coughing, grunting, barking, shrieking, stuttering, or repeating other people's words, your own words, or inappropriate or obscene words. Most people who have Tourette have only some of these symptoms, and they may vary over time, getting worse or better. With time, specific symptoms disappear and are replaced by others.

How did I get it?
The neurological disorder underlying TS is caused by a chemical imbalance in the brain. Why it occurs is still not known. Many cases appear to be hereditary, but in some cases, the tics may have been precipitated by the use of certain stimulant medications that curb hyperactivity.

How is it diagnosed?
Diagnosis is based on the classic symptoms of the syndrome, after other possible causes of the tics are ruled out. This may involve neurological evaluations and blood tests.

How is it treated?
Therapy depends on the severity of TS. Drugs available to reduce the tics include haloperidol and clonidine. However, these substances can have serious side effects, and none can completely eliminate all symptoms. People with TS are not mentally ill or any less intelligent than others. However, you can be made very uncomfortable by others who do not understand your disorder, producing secondary psychological problems. Psychological counseling may be needed to help you cope more effectively. Because TS may also cause compulsive rumination, distraction, and learning disabilities, children need a complete educational evaluation and may require special educational services.

Self-Care: Try to avoid undue physical or emotional stress, which may worsen symptoms. You can learn to suppress any one tic for several minutes or more, which may be useful in selected situations. However, in general, you need to learn to accept the disorder and explain it to those around you. Supportive counseling may be very helpful, either in private therapy or in a self-help group.

3

Lung and Breathing Disorders

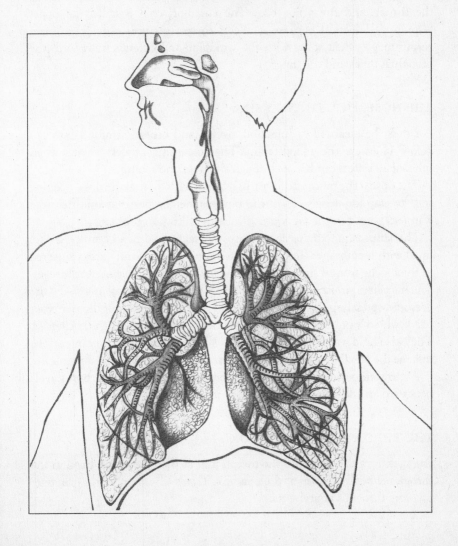

HOW THE RESPIRATORY SYSTEM WORKS

The respiratory system is crucial for life because it enables us to breathe. We think of breathing as essential because we get oxygen from the air by inhaling and get rid of carbon dioxide by exhaling. However, another important function of breathing is that it enables us to speak normally.

Most of the time, breathing is effortless and occurs without our even thinking about it. However, a variety of respiratory diseases can cause minor to major difficulty, either in getting sufficient oxygen into our system or in exhaling carbon dioxide and waste products.

The respiratory tract consists of an upper and lower respiratory system. The **upper respiratory system** includes the nose and mouth, the sinuses, the throat, and the voice box. The common cold is called an upper respiratory infection because it affects these structures only. The **lower respiratory system** starts with the windpipe and extends down into the bronchial tubes and the lungs.

THE NOSE, MOUTH, AND SINUSES

Air must be cleansed of infectious agents and other harmful substances before it enters the bloodstream. That cleansing process begins when inhaled air enters our bodies through the nose and mouth.

The **nose** is the more effective filter. Small hairs around the nasal opening start to trap impurities. Then the mucous membranes that line the nose warm and moisten the air and continue the filtration process.

The **sinuses** are empty cavities in your facial and head bones that are lined with membranes similar to those lining your nose and are connected to them. The frontal sinuses are behind your forehead, just above the eyes. The maxillary sinuses are on both sides of the nose, starting just below the eyes and spreading out to the cheeks. These air spaces help lighten your head, which would be extraordinarily heavy if bone filled these cavities. They also help warm and moisten air. When upper respiratory infections inflame the membrane lining of the sinuses, the result can be painful sinusitis.

Air entering the **mouth** is also warmed and moistened and then travels backward and downward toward the throat.

THE THROAT AND VOICE BOX

Passages from the nose and the mouth join at the base of the head in the **throat,** medically known as the pharynx. That's why your doctor may refer to a sore throat as pharyngitis.

At the base of the throat, the air passage divides again. One tube is the esophagus, which carries food to the stomach. The other tube contains the **larynx**, or voice box. It links to the windpipe, also known as the trachea. The epiglottis is a structure that permits air to enter the voice box, in order to form sound, but keeps out food and water. Occasionally, if you are talking while eating or eating rapidly, the epiglottis may fail and you get a bit of food or fluid "down the wrong pipe." If the food is large enough to block the windpipe, you can choke to death if it is not promptly expelled. If the food is tiny or if fluid has penetrated the trachea, it may move down into the lungs and cause a type of pneumonia referred to as aspiration pneumonia.

THE TRACHEA AND BRONCHIAL TUBES

The **trachea** and **bronchial tubes** look like an upside-down tree, with the windpipe as the trunk and the bronchial tubes as the multiple branches leading to the lungs. The trachea first branches into two large bronchial tubes. One goes to each lung, where it divides further.

These passages are lined with **mucous glands** and **cilia**. The glands secrete sticky substances that trap impurities in air and keep them from entering your system. The cilia are tiny hair-like structures that push the mucus up through the respiratory system toward the nose and throat. If the bronchial tubes become inflamed and fail to move mucus effectively, you may suffer with asthma or bronchitis.

THE LUNGS

In the **lungs**, the bronchial tubes branch into ever smaller offshoots, called **bronchioles**. These also are lined with mucous glands and cilia.

At the end of the bronchioles are the **alveoli**, millions of little balloon-like sacs. It is in the alveoli that the critical exchange of blood with gases occurs. The alveoli normally fill with air when you breathe in and then transfer oxygen to blood via the surrounding **capillaries**, the smallest of the blood vessels. The alveoli extract carbon dioxide and other gaseous waste from the blood and remove it from the body by contracting when you exhale. The elasticity of the alveoli is critical to normal function. If they lose their elasticity, they cannot force air out of the lungs when you exhale. This loss of elasticity causes emphysema.

The lungs are surrounded by the **ribs**. Attached to the ribs and below them is the **diaphragm**, a sheet-like muscle that separates the organs in the chest from those in the abdomen below. Movement of the ribs and the diaphragm is controlled automatically by the brain. This movement causes the lungs to expand and contract, moving air in and out of the respiratory system. When the diaphragm contracts, a vacuum is created, causing the lungs to expand and suck air into the system. When the diaphragm relaxes, the lungs contract and expel air out of the system.

This rhythmic inhalation and exhalation normally occurs at a regular, even pace. When you exercise and need more oxygen, you tend to breathe faster. Your heart rate increases, and your lungs extract oxygen from the air more rapidly.

SYMPTOMS AND SOLUTIONS

SHORTNESS OF BREATH

As long as you are breathing easily, you don't think much about it. When you do become aware of your breathing, it is usually because you are short of breath. Shortness of breath is the symptom people most commonly associate with a respiratory problem. Also known as breathlessness, it means that you are struggling to breathe or that you are uncomfortable and must labor for each gasp. Shortness of breath may mean nothing or it may be a sign of something seriously wrong.

In most cases, shortness of breath indicates a disease that directly affects the lungs, such as asthma, bronchitis, pneumonia, emphysema, and heart disease. Although shortness of breath by itself may be serious, it can be a sign of particularly severe problems when it occurs with such other symptoms as chest pain, coughing, wheezing, rapid gain or loss of weight, or spitting up blood.

Causes and Treatment of Shortness of Breath

Shortness of breath should not be confused with rapid breathing. Normal breathlessness can occur after you exercise, especially if you are out of shape. It also may occur if you become overheated or emotionally upset. In addition, you may breathe faster than usual when you begin moving around after a serious or long-term illness. However, such normal shortness of breath disappears after a few minutes' rest. If shortness of breath continues after resting, it may be a sign that something is wrong.

If shortness of breath occurs suddenly and is accompanied by persistent chest pain, especially if the pain radiates to your jaw, shoulder, or arm, it could be a **heart attack** (page 20). In this case, the breathlessness and pain

Shortness of breath after little or no exertion is never normal, regardless of your age or physical condition. If shortness of breath develops suddenly and is accompanied by any type of chest pain, get emergency care immediately. You may be having a **heart attack** (page 20) or may have a collapsed lung, also known as a **pneumothorax** (page 94).

• Call your doctor for instructions. Make it clear to whoever answers the doctor's phone that **this is an emergency.**
• If you can't reach your doctor immediately, call an ambulance. Again, make it clear that **this is an emergency.**
• If someone can get you to a hospital faster by car or taxi, get going. Don't try to go by yourself. You may collapse on the way.
• While waiting for help, remain quiet.
• Sit up rather than lie down.
• Take nothing to eat or drink.
• Take no medication unless it was previously prescribed and is urgently needed or you are told to do so by your physician or emergency medical personnel.

may be accompanied by sweating, dizziness, faintness, weakness, pallor, nausea, vomiting, palpitations, a fluttering sensation in the chest, or a feeling of impending doom. Immediate medical care in an emergency room is essential to help prevent death.

If shortness of breath occurs suddenly and is accompanied by chest pain that worsens when you inhale, you may have a collapsed lung. Also known as **pneumothorax** (page 94), this means that air has gotten into the space between the membranes that surround the lung. It may occur after an accident or for no apparent reason. Although the pain usually is felt on one side only, you may experience it as a tightness across the whole chest, which can mimic a heart attack. Or pain may be felt only at the base of the neck, near the shoulder, or lower down in the abdomen. Another indicator of pneumothorax is a dry, hacking cough. If the pneumothorax is severe, immediate medical care in an emergency room may be necessary to help prevent respiratory failure or circulatory collapse.

Shortness of breath after exercise or stress may also signal **angina** (page 14)—another indicator that the heart is not getting enough oxygen. If you know you have stable angina, your doctor has probably prescribed nitroglycerine tablets to be taken at such times. If you have never had such an attack, or if you experience any change in your anginal pattern, call your doctor immediately. Again, this may be a warning sign of heart attack.

Sudden breathing difficulty that is accompanied by wheezing, coughing, and a feeling of tightness or squeezing in the chest could signal **asthma** (page 86). Such problems usually begin after exercise or at night. Learn to avoid situations that trigger asthmatic attacks, and get prompt medical attention to treat those that occur. Even when asthma is being treated properly, a severe attack may be potentially fatal and warrant immediate emergency care.

The most common cause of a sudden episode of shortness of breath is **bronchitis** (page 88). It is accompanied by wheezing and coughing that produces sputum. If you also have a cold or the flu, it is probably acute bronchitis. Call your doctor because you may need antibiotics if it is determined that the cause is a bacterial infection. With proper care, your symptoms will resolve quickly.

If your shortness of breath, respiratory infection, and cough are accompanied by chills, shakes, and fever, however, you may have **pneumonia** (page 93). This is a more serious infection that is likely to need stronger or intravenous antibiotics and may require hospitalization. You will need more careful follow-up and have a slower recuperation.

Shortness of breath can develop so gradually that you may not be fully aware of the condition. Little by little, you may realize that you are breathless after only minor exertion, such as climbing a flight of stairs, or even after no exertion at all. This could be chronic bronchitis, especially if you are a smoker. If you have a "smoker's cough" that doesn't go away and you are always coughing up phlegm, make an appointment with your doctor for a complete evaluation.

Such a gradual development of shortness of breath, without any other symptoms, could signal **emphysema** (page 89). This is more likely if you get frequent respiratory infections. Prompt medical care is essential to help slow the course of this chronic disease.

Shortness of breath due to bronchitis, emphysema, or other lung diseases may be initiated or worsened by cigarette smoking. It is prudent to avoid smoking and, if you are already a smoker, to stop at once.

Gradual development of shortness of breath together with swollen ankles and weight gain may mean that you have **heart failure** (page 21). Your body retains fluid because your heart is not pumping effectively.

Shortness of breath may also signal tuberculosis or lung cancer, but their more prominent symptom is coughing, as discussed below.

Not all shortness of breath is caused by serious illness. Breathlessness may be caused by hyperventilation, which disturbs the normal balance of oxygen and carbon dioxide in your blood. Anxiety is likely to trigger this condition. If you experience sudden shortness of breath in a stressful situation, and it is accompanied by lightheadedness, sit down or lie down right away to prevent injury should you faint. Re-breathing your own exhaled air can restore the normal level of carbon dioxide in your blood. Breathe into a paper bag for a few minutes. If you experience such episodes repeatedly, see your doctor for a complete checkup. If no physical problem is found, you may wish to consider psychotherapy or relaxation training to learn how to cope with stress more effectively.

COUGHING

The second most common symptom of a respiratory problem is coughing. A chronic cough is not a disease in itself, but it is a sign that something is wrong with your breathing system.

If you have a persistent cough or repeated episodes of coughing, or if you can't explain even a single episode of coughing by any of the lifestyle causes discussed in this section, call your physician. This is especially important if you are also short of breath. Describe what is happening so that the doctor can decide whether you should be seen immediately.

Causes and Treatment of Coughing

Everybody coughs from time to time. The common **cold** (page 270) or **influenza** (page 280) might make you cough for as long as ten days to two weeks. However, don't take over-the-counter cough medicine for more than a week or two unless prescribed by your doctor. The medicine might suppress the cough, but the illness causing it might be getting worse.

If your cough hangs on longer than usual after a cold or flu, you may be developing a chronic cough. It doesn't matter that you cough only in the morning when you get up or in the evening when you lie down. It doesn't matter if you only cough during the fall or winter months. If you've been coughing for more than a few weeks, your cough is chronic and warrants medical attention.

The most common cause of a chronic cough is **smoking**. You should not ignore the cough just because it is a so-called cigarette cough. It might mean that your heavy smoking has damaged your breathing passages; you may be developing bronchitis, emphysema, or lung cancer. If you are a smoker, even if no disease is found to be causing your chronic cough, it is wise to quit. Smokers have a much higher risk of all types of respiratory diseases than nonsmokers.

As discussed earlier, under shortness of breath, coughing may be a symptom of asthma, bronchitis, emphysema, or pneumonia.

Another increasingly common cause of coughing is **tuberculosis** (page 288). TB has increased dramatically in the United States in recent years. Particularly suspect TB if your cough produces a foul-smelling or rust-colored sputum and if it is accompanied by fever, shortness of breath, or chest pain when you take a deep breath.

Perhaps the most feared respiratory disorder is **lung cancer** (page 90), and a chronic cough is often its most prominent symptom. However, lung cancer can also mimic other respiratory problems, with its same symptoms of shortness of breath, chest pain, and spitting up sputum or blood. In its later stages, lung cancer may cause fatigue, weight loss, and swollen lymph glands in the neck or armpits.

Not all coughing is caused by serious illness. A cough accompanied by sneezing, nasal congestion, and itchy nose and eyes may signal some type of **allergic rhinitis** (page 84). An allergic cause is most common during pollen-heavy months from spring through fall, although nasal allergies due to dust or mold may occur at any time of the year.

A cough accompanied by nasal congestion, as well as a headache and fever, but no itchiness, most likely indicates **influenza**, commonly called the flu (page 280).

CHEST PAIN

Although we usually think of chest pain as related to heart problems, and it is the most common warning of a heart attack, it also can signal severe respiratory disorders.

If you have any chest pain that lasts for more than a few minutes, or repeated episodes of chest pain, especially if it occurs when you take a deep breath, call your physician. This is especially important if you are also short of breath or have a cough. Describe what is happening so that the doctor can decide whether you should be seen immediately.

Causes and Treatment of Chest Pain

As discussed earlier, under shortness of breath, chest pain may occur in the presence of numerous cardiac and respiratory disorders, including heart attack, angina, tuberculosis, lung cancer, and pneumothorax.

If you experience chest pain only when you cough or breathe deeply, you may have **pleurisy** (page 92). The pain may be on both sides of the chest or only one side, if only one lung is affected. You will find yourself more comfortable if you take rapid, shallow breaths. Pleurisy is most likely to occur as a complication of a respiratory infection, such as pneumonia or tuberculosis, or of lung cancer. Or it may occur after a chest injury or inhalation of a foreign substance like asbestos. You may also suspect pleurisy if you have a predisposing condition, including lupus, rheumatoid arthritis, heart failure, or certain liver and kidney diseases. Immediate medical attention is needed to treat the underlying causes of the pleurisy.

NASAL CONGESTION

A stuffy nose that often alternates with a drippy nose can make you uncomfortable, but it rarely indicates a serious illness.

> If your upper respiratory symptoms seem worse, or last longer, than the problems discussed in this section, call your physician. You could be developing pneumonia or some other serious respiratory problem. Describe what is happening so that the doctor can decide whether you should be seen immediately.

Causes and Treatment of Nasal Congestion

If your stuffy nose is accompanied by sneezing and itching of the nose, eyes, or throat, suspect some type of **allergic rhinitis** (page 84). These symptoms could be triggered by hay fever or other respiratory allergy.

If nasal congestion is accompanied by a severe headache or aching on one or both sides of your nose, you are apt to have **sinusitis** (page 96).

If your stuffy nose comes on slowly and is accompanied by sneezing and a sore throat but no itchiness, it is probably the common **cold** (page 270). If you have a fever or headache, both are usually mild.

In contrast, the more sudden and severe onset of these symptoms is likely to indicate **influenza,** or flu (page 280). Although nasal congestion and sneezing may occur, it is less severe than in colds. Instead, headaches, muscle aches, dry cough, fatigue, and high fever are more likely.

Although the flu is usually a mild winter illness for most people, it can pose a severe threat for elderly people, children, and those with compromised immune systems. The worst of flu symptoms are over faster (in three to five days) than those of the typical cold (seven to ten days). However, feelings of weakness and fatigue can persist for weeks after the flu.

Repeated bouts of nasal allergy or infection accompanied by stuffiness and cloudy mucus may signify sinus infection. Your physician will take a sample of your nasal secretions for laboratory examination to determine the cause of the infection and the best antibiotic for treating it. If aggressive treatment with antibiotics, decongestants, and/or antihistamines does not halt the recurrent nasal problems, sinus irrigation or even surgery may be necessary.

COMMON DISORDERS OF THE RESPIRATORY SYSTEM

ALLERGIC RHINITIS is the medical term for allergies that cause nasal inflammation. The most common form is hay fever. Allergic rhinitis also occurs in response to pollens from weeds or flowers in the summer or fall; trees or grass in the spring; and molds, dust, feathers, or animal dander at any time of year.

What are the symptoms?
Sneezing, an alternately congested or "drippy" nose, and nasal itching are the most common signs of allergic rhinitis. Depending on your allergy, and your response, you also may have tearing and itchy eyes, a burning or itching throat, and a cough.

How did I get it?
Allergies are caused by a glitch in your immune system. You overreact to normal substances that never cause problems for most people. Such substances, called allergens, cause your body to release chemicals known as histamines. These in turn trigger a chain reaction leading to the symptoms characteristic of hay fever and other nasal allergies.

How is it diagnosed?
Your doctor usually can diagnose allergic rhinitis based on your description of your symptoms when considered in light of the time of year and situation

in which they arise. In some cases, skin testing will be performed to determine precisely what allergens trigger your problems.

How is it treated?
The most common treatment is antihistamine medication, which blocks the release of histamine and halts or prevents allergy attacks. New prescription antihistamines can avoid the drowsiness commonly associated with most over-the-counter antihistamines. Cromolyn sodium and beclamethasone, new drugs that you spray into your nose, prevent allergy symptoms by blocking the release of histamine. If an attack has already hit, decongestants can open a stuffy nose. If your allergic rhinitis is severe, you may consider immunotherapy—a series of injections over the course of a year or longer to desensitize your system to the offending allergens.

Self-Care: The best defense against allergic rhinitis is prevention. Try to avoid the substances that trigger your attacks. Stay indoors in the morning on high pollen count days. Let someone else do the dusting when you're not home. Use an air purifier or air conditioner, especially in your bedroom.

APNEA literally means an absence of breathing. The term is most commonly used to describe sleep apnea, a disorder in which you stop breathing briefly during sleep. Then, usually within a ten-second to three-minute interval, sleep lightens, you waken, resume breathing, and return to sleep. However, even when such episodes occur hundreds of times each night, you are not aware of the breathing cessation and awakening. In the morning, you have no recollection of these episodes. Years of apnea can cause hypertension, an irregular heartbeat, and lung problems. Sudden death while sleeping is also more common among people with sleep apnea, although apnea probably is not a factor in sudden death in infants.

What are the symptoms?
If you sleep with another person, your partner is apt to complain of the most common symptom: loud, intermittent snoring. Your partner also may report that you sleep restlessly. You have quiet periods when you don't seem to be breathing, followed by gasping or snorting when you waken and restart breathing. If you sleep alone, your only clues to apnea may be daytime sleepiness. Some people also have early morning headaches.

How did I get it?
The immediate cause depends on the type of apnea. In obstructive sleep apnea, the most common type, your airway is blocked due to the collapse of muscles in the throat. In central sleep apnea, respiratory centers in the brain shut down for unknown reasons. Mixed apnea includes both obstructive and central features. The underlying cause of apnea remains unknown, but it is more common in people who are overweight, who have nasal polyps or a deviated septum, or who have enlarged tonsils or adenoids.

How is it diagnosed?
Your sleeping partner may be able to report the classic symptoms, but you probably also will be evaluated in a sleep laboratory. This requires that you sleep overnight in an environment where you are monitored by health care professionals.

How is it treated?
Treatment depends on the severity of your disorder. Simply losing weight can reduce or eliminate mild to moderate obstructive sleep apnea. Another technique is sewing a pocket in the back of your nightclothes and inserting a ping-pong ball to prevent sleeping on your back, the position in which apnea usually occurs. For more serious problems, you may be given a continuous positive air pressure machine to use during sleep. You wear a mask that blows air into your nose, maintaining an open airway in your throat. For more severe cases, you may need surgery to widen the airway or to create an opening in your neck to allow airflow. This procedure is called a tracheostomy, and it involves placing a hollow tube in the hole at night to enable breathing.

> Self-Care: Do not take sleeping pills or tranquilizers, which are respiratory depressants. They can worsen your problem, making it more difficult both to breathe and to waken. These medications can place you at risk of sudden death during sleep.

ASTHMA is one of the most common chronic diseases, afflicting about 3 percent of the U.S. population. Technically known as bronchial asthma, it is characterized by problems in the bronchial tubes that make it difficult to breathe. Although most asthma patients develop the disorder in childhood and outgrow it as adults, it can arise at any time in life. Asthma is responsible for one-third of all school absences that result from a chronic disease.

Doctors do not know why the prevalence of asthma, and deaths caused by it, have increased by about 30 percent in the past decade.

What are the symptoms?
Asthma causes episodes of breathing difficulty accompanied by coughing, wheezing sounds, and a feeling of tightness or squeezing in the chest. The wheezing noise is produced by a narrowing and mucosal obstruction of the bronchial tubes. Coughing is your body's attempt to clear the airway. Coughing, especially at night or after exercise, is one of the earliest signs of bronchial asthma. The symptoms and severity vary widely from one person to another. You may have only occasional brief attacks, or you may have frequent attacks that last for ever longer periods of time.

How did I get it?
Asthma is caused by overresponsive bronchial tubes, and the tendency seems to be inherited. Your airways overreact to stimuli by narrowing. This narrowing is caused by spasm and contraction of the tiny muscles around the bronchial tubes, swelling of the lining of these tubes, and increased production of very sticky mucus that obstructs the bronchial tubes. What triggers these abnormal responses varies from person to person. One of the main causes is allergy, in which you are hypersensitive to substances that are harmless to most people. Pollens, dusts, molds, and animal hair are examples. Why allergies cause asthma in some people and not others is unknown. Many other factors can trigger an asthma attack, including exposure to strong odors like paints, perfumes, or chemicals in the workplace; respiratory infection; exposure to cold weather; excessive exercise; stress; or emotional upset. In some people, no specific cause of asthma can be found.

How is it diagnosed?
Your doctor will suspect asthma based on a report of your symptoms. Observing you during an attack can confirm the diagnosis, as can the findings from lung function tests, chest X-rays, blood tests, and laboratory analysis of your sputum. Your doctor will take a complete medical history to help determine what might be causing your asthma. You may need skin tests to assess your sensitivity to various substances.

How is it treated?
Asthma cannot be cured. However, antihistamines, decongestants, bronchodilators, and corticosteroids all may play a role in helping prevent

attacks or speeding their resolution. Medications that coat the mucous membranes in your nose can help prevent attacks. Drugs that are inhaled through the mouth can stop an attack by relaxing the spasm, easing inflammation, thinning the mucus, or opening the air passages. Other drugs taken by pill can help prevent attacks by forestalling allergies or relaxing the bronchial tubes.

> Self-Care: Try to avoid situations known to trigger your attacks, such as dusty environments, severe cold, or excessive exercise. If pollen is a problem, try to stay home in an air-conditioned room in the morning, when pollen counts are highest. Take preventive medications on the schedule recommended by your doctor, not just when you have an attack. See a physical therapist to learn healthier breathing patterns and postural techniques to drain your airways. If stress is a problem, learn relaxation techniques.

BRONCHITIS is an inflammation of the lining of the bronchial tubes. A brief attack is called acute bronchitis and usually accompanies a cold. Extended or frequent episodes are called chronic bronchitis. About 4 million Americans have chronic bronchitis, which they often neglect until it reaches an advanced stage. By then, your lungs may be seriously injured, making you more susceptible to life-threatening lung diseases and heart failure. Chronic bronchitis causes premature death for more than 5,000 Americans every year.

What are the symptoms?
When the bronchial tubes are inflamed, airflow to and from the lungs is partially blocked, and your breathing becomes labored and wheezy. You cough a lot, bringing up phlegm or sputum. This is called a productive cough. Chronic bronchitis can sneak up on you. If you are a smoker, your "smoker's cough" may get worse. As time goes on, the coughing and spitting last longer after colds and soon become an everyday part of your life. Symptoms are worse in the morning and evening and in damp, cold weather. In the most severe cases, you may be short of breath all the time.

How did I get it?
Acute bronchitis is usually caused by a respiratory infection and clears up quickly. The most common causes of bronchial irritation are air pollution and cigarettes. Most cases of chronic bronchitis occur in heavy smokers. In

other cases, the cause is unclear. Perhaps the bronchial tubes are first irritated by the bacteria or viruses that cause colds or influenza.

How is it diagnosed?
A complete physical examination must be supplemented by blood tests, chest X-rays, sputum analysis, and pulmonary function tests to diagnose chronic bronchitis. Your doctor also will perform tests to rule out tuberculosis and other possible causes of your symptoms.

How is it treated?
Antibiotics can quickly cure the bacterial infections that cause acute bronchitis, but no drug can cure chronic bronchitis. Changing your lifestyle may halt or slow the progression of chronic bronchitis if it is diagnosed early enough. If chronic bronchitis has become more severe, eliminating bad habits may at least reduce the impact of the disease on your life. You must eliminate all sources of irritation and infection in the nose, throat, mouth, sinuses, and bronchial tubes. See your doctor at the first sign of any respiratory infection. You may need immediate antibiotics. You may be advised to be vaccinated against influenza and pneumococcal pneumonia. If you have chronic breathing problems, you may be given a bronchodilator to help open breathing passages.

Self-Care: If you smoke, you must quit. If you are overweight, reduce to lower the workload on your heart and lungs. Take up a regular exercise regimen to develop aerobic stamina. Stay away from people who have colds. If you work or live in a polluted environment, consider changing your job or moving to a cleaner locale and one with a warm, dry environment. If you can't move, try to stay indoors when air pollution is severe.

EMPHYSEMA is one of the most common causes of shortness of breath in people over age 40. Also known as chronic obstructive pulmonary disease, or COPD, emphysema occurs when the balloon-like alveoli in the lungs lose their elasticity and are unable to absorb and expel air fully with each breath. As a result, you are not able to get enough oxygen or to rid yourself of carbon dioxide properly. This can lead to death due to respiratory failure.

What are the symptoms?
Emphysema usually begins very gradually, with shortness of breath only when you exert yourself. Over the course of months or years, breathlessness

worsens. You may have frequent respiratory infections. As your lungs become less efficient, your heart must work harder, which can lead to heart failure.

How did I get it?
All of the factors that cause emphysema are not fully understood. The greatest risk factor is probably smoking. People who have a history of bronchial irritation, asthma, allergies, lung infections, and exposure to air pollution are at greater risk. Also, some hereditary factors seem to be involved.

How is it diagnosed?
A complete physical examination must be supplemented by blood tests, chest X-rays, sputum analysis, and pulmonary function tests to diagnose emphysema. Your doctor will also listen to your chest while tapping it in a special way called percussion. Damaged alveoli yield a hollow sound in response to percussion.

How is it treated?
Emphysema cannot be cured. However, medical treatment and lifestyle changes can help slow its progression. To prevent lung infections, call your doctor at the first sign of any respiratory illness. You may be given antibiotics on a regular basis to prevent such infections. Drugs also may be prescribed to help open your airways. You may be sent to a respiratory therapist to learn special breathing techniques. If your emphysema becomes life threatening, you may qualify for a heart-lung transplant operation.

> Self-Care: If you smoke, quit. If you are overweight, reduce to lower the workload of your heart and lungs. Start a regular program of slow walking to develop aerobic stamina. Stay away from people who have colds. If you work or live in a polluted environment, consider changing your job or moving to a cleaner locale. If you can't move, try to stay indoors in an air-purified environment when air pollution is severe. Avoid travel to mountainous regions where the air is thin. Eat several small meals rather than one large one to avoid pressure from the stomach on your diaphragm, which can further impair your breathing.

LUNG CANCER is generally thought of as any malignancy that starts its growth in the lungs, in contrast to cancers that arise elsewhere and spread to the lungs, as so many do. A rare disease 50 years ago, lung cancer is now a leading cause of death in the United States. The most common type of lung cancer, accounting for more than 90 percent of cases, is carcinoma that arises in the bronchial tubes. This includes squamous cell (also known as epidermoid) carcinoma and adenocarcinoma, as well as the less common but more deadly small (or oat) cell carcinoma and large cell carcinoma. Alveolar carcinoma is a rare form of lung cancer that is less likely to grow rapidly and metastasize to other parts of the body.

What are the symptoms?
Lung cancer often mimics other lung problems. The symptoms include a persistent cough, aching chest pain, shortness of breath, and spitting up sputum or blood. Symptoms may develop very slowly. Some people have repeated bouts of bronchitis or pneumonia before they are diagnosed. In the later stages of the disease, you may be fatigued, lose weight, and develop swollen, tender lymph glands in your neck or armpits.

How did I get it?
How normal cells turn into cancer cells is not yet fully understood, but cigarette smoking is clearly the major cause of lung cancer. Continuing irritation from certain chemicals, radiation, viruses, air pollution, and other environmental and occupational hazards is believed to play a role in promoting or inducing some lung cancers. Also, people who are exposed over long periods of time to asbestos, chromium compounds, radioactive ores, and nickel are more likely to get lung cancer. However, the danger from pollutants and irritants is small compared to that from cigarette smoking. Smoking accounts for more than 90 percent of all cases in men and about 70 percent in women.

How is it diagnosed?
In addition to a complete examination, your doctor will likely order blood tests, laboratory examination of your sputum, chest X-rays, and a bronchoscopy. The latter test involves inserting a flexible tube down the throat to enable direct examination of the lung itself. Using the bronchoscope, the doctor can also perform a biopsy, extracting a small piece of the lung for laboratory examination.

How is it treated?
Treatment depends on the size of the cancer and whether or not it has spread. Surgery is often the first step, removing all or part of the lung in which the cancer is located. If the cancer is removed when the tumor is

small, you may be cured. Unfortunately, most lung cancer has spread by the time it is diagnosed. If the cancer is in both lungs or has spread to nearby lymph glands, radiation may be used to destroy or contain it. If the cancer has spread beyond these areas, chemotherapy may be best. In many cases, two or all three of these treatment methods may be used. Such therapy can often produce remissions, but in most cases the disease recurs. Less than 10 percent of lung cancer victims survive more than five years after treatment.

Self-Care: If you smoke, quit. This is the best way to prevent lung cancer and may enable your body to heal suspicious precancerous lesions. Even if you already have lung cancer, quitting smoking and keeping your environment as free of smoke and other pollutants as possible may help slow further growth of your cancer.

PLEURISY is an inflammation of the pleura, a thin, double layer of membrane that surrounds each lung. When fluid seeps into the thin space between these layers, the condition is called pleural effusion. Once relatively common problems, pleurisy and pleural effusion have become somewhat unusual because their primary cause is now easily treated. However, if pleurisy does not receive prompt therapy, it can become life threatening.

What are the symptoms?
When you develop pleurisy, breathing deeply or coughing causes pain because the pleura are no longer able to lubricate the lungs properly as they expand and contract. You may try to make yourself more comfortable by taking rapid, shallow breaths. If only one lung is affected, the pain will occur on only one side. If pleural effusion develops, the pain may disappear because of the fluid seepage, but your condition has actually worsened. In this instance, you are likely to become short of breath. Depending on the underlying cause, you also may develop a fever.

How did I get it?
The most common cause of pleurisy used to be unchecked infections, such as pneumonia and tuberculosis. As antibiotics have largely conquered bacterial infections, pleurisy arises less frequently. Other possible causes include injuries to the chest or inhalation of a foreign substance like asbestos. In addition, pleurisy may arise as a complication of some other disease. Predisposing disorders include lung cancer, lupus, rheumatoid arthritis, heart failure, and certain liver and kidney diseases.

How is it diagnosed?
As part of a complete examination, your doctor will listen to your chest with
a stethoscope, seeking sounds characteristic of pleurisy. A chest X-ray is also
likely to be needed. If you have pleural effusion, your doctor will want a
needle aspiration performed to obtain a sample of the fluid. The sample is
obtained by inserting a hollow needle through your back into your lungs.
Laboratory examination of the fluid can assist in diagnosis.

How is it treated?
To ease your discomfort, your chest may be wrapped with elastic bandages,
and aspirin or a stronger analgesic may be prescribed. Then your doctor will
seek to diagnose and treat the underlying condition causing the pleurisy.
For example, if you have an infection, you will be given antibiotics. If your
pleurisy is a complication of lupus or rheumatoid arthritis, you will be given
immunosuppressive drugs to help relieve the inflammation. If you have
heart failure, you will need diuretics and other medications to strengthen
the action of your heart. If you have pleural effusion, the fluid may be drained
in a process similar to the one used to take a sample of the fluid for diagnosis.
With proper treatment, pleurisy usually disappears within a week or two.

> Self-Care: In order to help prevent pneumonia, you will be encouraged
> to cough regularly. Coughing will be less uncomfortable when you sit
> up and hold a pillow firmly against your chest.

PNEUMONIA is an inflammation of the lungs in which fluid accumulates
in the alveoli and impairs their ability to function. Although pneumonia
can strike anyone, some people are at greater risk: those with chronic lung,
heart, or kidney disease or diabetes; the elderly; people who smoke, drink
excessively, or have inadequate nutrition; and those who are severely
overweight. If you have any symptoms of pneumonia, get medical attention
immediately because the illness can be fatal.

What are the symptoms?
Pneumonia may follow a cold, flu, or other upper respiratory infection.
Chills and fever develop, with temperature rising as high as 105° F. You feel
weak and experience muscle aches and appetite loss. Breathing becomes
difficult and is complicated by a cough. As the illness progresses, the cough
produces sputum, ranging from green to yellow to rusty in color. If left
untreated, the lung infection can spread to other parts of the body, including

the joints, ear, heart, brain, or bloodstream. In the brain, infection can cause meningitis.

How did I get it?

The most common cause of pneumonia is infection with a bacteria, virus, or fungus. Pneumococcal pneumonia is the most common type of bacterial pneumonia and continues to be a leading cause of death around the world. *Pneumocystis carinii* is an organism that causes a pneumonia called PCP in people with weakened immune systems, such as those with AIDS. Pneumonia also may be caused by chemical damage to the lungs after inhaling a poisonous liquid or gas, or by blockage of a section of the lung after getting a tiny bit of food or fluid down the wrong pipe.

How is it diagnosed?

As part of complete physical examination, your doctor will listen for certain chest sounds characteristic of pneumonia. A chest X-ray can confirm the diagnosis. Blood tests and laboratory examination of your sputum can help identify the agent causing the infection.

How is it treated?

If bacterial infection or PCP is diagnosed, your physician will prescribe antibiotics to cure it. Antifungal drugs are also given to those with PCP. Viral pneumonia does not respond to antibiotics and, although it can be dangerous, most cases heal on their own. To help reduce fever, aspirin and cool sponge baths may be recommended. Immediate bed rest is essential. Also, drink plenty of fluids, especially fruit juices. You must be carefully monitored because pneumonia can become very severe in just a few hours. In such cases, you may have to be hospitalized and given oxygen to help you breathe. Recovery may take from ten days to three weeks, depending on your general health.

Self-Care: A vaccine against pneumococcal pneumonia is available to help protect those at special risk. If you have a chronic disease or are 50 years of age or older, discuss vaccination with your physician.

PNEUMOTHORAX occurs when air gets into the space between the double-layered pleural membranes that surround each lung. Because of the pressure of this air, the lung cannot expand normally. This condition is called collapsed or compressed lung: All or part of the lung is emptied of air.

Depending on the cause and severity of the pneumothorax, it may be a mild condition that you barely notice and that heals itself, or it may be severe and rapidly become life threatening. If pneumothorax is severe and untreated, it can cause shock, respiratory failure, and circulatory collapse.

What are the symptoms?
The primary symptoms are shortness of breath and chest pain. The pain ranges from mild discomfort, to general tightness across the chest, to a sudden, sharp pain. The pain usually occurs on one side only, although you may feel it higher up, at the base of the neck or near the shoulder, or lower down in the abdomen. Sometimes you get a dry, hacking cough. Young people in otherwise good health may have few symptoms, even in the presence of a large pneumothorax. Older people, especially those with chronic bronchitis or other lung problems, may have severe symptoms even with a small pneumothorax.

How did I get it?
The most frequent cause of pneumothorax is a chest injury causing a hole in the pleura. This may occur due to internal injury or penetration by an external object. Among people who are on respirators, the trauma may be caused by having air accidentally forced into the lungs and rupturing the pleura. Less common is spontaneous pneumothorax. It may occur in otherwise healthy young people due to a congenital weak spot on the lung. This is more likely if you engage in a sport like diving or high altitude flying, which involves changing air pressure. Spontaneous pneumothorax also may occur in people who have other lung diseases, such as emphysema, asthma, or tuberculosis.

How is it diagnosed?
Your doctor will listen to your chest with a stethoscope for sounds characteristic of pneumothorax. If the pneumothorax is small, these sounds may not be easily detectable. However, X-rays usually can spot even a small one.

How is it treated?
A small, spontaneous pneumothorax typically requires no treatment other than rest. Your doctor will take new X-rays in a few days to make sure that the air in the pleural space has been reabsorbed by your body and that your lung has returned to normal size and function. If the pneumothorax is larger, healing may take several weeks. To speed the process, or for a more severe pneumothorax, your doctor may attempt to drain the air out. This is done

by making a small incision in your chest and inserting a flexible tube called a catheter. To remove the air, suction is applied to the catheter, much like sucking on a straw. In another technique, one end of the catheter is placed in a bottle of water, allowing the air to seep out gradually. In rare cases, pneumothorax becomes a medical emergency and surgery must be performed immediately to remove the air.

> Self-Care: Wear a seat belt whenever you are in a car to reduce the risk of pneumothorax if an accident occurs.

SINUSITIS is the inflammation of mucous membranes in the sinuses, the open cavities just above and around the eyes, and on either side of the nose. Sometimes called sinus headache, sinusitis is an uncomfortable but very common problem that occurs most often after a cold or in those who have allergies with nasal symptoms.

What are the symptoms?
The most common symptom is a severe headache just above the eyes that may occur in conjunction with aching pain on either side of the nose. In the worst cases, your whole face and head may even seem to ache. Some people also experience dizziness or nasal congestion. The pain may be worse in the morning, when you get out of bed. Sometimes pain can be alleviated by holding your head in a certain direction.

How did I get it?
The underlying cause is usually an infection by a virus, as from a cold, or by a bacteria, perhaps from a tooth abscess. Irritation of the nasal passages from allergies, smoking, pollution, or other causes also can predispose you to sinus aggravation. The infection or irritation leads to inflammation of the sinus membranes, which produces swelling and closes the passages. Because they cannot drain, painful pressure builds up in the sinuses. For unknown reasons, some people are prone to sinusitis. However, sinusitis is more common among those who live in temperate or cold climates, where respiratory infections are more frequent. Heat and lack of humidity in overheated homes and offices produce swollen, dry nasal membranes, which are predisposed to infection.

How is it diagnosed?
Your doctor usually diagnoses sinusitis based on your description of symptoms and an examination of your mouth and nasal cavity. If there is any doubt, an X-ray can be done.

How is it treated?

Therapy depends on what is causing the infection. If it is bacterial, antibiotics will be prescribed; if viral, antibiotics won't help. If your problem is related to an allergy, you may need an antihistamine. Whatever the cause, your physician may recommend decongestant tablets, nose drops, or a nasal spray to shrink the swollen mucous membranes. If sinusitis persists, a minor operation may be recommended to drain the sinuses. This is done with a local anesthetic in the doctor's office. Instruments are inserted through the nasal openings so that no external incision is needed. Drainage usually provides prompt pain relief. Material removed from the sinuses may be sent for laboratory analysis to determine the cause of the infection and the best way to fight it. In rare cases, when severe pressure builds in the area above the eyes, sinusitis can be dangerous and requires immediate sinus drainage.

Self-Care: During a sinusitis attack, try to avoid going outside in extremely cold weather. If you must, cover your face with a scarf so that you rebreathe your own warm air to a certain extent. Use a humidifier or take frequent hot showers, inhaling the steam, to help open your nasal passages. Never use decongestant nasal sprays or drops for more than three days; overuse can seriously impair normal nasal function, causing a rebound effect and worse congestion. If you have high blood pressure, don't use oral decongestants without your doctor's approval because they can raise pressure unexpectedly.

4

Bone, Joint, Muscle, and Tendon Disorders

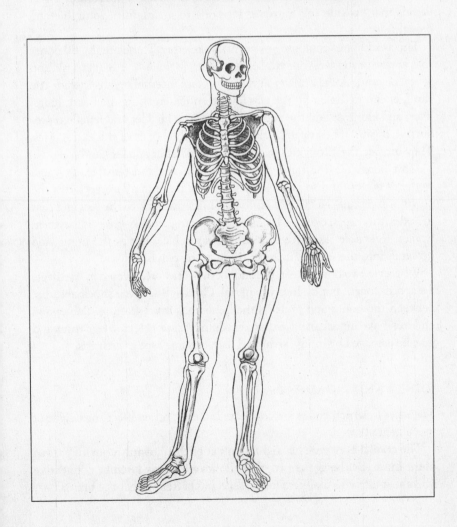

HOW THE MUSCULOSKELETAL SYSTEM WORKS

BONES AND CARTILAGE

The **skeletal system** is composed of the **bones**, **ligaments**, and **tendons**.

The normal human body contains 206 bones. Bones give your body form and enable you to stand upright. Although we think of bone as "hard as a rock," our bones change everyday of our lives. As some cells are added, others die. The normal result is a continuing increase in bone density until the middle to late 30's. Then, as metabolism changes, bone strength decreases. Bones serve as the body's storehouse for certain minerals, such as calcium. Further, like all other living tissue in the body, bones contain blood vessels that provide the nutrients for bone to maintain ongoing life and growth.

The **axial** bones compose your central skeleton. These are the 80 bones that encase or support your vital organs. They include your skull, trunk, and spinal column. Axial bone groups that protect internal organs include the **skull**, encasing the brain; the **ribs** and **sternum**, encasing the heart, lungs, liver, and kidneys; and the **pelvis**, encasing the bladder and female reproductive organs. The **appendicular** bones are the bones of the extremities. They include the 126 bones in your arms and hands and legs and feet.

Most bones are the same shape in both males and females, although women's bones tend to be slightly smaller. The primary exception is the pelvis or hip bone—a circular bone that links the back to the legs and that includes the hip sockets. The circular opening in this bone is larger in women to enable the birth of a baby. As the baby leaves the uterus and descends into the vagina, it passes through the pelvis.

Wherever two bones meet, the ends of the bones are covered by **cartilage**, a smooth, tough, but cushiony material. Cartilage acts as a shock absorber between the bones and protects the bone ends from pressure. Babies and children have more cartilage than do adults. As we age, cartilage thins and may be damaged by injury, wear and tear, or some type of arthritis.

JOINTS AND LIGAMENTS

The ways in which bones are connected to each other affect the degree of movement allowed.

The **cranial** bones are not tightly knit at birth, allowing room for growth of the brain. By the age of two, these bones are nearly fused by connective fibers that allow virtually no movement and better protect the brain.

The 26 bones that form the spinal column or back bone are called **vertebrae** (singular, **vertebra**). The vertebrae are circular bones, flat on top and bottom, and separated by spongy disks of cartilage and fibrous tissue. Although relatively little movement can occur between one vertebra and another, the cumulative movement along the length of the spine allows for considerable flexibility.

More commonly, the sites where bones meet form **joints** to facilitate greater movement. The two main types of joints are the ball-and-socket and the hinge.

For example, the ball at the top of the thigh bone fits into the socket of the pelvis bone to form the hip. The shoulder is also a ball-and-socket joint. These joints allow motion in all planes, including rotational twisting. The elbow and the knee are hinge joints. They allow full motion in only one plane—backwards and forwards—and relatively little lateral or rotation motion.

The stability of a joint is provided by the conformity of the two bones at the joint, the alignment of the joint surfaces, and the surrounding ligaments. **Ligaments** are bands of fibrous tissue that bind bones together.

At each joint, the bone ends, cartilage, and sometimes the ligaments are enclosed by a thin capsule called the **synovial membrane**. This membrane produces a thick liquid called **synovial fluid** that provides lubrication within the joint. In conjunction with joint structure and cartilage, the fluid further facilitates smooth and easy joint movement.

TENDONS AND MUSCLES

Tendons are the fibrous tissue that link muscles and bone. **Muscles** are composed of tissues that contract when stimulated by nerves. Skeletal muscles enable bone movement and are always attached to two or more bones. Usually, several muscles act in concert, some of them relaxing and elongating and others contracting. Leg muscles are among the most powerful in the body. Other muscles are responsible for much finer movements.

The skeletal muscles are voluntary; that is, they are under our conscious control. When we want to move an arm, our brain sends a message along nerves to the appropriate muscles to relax or contract, causing movement. There are also involuntary muscles, such as those of the heart and those of the esophagus and intestines that propel food through the gastrointestinal tract. We don't have to think about these actions for the muscles to act.

Because bones, joints, and their supporting structures allow movement only within a specified range, they are at risk for injury if they are stretched, bent, twisted, or otherwise subjected to excessive physical pressure. Improper use of these structures, or damage to any one due to trauma or disease, can cause pain and disability.

SYMPTOMS AND SOLUTIONS

BACKACHES

Backaches are among the most common human ailment. They may disable eight out of ten people at some time during their life. Tumors, congenital malformations, infections, kidney disease, muscle inflammation, and pelvic and abdominal disorders, as well as other problems like bad posture, overweight, and trauma, can cause backache and require medical treatment.

Causes and Treatment of Backaches

Sudden low back pain usually results from exercise or injury. If you have had a minor sports injury, are a weekend athlete who overdid it, or have been shoveling snow or moving heavy objects, and your pain is mild to moderate, you probably have a **sprain** or **strain** (page 125). Complete bed rest on a very firm mattress is the best treatment. Warm, moist compresses and aspirin or ibuprofen, as tolerated, can ease your discomfort. If pain becomes severe or does not respond to self-care within a day or two, call your doctor. You may be given stronger medication to relieve pain or relax your muscles. If the damage has been severe, hospitalization may be necessary for traction, and a supportive brace may be needed during healing.

Chronic back or neck pain is often caused by a **ruptured disk** (page 122). The pain may begin suddenly or gradually, is centered in one spot on the spine or in the leg, and is worsened by movement, coughing, or laughing. You also may experience numbness or tingling in the leg or foot. Although self-care is the mainstay of treatment, severe ruptures may require traction or surgery.

Pain in the lower back that shoots down your leg, especially if you are over 35, is probably **sciatica** (page 70). Although it is often related to a disk problem, sciatica is actually caused by any pressure, injury, or inflammation affecting the sciatic nerve. Bed rest usually helps, but if pain is persistent, make an appointment with your doctor to determine the underlying cause and to get relief.

Mild back pain in postmenopausal women is often ignored but should be heeded. It is often an early sign of **osteoporosis** (page 120). If you notice that you are getting shorter, osteoporosis is the likely cause. Bone scans can determine if you have a problem long before shrinkage occurs, and treatment with calcium, estrogen, or other drugs can often halt further bone degeneration.

If you have sudden severe back pain after a fall or injury and have difficulty moving any limb, feel numbness or tingling in any limb, or can't control your bladder or bowels, you may have damaged your spinal cord.

• Don't move at all.
• Have someone call your doctor for instructions. Make it clear to whoever answers the doctor's phone that **this is an emergency.**
• If you can't reach your doctor immediately, call an ambulance. Again, make it clear that **this is an emergency.**
• While waiting for help, remain absolutely quiet.
• Take nothing to eat or drink.
• Take no medication unless it was previously prescribed and is urgently needed or you are told to do so by your physician or emergency medical personnel.

Most backaches are far less severe. However, if you have a persistent backache, or if you can't explain a single episode of moderate to severe backache by any of the lifestyle causes described in this section, call your physician. Describe what is happening so that the doctor can decide whether you should be seen and when.

If mild backache occurs in a teenager, observe the youngster's posture. If one shoulder is slightly lower than another, or if you can observe spinal unevenness when the youngster leans over, it could be **scoliosis** (page 124). Prompt orthopedic evaluation is important to determine whether treatment should be given to normalize any curvature of the spine.

Most chronic low back pain is not due to any disease or hidden abnormality. Rather, it results from how we live. If you are overweight, sleep on a very soft mattress, have poor posture, or frequently carry heavy things, try changing your lifestyle to eliminate your back pain. Start a regular exercise program to build muscle strength. Stand tall, with your back as straight as possible and your abdomen tucked in. Sit well back in chairs, again with your back straight. When standing in one place for a long time, put one foot up on the rung of a chair or other object to relieve back stress. Try to vary your position throughout the day. Lift things by stooping, bending your knees, and keeping your back straight. Hold objects close to your body. In bed, sleep on your side with knees bent or on your back with a pillow under your knees—never on your stomach.

JOINT AND LIMB PAIN AFTER INJURY

Causes and Treatment of Joint and Limb Pain after Injury
Sprains and strains (page 125) are the most common cause of pain at the site of an injury. You will notice swelling and tenderness developing quickly and possible bruising under the skin, later followed by a black-and-blue bruise.

Strains, also called pulled muscles, are most likely to occur in the thigh, the arm, and the back. A sprain involves the wrenching of a joint beyond its normal range of motion and a tear of the ligament that holds it in position. Any joint can be sprained, although those most susceptible are the ankle, the knee, and the fingers.

NONINJURY JOINT AND LIMB PAIN

A great deal of joint pain is caused by some type of arthritis. The word *arthritis* literally means inflammation of a joint. It is applied to many different illnesses in the family of rheumatic diseases. There are more than 100 different types of rheumatic disease, which is the general term given to problems that cause pain in joints, bones, muscles, tendons, or ligaments.

Causes and Treatment of Noninjury Joint and Limb Pain
If you are over 45 years of age and gradually develop recurrent discomfort in one or a few joints, it could be **osteoarthritis** (page 118). This is more likely if the pain is always in the same joints, if it is in your fingers, hips, or knees, and it does not affect the same joints on both sides of the body. You may have mild morning stiffness that is eased by activity. If you have anything more than mild discomfort that is alleviated by aspirin or acetaminophen, call your doctor. Older people no longer need suffer with this degenerative form of arthritis. Treatment regimens are available to keep you comfortable and active.

If you have sudden joint or limb pain after a fall or injury and the pain is so severe that you cannot use the involved part (such as being unable to stand), if the joint or limb is misshapen, if bone protrudes through the skin, or if you can't move the joint through its normal range of motion, you may have ruptured a ligament or muscle or fractured a bone.

- Don't try to move the limb at all.
- Call your doctor for instructions. Make it clear to whoever answers the doctor's phone that **this is an emergency.**
- If you can't reach your doctor immediately and the affected bone or joint is your hip or in your leg, call an ambulance. Again, make it clear that **this is an emergency.**
- If you can't reach your doctor immediately and the affected joint is in your shoulder, arm, or hand, and someone is available to take you to a hospital, follow instructions for splinting under **fractures** (page 114). Then head for a hospital emergency room by car or taxi. If no one is available to help you, call an ambulance.
- Take nothing to eat or drink.
- Take no medication unless it was previously prescribed and is urgently needed or you are told to do so by your physician or emergency medical personnel.

Most joint and limb injuries are far less severe. However, even if you think the injury is mild and you proceed with self-care, reevaluate your situation a day or two after the injury. If you need more than a mild painkiller (aspirin or acetaminophen) to ease discomfort, if you are still limping, or if even moderate pain or swelling persists for more than two or three days, call your doctor. Describe what is happening so that the doctor can decide whether you should be seen immediately.

If you are under 45 and gradually or suddenly develop recurrent discomfort in one or a few joints, it could be **rheumatoid arthritis** (page 121). This is more likely if the pain is always in the same joints, the joints are warm and swollen, and the pain is symmetrical, affecting the same joints on both sides of your body. You also may experience more fatigue than usual and may have morning stiffness that is eased by activity. Such symptoms warrant prompt evaluation by your doctor. Rheumatoid arthritis requires a comprehensive treatment program to help prevent joint deformity and disability.

RICE TO THE RESCUE

RICE stands for *R*est, *I*ce, *C*ompression, and *E*levation. The acronym helps you to remember how to treat minor strains and sprains at home.

• *Rest* by not using the damaged joint or limb. If the arm or hand is affected, put it in a sling so that you won't use it for 24 hours. If the leg or foot is affected, settle yourself in a comfortable chair or bed for the same period.
• *Ice* means apply frequent ice packs. For example, apply ice for 10 to 15 minutes out of every hour for the first day or two, except when you're asleep.
• *Compression* means binding the area gently to support the injury and minimize swelling. Use a stretch bandage, but avoid wrapping it so tight that you interfere with circulation.
• *Elevation* also helps to reduce swelling and further enforces rest. Use pillows to elevate the injured part above the level of your heart.

If you are a woman and your joint pain wanders—that is, the pain occurs in different joints at different times—and especially if you have severe fatigue and a low-grade fever at night, it could be **lupus** (page 116). You also may sometimes have a blush or rash on the center of your face (on both sides of your nose), oral ulcers, or hair loss. Because lupus is potentially life threatening, you need to be under the regular care of a rheumatologist.

If pain is limited to one joint, has not resulted from injury, and is particularly severe when the joint is moved, it could be **bursitis** (page 111). It may develop gradually or suddenly. The area over the pain may be warm and tender, and you may see a small bulge where the sac-like bursa has filled with fluid. The affected joint needs complete rest and should be evaluated by a doctor. In severe cases, fluid may be withdrawn from the bursa.

If pain is limited to one joint, has not resulted from injury, starts suddenly,

---

Joint and limb pain is never normal. If you have any persistent joint or limb pain, or if you can't explain a single episode of moderate to severe pain by any of the lifestyle causes discussed in this section, call your physician. Describe what is happening so that the doctor can decide whether you should be seen immediately.

and is exquisitely painful, it could be **gout** (page 115). The overlying skin is likely to be shiny, red, tender, and warm. Gout is more likely to occur in the big tow, knee, or elbow. If left untreated, a first attack will likely subside within a week, but your doctor can give you medication to reduce pain within 12 hours and banish it within two days. For recurrent attacks, you need ongoing medication to reduce their frequency and severity, as well as a modification of your diet.

If pain is limited to your fingers or wrist, and especially if it is accompanied by tingling or numbness in all fingers except your pinkie or by weakness in the hand or swollen fingers, it could be **carpal tunnel syndrome** (page 112). This is more likely if pain occurs at night and if your daily activities involve a lot of hand use, such as working at a computer. You will probably need a wrist splint and anti-inflammatory medication. If modifications in your work environment don't help, surgery may be necessary.

If pain seems to be over but not in a joint, develops gradually, and is accompanied by swelling but no redness or warmth, it could be **tendinitis** (page 126). Pain is likely to worsen with movement. Again, you will probably need to modify your activities and give the joint considerable rest for this condition to heal. In rare cases, the tendon ruptures and surgery is needed.

If pain is limited to your jaw joint, develops gradually, and is worse when you awaken in the morning, it could be **TMJ syndrome** (page 128). The pain may be accompanied by a headache and is more common in tense people who grind their teeth. Both your dentist and your physician may participate in the diagnosis and treatment of your problem.

Deep pain, swelling, and tenderness in the calf or thigh in the absence of exercise may indicate **phlebitis** (page 33), an inflammation of a vein that requires an immediate call to your physician. Phlebitis can lead to the formation of a blood clot, also called a thrombus. The clot adheres to the wall of the vein and partially or completely blocks the flow of blood. Pain in the calf or thigh accompanied by skin redness, warmth, and swelling, as well as chest discomfort or rapid breathing or pulse, may indicate the presence of a thrombus. Immediate medical attention is necessary because this condition can be life threatening if the clot breaks free and travels through the bloodstream to lodge in the lungs.

LEG CRAMPS

Leg cramps are very common. Most often, they are just minor and temporary and easily banished with a few simple techniques. In other instances, leg cramps may be a sign of serious illness and warrant consultation with your physician.

If you have persistent leg cramps, or if you can't explain a single episode of moderate to severe cramps by any of the lifestyle causes discussed in this section, call your physician. Describe what is happening so that the doctor can decide whether you should be seen immediately.

Causes and Treatment of Leg Cramps

Leg cramps that occur *after exercise or at night while resting* are the most common type and usually are not a problem. These cramps occur when a muscle goes into intense contraction and then does not relax normally. This can be a quick squeeze/release in seconds—a jolt that's called a spasm—or a tightening, in your calf muscle, for example, for as long as a minute or two that interferes with function. Doctors know very little about what causes these cramps, although they sometimes arise from muscle fatigue due to overuse.

When these cramps hit, the muscle knots up and you can feel it tense and harden with your hand. If left alone, the muscle will eventually relax, a process that can mean minutes of suffering, which can feel like hours. For faster relief, immediately stretch the muscle gently in the opposite direction of the contraction.

• If the cramp is in the calf with the ankle being forced down into a ballerina's point, flex the foot upward or stand up.
• If the cramp is in the sole of your foot and your toes are curling under, take hold of them and gradually stretch them back up.
• If the cramp is in the front of the thigh, bend your knees and squat.
• If the cramp is in the back of the thigh, sit on the floor with your feet straight out in front of you and stretch your arms out toward your toes.

Cramps that occur *during exercise* and that go away after resting may be due to fatigue but are more likely to be a sign of a more serious problem and possibly even major illness. However, these problems are related not to your musculoskeletal system but to your circulatory system—and both are likely to improve with exercise that enhances your circulation.

If you experience mild to moderate heaviness, aching, or crampy feelings in your calves when you have been standing or walking for long periods and you can actually see some veins standing out in your leg, it is probably **varicose veins** (page 36). The discomfort should ease after you sit down for awhile. Elastic support hose may be helpful if you must be on your feet a great deal. In some cases, it may be necessary to have the abnormal veins removed.

If you have discomfort that ranges from a tired feeling to a crampy ache to severe pain in your calves, thighs, or buttocks that occurs while you are walking or exercising, and pain worsens markedly if you walk rapidly or uphill, it could be **intermittent claudication** (page 30). The pain should disappear after one to five minutes of rest. As the problem worsens, the distance you can walk before pain occurs gradually decreases. Intermittent claudication is caused by atherosclerosis and warrants comprehensive treatment by your physician and a change in your lifestyle.

MUSCLE WEAKNESS

Muscle weakness may be felt as a heaviness in your limbs, an inability to lift objects or walk normally, or a failure of any other part of the body controlled by muscles, such as a drooping eyelid or difficulty in swallowing.

If you have any persistent muscle weakness, or even weakness that comes and goes without explanation, call your physician. Describe what is happening so that the doctor can decide whether you should be seen immediately.

Causes and Treatment of Muscle Weakness

Muscle weakness most often is caused by a problem in the **brain;** the **central nervous system,** including the nerves in the spinal cord; or the **peripheral nervous system,** the nerves in the arms and legs. (See pages 40–41.)

When muscle weakness is observed in a little boy, it could be Duchenne **muscular dystrophy** (page 117). The youngster develops a waddling, ducklike walk, keeping his feet wide apart. He has progressive difficulty walking, especially climbing stairs, and lifting objects. Although muscular dystrophy cannot be cured, medical attention is needed to help the youngster to be comfortable and to assist the parents in family planning because this is an inherited disorder.

COMMON DISORDERS OF THE
MUSCULOSKELETAL SYSTEM

ANKYLOSING SPONDYLITIS (AS) is a severe form of arthritis that primarily affects the spine, although other joints and organs may be involved. It is an inflammatory disorder that can be seriously painful and crippling. AS usually strikes between the ages of 20 and 40, and men are afflicted three times as often as women. This chronic disease cannot be cured, but effective treatment is available.

What are the symptoms?
The major symptom is back pain, especially at night, and back stiffness upon rising in the morning. Sometimes joints in the hands and feet may be painful, particularly in women and children. You may find yourself seeking to relieve back pain and muscle spasm by adopting a slightly bent-over posture. Some people also experience fever, fatigue, loss of appetite, weight loss, and red or painful eyes. AS can also damage the lungs, skin, muscles, and heart. The disease sometimes flares or goes into remission for unknown reasons. Both changes are usually temporary.

How did I get it?
Doctors still don't know exactly what causes AS, but both genetic and environmental factors seem to be involved. If you are born with the genetic predisposition, a virus or some other environmental agent seems to trigger the disorder.

How is it diagnosed?
Diagnosis is based on a complete physical examination, your report of your symptoms, blood tests, and X-rays.

How is it treated?
Aspirin is the anti-inflammatory drug most commonly prescribed for AS, but it must be taken in high doses on a regular schedule—not just when you have pain—to have long-term beneficial effects. If aspirin doesn't help, your doctor may prescribe one of the newer nonsteroidal anti-inflammatory drugs, such as naproxen, sulindac, diclofenac, indomethacin, phenylbutazone, or oxyphenbutazone. Corticosteroid ointments may be prescribed for eye problems, and injections of corticosteroids may help particular joints. Oral corticosteroids are rarely prescribed. For those with severe AS, physi-

cians may recommend more potent drugs such as sulfasalazine, which may slow the disease down but has potentially serious side effects. Complete treatment of AS also requires learning how to protect affected joints by doing daily tasks in new ways and doing special exercises to strengthen muscles and maintain joint mobility. Exercises must be done daily to maintain good posture and prevent deformity. If the spine becomes deformed, surgery may be required.

Self-Care: Take a hot bath or shower first thing in the morning to ease back stiffness. Always take aspirin and other nonsteroidal anti-inflammatory drugs with meals in order to help prevent stomach irritation. Try to sleep on a hard mattress on your stomach, without a pillow, to keep your back straight and muscles strong. Deep breathing and swimming can help you maintain flexibility in your chest and rib cage.

BURSITIS is a rheumatic disease involving the bursa, the soft, thin sac or pouch located around a joint, such as the knee, shoulder, or elbow. The bursa contains a small amount of lubricating fluid that helps make joint movement smooth. Bursae are usually located between the skin and underlying bone or between tendons and bone. If the bursa becomes inflamed, bursitis occurs. Although the bursa of any joint in the body can be affected, the ones most commonly affected are those deep in the shoulder, the knee ("housemaid's knee"), the elbow, and the hip. Acute bursitis is a fairly common condition that may respond to simple self-care. Even chronic bursitis usually clears up after a year or two.

What are the symptoms?
Bursitis causes pain, swelling, and inflammation around the joints. The first sign usually is severe pain when the joint is moved. The area may be warm and tender, and surrounding muscles may be tense. Sometimes so much fluid has accumulated in the bursa that it can be felt or seen as an enlarged sac. Sometimes an acute bursitis attack fails to clear completely and becomes chronic. Although pain is not as severe, joint movement may become limited, and flareups of acute bursitis may occur.

How did I get it?
The most common causes of bursitis are excessive or improper use of the joint or joint injury. Sometimes the condition may be caused by a general body disorder, such as rheumatoid arthritis, gout, or an infection.

How is it diagnosed?
Your doctor usually can diagnose bursitis based on a physical examination. If your swellings are particularly painful and red, blood tests may be performed to rule out other possible causes, such as infection. In some cases, X-rays are also necessary.

How is it treated?
Complete joint rest is essential. Take aspirin or ibuprofen to ease pain and help reduce inflammation. Ice packs help reduce swelling. As soon as acute pain eases, start gentle exercise to return the joint's full range of motion. This helps prevent the formation of adhesions, which can lead to chronic disability. If rest and self-care don't yield improvement within a few days, or if pain is severe, call your doctor. Therapy may include drawing fluid out of the bursa by needle aspiration or injecting a steroid drug directly into the bursa. Healing of chronic bursitis may be expedited with heat treatments, physiotherapy, and medication. In extreme cases of chronic bursitis, surgery may be done to remove calcium deposits in the bursa, to eliminate adhesions, or to remove the bursa itself. This surgery seldom requires more than 24 hours in the hospital.

> Self-Care: A bag of frozen peas can be an effective ice pack because it can flex over the joint. (But never eat the peas after the bag has been frozen and thawed more than once.) Avoid heating pads—heat only makes acute bursitis pain worse. Minimize any activities that seem to worsen your condition.

CARPAL TUNNEL SYNDROME is an increasingly common disorder. The carpals are small bones in the wrist that, together with a ligament just beneath the skin, form a tunnel. Passing through that tunnel is the median nerve, which provides sensation to the fingers and muscle control to the thumb. If inflammation and swelling occur in the wrist joint, muscles, or tendons surrounding the area, the result may be significant discomfort in the hand, wrist, and arm—called carpal tunnel syndrome.

What are the symptoms?
When nerve communication to the hand is impeded, the most common symptoms are pain, tingling, or numbness in all the fingers except the pinkie. When the median nerve is placed under pressure, the primary symptom is shooting pain in the wrist and arm. Symptoms may worsen at night and even awaken you from sleep. You also may experience weakness

in the hand and an inability to grasp properly. Your fingers may swell, or the skin on your hand may seem pale because of impaired blood flow. Symptoms may come and go over a period of months or years. If the underlying cause is not resolved, pain may eventually become severe and chronic.

How did I get it?

This disorder has been in the news a great deal because of its relationship to the repetitive stress injury that may be caused by long hours spent at a computer. However, it may be caused by any job that requires firm grasping, or by other wrist injuries. Arthritis, diabetes, thyroid problems, or other diseases that cause joint or hand swelling may also be involved. Even pregnancy or the use of birth control pills may cause hand swelling and trigger the syndrome.

How is it diagnosed?

An orthopedist diagnoses the disorder based on complete history and examination, including an analysis of what types of movement cause symptoms. X-rays and other tests may be required to rule out other potential causes of your pain.

How is it treated?

If an underlying disease is contributing to the problem, getting that disorder under control may alleviate or cure carpal tunnel syndrome. In the mean-time, your doctor may prescribe aspirin or ibuprofen to reduce inflammation and swelling. In some cases, steroid drugs may be injected directly into the wrist. The use of a splint can hold the wrist straight and help reduce pain. If your problem is related to job or home activities, a physical or occupa-tional therapist can help you learn how to adjust your activities to reduce wrist stress. There are workplace specialists who can analyze the conditions that may be causing your problem. If such conservative measures fail, a surgical procedure called carpal tunnel release may be necessary. This is usually done on an outpatient basis. Special exercises are needed to restore normal hand motion, which usually returns after about two months.

Self-Care: To prevent or alleviate carpal tunnel syndrome, analyze how you do your daily work. Try to reduce stress and bending of your wrists. If you work at a computer, use a wrist support. Take frequent breaks to exercise your wrists and hands. At the first sign of symptoms, consult your doctor and consider the use of wrist splints.

FRACTURES are breaks in bones. The most common types of fractures, in increasing order of severity, are simple and hairline fractures, in which the bone is broken but does not damage surrounding muscle and other tissue; compound fractures, in which sharp edges of bone damage surrounding tissue and often protrude through the skin; comminuted fractures, in which some bone is crushed; and dislocation fractions, in which a broken bone is also dislocated at its socket, such as at the shoulder or hip.

What are the symptoms?
A fracture causes moderate to severe pain and usually produces rapid swelling. In the absence of other symptoms, a lay person may find it impossible to differentiate a simple fracture from a severe sprain or strain. Sometimes, the injured part can be seen to be out of normal alignment. In other cases, you may be unable to use the affected part. Less commonly, the bone may protrude through the skin.

How did I get it?
Normally, fractures are caused by some accident or injury that puts excessive force on a bone. However, in elderly people who have osteoporosis, fractures may occur spontaneously or from only minor pressure.

How is it diagnosed?
A complete orthopedic examination and X-rays are necessary to identify a fracture.

How is it treated?
First the bone is realigned in proper position. Depending on the severity of the fracture, you may be given general anesthesia during the procedure. In some cases, the realignment is done by external manipulation. In others, an incision is made to ensure proper positioning. Then the bones are immobilized until properly healed. This usually requires application of an external cast that is worn for several weeks to several months. Sometimes an operative procedure is performed to insert surgical screws or plates and to immobilize the bone internally. You can start using the limb within a few days after such procedures.

Self-Care: If fracture is suspected, do not try to move the affected part. Rather, devise a splint to immobilize it, using a board, broom handle, or tightly rolled newspaper as the splint. Pad it with towels or clothing, and then tie it snugly to the part above and below the area of suspected injury. Do not tie it too tightly or circulation will be impaired. Do not try to use or stand on the limb. Obtain immediate transport to a hospital emergency room.

GOUT is a rheumatic disease that can cause exquisite joint pain, most commonly in the big toe. It afflicts about one million Americans and is more common in men than in women. Once thought of as a problem caused by overindulgence in food or drink, gout is now better understood as usually related to a metabolic defect that leads to uric acid crystal deposition in the joint and subsequent pain.

What are the symptoms?
Although the most common sites of gout attacks are the big toe, the knee, hands, or elbows, they can occur in any joint. When gout hits, inflammation causes intense pain. The joint becomes extremely tender and warm, and the skin over the joint may appear red or almost purple. In your first attack, only one joint is likely to be affected. Later attacks may affect several joints. Some people also develop fever, chills, fatigue, and a rapid heart beat. Although the first few attacks may last only a few days, untreated gout may persist for weeks.

How did I get it?
Gout usually derives from an inherited tendency to abnormal metabolism of food substances called purines. However, it also may be triggered by diuretics used to treat hypertension or by other causes of dehydration. When the metabolism runs amok, the levels of uric acid, a normal body waste product, rise dramatically in the blood and urine. Gout may be due to overproduction or underexcretion or uric acid or to both. As uric acid builds up, needle-like crystals form, settle in the joints, and precipitate gout attacks.

How is it diagnosed?
The symptoms of gout are so characteristic of the disorder that a rheumatologist usually can diagnose the disease based on a physical examination and your description of symptoms. Urine and blood tests can confirm the diagnosis, in conjunction with analysis of the joint fluid.

How is it treated?
A first attack will most likely be treated with indomethacin or colchicine, which can reduce symptoms within 12 hours and eliminate them within

two days. If attacks recur, the goal of therapy will be to prevent or treat painful attacks, as well as to avoid uric acid buildup in the body, because this also can cause kidney damage. Colchicine, allopurinol, probenecid, or other drugs are prescribed to reduce the incidence of attacks. Nonsteroidal anti-inflammatory drugs may be used to reduce symptoms, such as indomethacin, ibuprofen, naproxen, or tolmetin.

> Self-Care: Do not take aspirin; it slows down the excretion of uric acid. Drink a lot of water and other fluids to help control uric acid levels. Because some foods may precipitate gout attacks, your doctor may recommend dietary changes to reduce your intake of foods high in purines. Anchovies, sweetbreads, liver, kidney, and alcohol, especially wine, are examples of such foods. Attacks may also be triggered by stress, fatigue, or infection.

LUPUS refers to systemic lupus erythematosus, or SLE. It is a chronic rheumatic disease that can affect organs throughout the body. Lupus strikes women about ten times as often as men. It is most likely to occur in young adults in their 20's and 30's, although it can develop at any time from infancy through old age. Although it is a mild disease for many people, lupus can be serious and even life threatening. Symptoms may come and go without any clear reason. After some years, the disease may vanish in some people or become severe in others. A milder form of the disease, called discoid lupus erythematosus, affects only the skin.

What are the symptoms?
Lupus is a highly variable disease. Although the most common symptoms are fatigue and joint pain, it has no definite pattern. You also may have a low fever, hair loss, weakness, weight loss, dry mouth, muscle aches, swollen glands, loss of appetite, nausea, and mouth ulcers. About half of all people with lupus get a butterfly-shaped rash over the nose and cheeks. It may range from a blush, to mild scaliness, to a blistery eruption. In some people, symptoms worsen after sun exposure. Lupus may also cause severe headaches, anemia, inflammation of the lining of the heart or lungs, and kidney problems.

How did I get it?
Doctors don't know exactly what causes lupus, but both genetic and environmental factors seem to be involved. If you are born with the genetic predisposition, a virus or some other environmental agent seems to trigger

the disorder. Lupus is an autoimmune disease. This means that the body's immune system, which is supposed to defend against outside invaders like viruses, goes out of kilter; it attacks healthy connective tissue throughout your body.

How is it diagnosed?
Because symptoms are so variable, lupus can be difficult to diagnose. An important part of your medical evaluation will be blood tests. Your doctor will want to know if your body is producing antibodies to your own tissue.

How is it treated?
Although doctors still cannot cure lupus, most patients can have normal lives with proper treatment. Because lupus varies so, there is no one guaranteed treatment program for everyone. You and your doctor may have to experiment with several drug regimens over a period of months to find the right one for you. Those with relatively mild illness may be controlled with aspirin or other nonsteroidal anti-inflammatory drugs to suppress inflammation that causes the pain of lupus. Drugs long used to fight malaria may be prescribed to increase resistance to sun exposure and help prevent rashes and joint pain. For more severe problems, your doctor may prescribe corticosteroids, the most potent anti-inflammatory drugs, or drugs used in transplant medicine to suppress the action of the immune system. Because these two categories of drugs can have severe side effects, people taking them must be carefully monitored with frequent blood and urine tests.

Self-Care: To cope with fatigue, get at least eight or nine hours of sleep at night and balance your day with one or more half-hour rest breaks between periods of activity. Try to avoid stress, which can trigger flareups. Learn relaxation techniques to practice during your rest breaks. If your symptoms are worsened by the sun, avoid exposure in midday and always use sunscreens and brimmed hats. Because dry mouth increases your risk of caries and gum disease, get scrupulous dental care. Aspirin and other nonsteroidal anti-inflammatory drugs should always be taken with meals to help prevent stomach irritation.

MUSCULAR DYSTROPHY, also known as MD, is a term used to describe a group of disorders that cause deterioration of the muscles that control body movement. The most common type is Duchenne muscular dystrophy, which affects only boys and usually begins in early childhood.

What are the symptoms?
At the onset of Duchenne MD, the youngster develops a waddling, duck-like walk, with his feet wide apart. He has progressive difficulty walking, especially climbing stairs. As other muscles are affected, the child has difficulty lifting things or even raising his hands over his head. When facial muscles are affected, he may find it difficult to close his eyes or whistle. Although the muscles are deteriorating, they may look larger than normal as fat replaces muscle tissue. With time, deformities occur and the youngster becomes confined to a wheelchair. Complications of the disease, such as pneumonia, are often fatal before adulthood.

How did I get it?
All types of muscular dystrophy are genetic disorders that are inherited. Although only boys get Duchenne muscular dystrophy, the genes are passed by the mother.

How is it diagnosed?
If MD is suspected, tests will be done to rule out other possible causes of the muscle weakness, such as nerve disorders. Examinations may include an electromyogram to measure muscle activity and a muscle biopsy. The diagnosis can be confirmed with a blood test.

How is it treated?
No treatment is available to cure or slow the progress of MD. Therapy is aimed at making the child more comfortable and helping him remain active as long as possible. This may include physical therapy and the use of canes or braces. In some cases, deformity can be corrected with surgery.

Self-Care: Women whose families have a history of Duchenne muscular dystrophy may wish to consider genetic counseling to determine whether they are carriers of the gene that causes the disorder. If they do, there is a 50 percent chance that any male offspring will have the disease. Tests can be performed during pregnancy to determine whether the fetus is affected.

OSTEOARTHRITIS is the most common form of arthritis, afflicting some 16 million Americans. It is also called degenerative joint disease and the "wear and tear" disease. Osteoarthritis most often afflicts those over 60 years of age, but younger people who do a lot of repetitive motion are also at risk. Although osteoarthritis cannot be cured, much can be done to prevent pain and disability.

What are the symptoms?

Osteoarthritis can be so mild that some people never have symptoms. For most, the major symptoms are pain, which can range from mild aching to severe discomfort, and loss of mobility, especially in the morning, due to joint stiffness. Among older people, osteoarthritis usually afflicts the weight-bearing joints, such as the hips, knees, and spine, as well as finger joints. In younger people, the location depends on joint damage. Commonly involved are the elbow joints of tennis players and pneumatic drill workers, the ankles of ballerinas, the knees of football players and runners, and even the hands of knitters.

How did I get it?

Osteoarthritis appears to be caused by damage to cartilage, the rubbery shock absorber that surrounds and protects bone ends. Pain occurs as the smooth cartilage surfaces and joint fluid that enable joints to move freely are worn away. What starts the destructive cycle still is unknown, although some people may inherit a predisposition to it. The damage may be caused by the weight-bearing stress of obesity, the wear and tear of a lifetime of movement, or by trauma. The more frequently and joltingly any repetitive movement is done, the more likely it is to cause joint injury that can lead to osteoarthritis.

How is it diagnosed?

Diagnosis is usually based on a physical examination and your report of symptoms. In some cases, your doctor may order X-rays and blood tests to rule out other possible causes of joint pain.

How is it treated?

Aspirin is the drug most commonly prescribed for osteoarthritis, but it must be taken regularly, as recommended by your physician. If aspirin doesn't help, your doctor may prescribe a nonsteroidal anti-inflammatory drug such as ibuprofen or naproxen. Complete treatment also may involve learning how to protect the affected joints by doing daily tasks in new ways and performing special exercises to strengthen muscles and maintain joint mobility. For more severe cases, heat treatments and resting splints may be needed. A badly damaged joint can often be replaced surgically.

Self-Care: Take a hot bath or shower first thing in the morning to ease joint stiffness and help you get moving. Aspirin and other nonsteroidal anti-inflammatory drugs should always be taken with meals to help prevent stomach irritation. If you are overweight, reduce to ease the burden on your joints. Avoid exercise like jogging or high impact aerobics, which place excessive stress on joints. Walking, swimming, and low impact aerobics are better choices.

OSTEOPOROSIS causes bone to become fragile and easily breakable, due to loss of mineral and protein components, especially calcium. As metabolism changes, bone strength decreases. The process is faster in women than in men, and it accelerates in the decade or two after menopause. When bone becomes so light that fractures occur with little or no pressure, the condition is called osteoporosis. It can be the scourge of aging, especially among women, causing bone fractures and even fatal complications.

What are the symptoms?
The earliest symptom is the mild back pain that many women ignore when they should seek medical attention. As tiny bones in the back break, others become depressed, decreasing height and leading to the commonly seen "dowager's hump." If left untreated, osteoporosis can cause even more serious fractures of the spine and hip, which can lead to permanent disability.

How did I get it?
The most common form of osteoporosis is believed to be caused by low levels of estrogen in women after menopause. Hence, women over the age of 45 are the primary victims. More than 5 million American women—25 percent of those over 45—have osteoporosis. Men show the signs of osteoporosis a decade later. Demineralization of bone can also be caused by a variety of other problems, such as Cushing's disease, liver disease, or long-term use of high-dose steroids.

How is it diagnosed?
Diagnosis is based on special X-rays called bone scans. Some doctors recommend that women have a baseline scan at menopause, then repeated six months to a year later, to help them decide whether or not to take estrogen replacement therapy.

How is it treated?
Current therapies may be able to stop the progression of osteoporosis, but they cannot repair damage already done. That's why prompt diagnosis and treatment are essential. Treatment is aimed at slowing down bone loss. It may include increasing calcium intake, through diet and supplements, as well as supplements of vitamin D and/or fluoride, which affect bone metabolism. Estrogen replacement therapy in postmenopausal women may be able to prevent or halt the development of osteoporosis.

Self-Care: To help prevent osteoporosis, practice tactics for building bone density in youth and middle age. These include weight-bearing exercise, because a sedentary lifestyle contributes to bone loss, and a diet high in calcium. Calcium-rich foods include milk and milk products, green leafy vegetables, and seafood.

RHEUMATOID ARTHRITIS (RA) is one of the most severe forms of arthritis, afflicting some 7 million Americans. An inflammatory disorder that can be seriously painful and crippling, RA usually strikes between the ages of 20 and 45, although it can even begin in childhood. Women are afflicted three times as often as men. This chronic disease cannot be cured, but effective treatment is available.

What are the symptoms?
The major symptom is joint pain. Although sometimes only a few joints are affected, they are symmetrical; that is, the same joint—the wrist or the knee, for example—is affected on both sides of the body. In other cases, widespread joint pain may feel like a bad toothache all over the body. In addition, you may suffer weight loss, fatigue, joint stiffness, and deformity. RA also can damage the lungs, skin, blood vessels, muscles, heart, and eyes. The disease sometimes flares or goes into remission for unknown reasons. Both changes are usually temporary.

How did I get it?
Scientists don't know exactly what causes RA, but both genetic and environmental factors seem to be involved. If you are born with the genetic predisposition, a virus or some other environmental agent seems to trigger the disorder. RA is an autoimmune disease. This means that the body's immune system, which is supposed to defend you by killing outside invaders, goes out of kilter. It attacks and destroys healthy tissue—starting with the

synovial membrane that surrounds the joint, extending to the rubbery cartilage that protects bone ends, and even affecting the underlying bone.

How is it diagnosed?
Diagnosis is based on a complete physical examination, your report of your symptoms, blood tests, and X-rays.

How is it treated?
Aspirin is the anti-inflammatory drug most commonly prescribed for rheumatoid arthritis, but it must be taken in high doses on a regular schedule—not just when you have pain—to have long-term beneficial effects. If aspirin doesn't help, your doctor may prescribe one of the newer nonsteroidal anti-inflammatory drugs, such as ibuprofen, naproxen, fenoprofen, tolmetin, sulindac, or indomethacin. For those with severe RA, physicians may recommend more potent drugs that seem to slow the disease down. They include methotrexate, gold compounds, penicillamine, hydroxychloroquine, sulfasalazine, corticosteroids, and other immunosuppressive drugs. Unfortunately, these drugs all have potentially serious side effects. Complete treatment of RA also requires learning how to protect affected joints by doing daily tasks in new ways and doing special exercises to strengthen muscles and maintain joint mobility. Because medication may not provide total pain relief, hot or cold compresses and other physical therapy techniques may also be needed. If a joint becomes badly damaged, surgery may be required to remove the damaged tissue, stabilize the joint, or to replace it completely with an artificial joint.

Self-Care: Take a hot bath or shower first thing in the morning to ease joint stiffness and help you get moving. Aspirin and other nonsteroidal anti-inflammatory drugs should always be taken with meals to help prevent stomach irritation. If you are overweight, reduce to ease the burden on your joints. To cope with fatigue, get at least eight or nine hours of sleep at night and balance your day with one or more half-hour rest breaks between periods of activity. Try to avoid stress, which can trigger flareups. Learn relaxation techniques to practice during your rest breaks.

RUPTURED DISK is also called a slipped, herniated, or prolapsed disk. These terms refer to a disorder of the spongy sacs that serve as shock absorbers in the spine. The backbone is made up of bones called vertebrae. These bones support the weight of the entire upper portion of your body. In between each vertebra is a soft, spongy disk that lets the spine bend and curve. The disks absorb shock from any jarring, pressure, or sudden movement change. Each disk is composed of a strong, fibrous outer layer of tissue that is filled with a softer spongy material.

What are the symptoms?

Discomfort may begin gradually or suddenly. It's always worse when you move and also may be worsened by coughing or laughing. Depending on the location of the rupture, pain can occur anywhere along your spine. You may have an aching neck that you cannot straighten without marked pain. Or you may have a searing pain at the base of your back. You also may have pain, numbness, or tingling radiating down an arm or a leg. You may be unable to walk, much less do any heavy physical work. The pain may even force you to go to bed.

How did I get it?

When enough pressure is placed on a disk, the outer tissue can tear, allowing the spongy inner portion to bulge into the spinal canal. The expression "slipped disk" refers to this bulging process. As this material bulges out, it presses on nerves in your backbone. Although a ruptured disk sometimes occurs in young adults, it occurs more often in those 45 years or older. As we grow older, the disks begin to lose some of their fluid. This drying out can cause degeneration of the disks, placing them at greater risk of rupture because they can no longer withstand shocks and sudden change of movement. Even something as minor as sneezing, slipping on a rug, or picking up a book from an awkward position can cause the disk to rupture.

How is it diagnosed?

Your doctor will suspect a ruptured disk based on your description of symptoms. The diagnosis can be confirmed with a back X-ray. The severity of the problem may be better defined with special imaging techniques, such as a CAT scan or magnetic resonance imaging (MRI).

How is it treated?

Therapy depends on the location of the rupture and the severity of your discomfort. If it is in the neck, you may have to wear a supportive collar for several weeks. If it is lower down, a supportive medical corset may be recommended. In either case, you will probably be told to spend one to several weeks in bed, with a piece of plywood under your mattress to firm it up. Such conservative treatment usually leads to recovery within a few weeks. If your problem is more severe, traction at home or in a rehabilitation therapy unit may be necessary. If your pain becomes chronic, or if there is any loss of movement in the leg or foot, more aggressive care may be appropriate. Some doctors try to dissolve the bulging disk material with injections of an enzyme called chymopapain. Others recommend surgery to remove the ruptured disk. If the ruptured disk is lower down on the back and is causing pressure leading to incontinence or urine retention, immediate surgery will be needed.

Self-Care: Taking hot baths or applying heating pads to your back may ease muscle spasm and pain. When lying on your back, you may be more comfortable with a small pillow under your knees. Some people get relief by lying on their sides in a fetal position. After surgery or recovery, you should do exercises that strengthen back and stomach muscles and stretches for suppleness.

SCOLIOSIS means abnormal curvature of the spine. Many people have a minor degree of such curvature, but it is usually barely noticeable and does not impair posture and function. When it is severe, scoliosis can interfere with normal posture and gait. If left to progress without treatment, it can compromise lung function, because the chest wall on one side may be compressed.

What are the symptoms?
A minor curvature may not be noticeable, although even minor curvatures may keep your clothes from hanging straight. You may look as if one shoulder is slightly lower than the other. As a curvature progresses, you may get backaches. In more severe cases, the upper body seems compressed and a bulge from the spine may be observed on the back.

How did I get it?
The most common type of scoliosis arises for unknown reasons and usually develops between the ages of 5 and 15, most often in girls. It may also be caused by polio, tuberculosis, or such congenital defects as the absence of half a vertebra, unequal leg length, or faulty function of a hip joint.

How is it diagnosed?
If the curvature is not pronounced, it may not be spotted until a checkup during which the doctor asks you to bend over. In that position, any curvature becomes more noticeable. If scoliosis is observed, you will need

X-rays of the spine and careful measurement of the degree of curvature. Even if the curvature is minor, your doctor may want to repeat X-rays from time to time to observe any progression.

How is it treated?
Treatment depends on the cause and severity of the curvature. Most cases are minor and require little if any treatment. For example, if the cause is unequal leg length, using a shoe lift for the shorter leg is all that is necessary. In other cases, physical therapy can help you improve posture and improve the strength of back muscles. If the scoliosis is the type that can progress to become a serious deformity, prompt intervention is vital. Youngsters may need to wear a brace on the torso to gently nudge the spine into normal position, thus avoiding surgery and deformity. After adolescence, the spinal column becomes less responsive to bracing, and surgery may be needed to correct any deformity that develops.

Self-Care: Although many youngsters adapt easily to brace treatment for several months to a year, others find the disorder and its treatment a serious threat to their self-image. Extra effort should be made to boost the child's self-esteem by recognizing achievement in any area. In some cases, supportive counseling may be necessary.

SPRAINS AND STRAINS are two different types of orthopedic injury with similar symptoms and first-aid needs. Also called a pulled muscle, a strain occurs when a muscle is overstretched and some muscle and tendon fibers are torn. A sprain involves the wrenching of a joint beyond its normal range of motion and a tear of the ligament that holds it in position. Strains are most likely to occur in the thigh, the arm, and the back. Any joint can be sprained, but those most susceptible are the ankle, the knee, and the fingers. The potential for permanent disability is greater with severe sprains.

What are the symptoms?
The primary symptoms of a strain or sprain are pain at the moment of injury, followed by the development of swelling and tenderness and black-and-blue marks near the injury. A mild, grade I injury involves tearing of fewer than 30 percent of the fibers of the involved muscle or ligament, yielding an achy pain that lasts from a few hours to a day. A moderate, grade II injury involves tearing about half of the fibers of the muscle or ligament; there may be considerable swelling and pain within a few hours, and it may be longer lasting. A severe, grade III injury involves complete rupture of a muscle

or ligament and is so uncomfortable that you are not likely to walk away from it.

How did I get it?

A strain occurs when the muscle is damaged by pulling or overstretching. It is likely to occur when you do very vigorous exercise to which you are unaccustomed, especially without adequate warm-up stretches and exercise. Some muscle fibers are torn, internal bleeding occurs, and the muscle contracts markedly. In sprain, the ligaments that hold the bones of joints together are damaged. A sprain is likely to occur when excessive demands are placed on a joint or it is twisted beyond its range of motion, as may happen when you land on your foot with your ankle twisted. Some ligament fibers are torn, internal bleeding occurs, and the function of the joint may be impaired.

How is it diagnosed?

Examination by an orthopedist and X-rays may be necessary to assess the extent of damage.

How is it treated?

Minor sprains and strains are best treated at home. For persistent discomfort, your doctor may prescribe a painkiller and, possibly, a muscle relaxant. You may be given crutches to avoid weight bearing on an injured leg or a sling for an injured arm. A severe sprain may be placed in a cast for several weeks. If a muscle or ligament has been ruptured, surgery may be necessary. You also may be referred to a physical therapist for restoration of motion and strength.

Self-Care: For minor sprains and strains, use RICE (Rest, Ice, Compression, Elevation; page 106) for the first two days. Then switch to soaks of warm water several times a day to promote circulation.

TENDINITIS is irritation and inflammation of tendons, the fibrous bands of tissue that connect muscles to bones and facilitate muscle action. Tendons do not contract or do the same work as muscles. Rather, they transmit the power of the muscle contraction to the right spot on the bone so that the muscle may do its work properly. Because tendons usually cross over a joint before connecting to a bone, the most common areas affected by tendinitis are the shoulder, elbow, wrist, knee, and ankle, as well as the feet and hands. When the elbow is involved, the condition is often called "tennis elbow." However, both tennis and nontennis players may suffer from the problem.

What are the symptoms?

The signs of tendinitis are primarily swelling and pain where the affected tendon is located, especially upon movement. Certain movements may be especially painful, and certain spots over the joints may bring pain when pressed. There is no redness or increased warmth over the areas involved, unless other problems are present. However, when tendons rupture, there is immediate swelling.

How did I get it?

Overuse or misuse of muscles may place extreme tension on a tendon and cause injury. Trauma or direct injury to the tendon can also bring on tendinitis. Calcification of the injured tendon may cause further discomfort after the original injury is healed. An activity performed repeatedly, especially if it is not done smoothly, can trigger tendinitis. Aging causes tendons to lose their resistance to damage more readily, but tendons can be injured at any age.

How is it diagnosed?

Examination by an orthopedist and, sometimes, X-rays may be necessary to make the diagnosis.

How is it treated?

The first step in treatment is reducing or stopping the particular activity that causes the pain. Slings, supports, or crutches can help reduce stress on the area. Medication to reduce inflammation may be given orally, locally by injection, or in combination. Local application of heat or alternating hot and cold packs may be recommended. If pain is severe, you may need prescription analgesics. Tendinitis may take several months or more to heal. Unless tendon rupture occurs, surgery is rarely needed.

Self-Care: Most people can control their tendinitis problems with the treatment procedures just described. However, some changes in your activities may be indicated. If the tendinitis derives from your participation in tennis or another sport, you may want to hire a "pro" to analyze your form and make suggestions to reduce stress.

TMJ SYNDROME is the term used to describe the facial pain and related difficulties caused by malfunction of the temporomandibular joint and certain surrounding muscles. The TMJ is one of two joints that connect the lower jaw to the skull, and it plays a pivotal role in chewing. The condition is also called myofascial pain dysfunction syndrome.

What are the symptoms?
The primary symptom is pain or tenderness of the joint or jaw muscles. It is felt most intensely on the upper cheek, about three-quarters of an inch in front of the center of the ear. You may also have headaches on the side of the affected jaw. Pain and headache may be particularly noticeable when you just awaken. You may also have difficulty chewing and opening your mouth, or hear clicking or snapping noises when you are eating or otherwise moving your jaw.

How did I get it?
Although the immediate cause is believed to be a dislocation of the joint, the underlying causes can be more diverse. For example, poorly aligned teeth, dentures that don't fit properly, various types of arthritis, or an accident can damage the jaw and cause the syndrome. However, in most cases, stress is a primary factor. Most people with TMJ clench or grind their teeth, especially in their sleep, causing local muscles to become fatigued and go into spasm.

How is it diagnosed?
The condition is diagnosed largely on the basis of your symptoms. X-rays of the jaw rarely show deformity, especially in the early stages. An MRI scan can be helpful in ruling out other possible causes of your pain.

How is it treated?
Both your doctor and your dentist may play a role in treatment, depending on the cause of the problem and your response to therapy. If TMJ is related to rheumatoid arthritis, treatment of the disease may help the syndrome. If it is caused by poorly aligned teeth, orthodontia will be needed. If your dentures don't fit properly, you will also need dental care. However, treatment usually is devoted largely to resting your jaw and breaking a habit of tooth grinding or clenching. This may include eating a soft diet requiring little chewing, taking a tranquilizer to relax you and your muscles, and taking a nonsteroidal anti-inflammatory drug to reduce inflammation. Relaxation techniques and psychotherapy may be advised to help you learn

to cope more effectively with stress. If all else fails, your dentist may recommend a specially made night appliance to prevent tooth grinding.

Self-Care: Try to become more aware of when you clench your jaw or grind your teeth. Ask people close to you, such as roommates or a spouse, to tell you if they notice you doing it. Consciously learn to relax your jaw. Try to make more time for overall relaxation in your life. Regular exercise is an effective means of easing tension.

5

Reproductive and Sexual Disorders

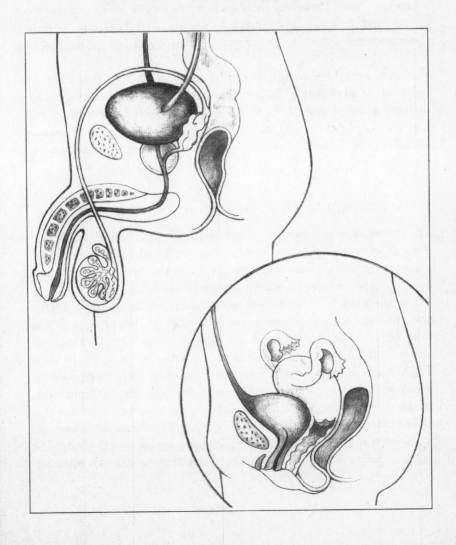

HOW THE REPRODUCTIVE SYSTEM WORKS

Human reproduction is an intimate partnership. The male manufactures **sperm,** the cells that carry his genetic material. Sperm are normally delivered into the female reproductive system during sexual intercourse. The female provides **ova,** the eggs that carry her genetic material and that are fertilized by sperm. The female body prepares for pregnancy every month during the fertile years from puberty to menopause. In months when conception does not take place, those preparations are discarded by the body through menstruation. When conception does take place, the woman's body nourishes the fetus until it comes to term and birth occurs.

Each partner has a corresponding set of glands, the **testes** in men and the **ovaries** in women, structures where sex hormones are manufactured and the reproductive material—sperm or ova—are prepared for conception. Beyond these similarities, the systems are rather different and are discussed separately.

Beyond reproduction, human genitals have an additional function as organs of sexual pleasure. The normal range of human experience includes deriving sexual pleasure alone through masturbation or with a partner in heterosexual or homosexual relationships. A brief review of human sexuality follows the discussions on female and male reproductive structure and function.

FEMALE REPRODUCTIVE STRUCTURE AND FUNCTION

The **uterus,** or womb, located in the lower abdomen, is about the size and shape of an inverted pear. Its muscular walls are lined by the endometrium, a membrane that thickens every month during the reproductive years, in order to prepare a supportive environment for the fetus.

Extending from the top of the uterus are the two **fallopian tubes.** Each is about four inches long and opens at its end with finger-like projections that reach out to the adjacent **ovary.** Each ovary, about the size and shape of an almond, contains hundreds of thousands of immature eggs, also called ova. Together, the two ovaries store twice that number. The ovaries produce the female sex hormones, estrogen and progesterone, and ripen eggs for monthly release during ovulation. Normally, only one egg is released each month.

The base of the uterus, the **cervix,** is a donut-shaped structure connected to the **vagina,** a ridged, soft-walled passage that leads out of the body. The vagina is lined with a thick mucous membrane that is constantly bathed by secretions that contain mucus, water, proteins, and salt. These secretions help wash out of the vagina sloughed-off superficial cells from the uterus and vaginal walls, microorganisms and the debris they produce, menstrual blood, seminal fluid, and the remains of contraceptives and other substances that may have been introduced into the vagina.

Vulva is the term used to describe the external female genitals. These include two sets of vaginal lips, known as the **labia minora** and **labia majora,** which enclose the vaginal opening. Nestled at the front of the labia minora is the **clitoris,** an exquisitely sensitive cluster of tissue. The **mons pubis** is a pad of fatty tissue just in front of the vulva on which female pubic hair grows during the reproductive years.

The **breasts** are composed of fat, connective tissue, and milk-producing mammary glands. In the center of each breast is a **nipple,** surrounded by a darkened area of skin called the **areola.** When a woman becomes pregnant, the mammary glands become active to prepare for breastfeeding. Milk produced in the breasts is carried to the nipple in special milk ducts.

Menstruation and Conception

Menstruation is the process by which the female uterus discards the extra blood supply and the uterine lining that accumulate each month in preparation for pregnancy. The menstrual cycle varies from woman to woman— from as short as 20 days to as long as 40 days—but it averages about 28 days. In such an average cycle, days 1 through 5 usually are the period during which menstruation occurs. This period, together with the next eight days, is called the preovulatory period.

As soon as one menstrual period ends, preparation for the possibility of pregnancy begins again in the uterus. Hormones signal the body to build a thick lining and increase blood supply in order to be ready to receive a fertilized egg. Ovulation usually occurs around the fourteenth day of the cycle. The ovaries release an egg which travels through the fallopian tubes toward the uterus. If sexual intercourse takes place at this time, the egg may be fertilized by the sperm. The fertilized ovum normally travels through a fallopian tube to the uterus and attaches itself to the thickened lining of the uterus. Hormones continue to signal the uterus to build up the uterine wall to nourish the growing egg.

If fertilization does not occur, the days after ovulation are called the postovulatory period. During this time, the unfertilized egg simply disintegrates in the uterus. Hormones signal the uterus that the nest it has been building is not needed this month. Because the extra lining and blood are not needed, they are simply shed and passed out of the body through the vagina. This is the process of menstruation.

Regular menstruation is a sign of good health. Although a woman may feel some physiological changes in her body around the time of menstruation, none is harmful. In most women, slight cramping or a sensation of heaviness in the pelvis may occur. A fullness in the breasts may be experienced, or a mild pain in the lower back. Some women may feel tense or irritable just before menstruation.

Pregnancy and Birth

The hallmark sign of pregnancy is a missed menstrual period. However, because many factors may cause a late period—even anxiety over pregnancy—testing may be performed to confirm it. Home pregnancy tests search for certain hormones in your urine; they may be able to detect pregnancy as early as two weeks after conception. Other early signs of pregnancy include breast tenderness, a feeling of nausea in the morning or at other times of the day, and changes in your food tastes. As soon as you suspect you are pregnant, you should see an obstetrician to begin regular prenatal care.

Pregnancy normally lasts about 38 weeks. It is common to call each three-month period a trimester. Your due date is calculated as 40 weeks from the first day of your last menstrual cycle. During the nine months of pregnancy, the uterus expands to hold the growing fetus. The fetus is connected to the mother by the **umbilical cord,** which links it to the **placenta,** a spongy structure that grows in the uterus during pregnancy and through which the fetus derives nourishment from the mother. Fetal blood flows into the placenta, where it absorbs nutrients from the mother's blood and expels waste products. The growing baby, the placenta, and certain body changes all contribute to a normal weight gain of anywhere from 10 to 35 pounds during pregnancy.

During the first trimester, the developing organism is called an **embryo**. This is the period of most rapid development, although the embryo is only about two inches long at the end of this period and there is little obvious change in the shape of the mother's body. The heart is formed by the end of the first month, the eyes and ears are apparent by six weeks, and the head and limbs are recognizable by the end of the second month.

At the beginning of the second trimester, the uterus has usually expanded to the point that the woman can feel a bulge in her abdomen. The developing organism is called a **fetus** during this period of pregnancy, and

ABORTION is the removal of the fetus and the placenta from the uterus in order to terminate a pregnancy. Although abortions up to 24 weeks of gestation are very safe, some risks of physical and emotional complications may be present and expert advice should be sought.

The most common technique for abortion in the first trimester is vacuum aspiration: dilating the cervix and suctioning the contents of the uterus. The procedure takes less than 15 minutes and is usually performed with a local anesthetic as an outpatient procedure. This technique has largely replaced the old dilation and curettage (D&C) in which the cervix is dilated and a curved knife called a curette is used to scrape out the uterine contents.

Pregnancies of four months and beyond require either a dilation and evacuation (D&E) with general anesthesia or an instillation procedure with local anesthesia. A D&E, which takes less than an hour, is similar to but more extensive than a D&C. It involves dilation of the cervix and evacuation of the uterine contents by a combination of suction and curettage and, possibly, use of forceps to assist in removal of the fetus.

In women for whom D&E is not appropriate or available, an induction or instillation abortion is required. Premature labor is induced by injecting saline or some other fluid through the abdomen into the amniotic sac. Because instillation abortion involves labor and delivery, and may last as long as 24 hours, it is the most uncomfortable form of abortion both physically and emotionally. If this technique is not possible, a hysterotomy may be performed. This procedure is similar to a Cesarean birth in which the baby is removed through an abdominal incision.

the mother begins to feel it moving around in the uterus. Toward the end of this trimester, the mother's navel may begin to protrude.

If the pregnancy is unwanted, abortion should ideally take place in the first trimester but no later than the end of the second trimester.

In the third trimester, as the fetus grows larger, it may press against the mother's diaphragm and make breathing difficult. During this period, the breasts continue to enlarge and may become tender. By the end of the trimester, the baby usually settles in an upside-down position, with the head low in the mother's pelvis. When this occurs, breathing becomes easier, but there may be more frequent urination as the fetus presses on the bladder.

CESAREAN BIRTH, also known as a Cesarean section, is the surgical delivery of a baby through an incision in the mother's abdomen. A Cesarean may be chosen

• If rapid delivery is necessary because mother or baby appear to be at risk, especially due to prolonged labor
• If a breech birth (buttocks or feet rather than head first) is underway
• If a vaginal delivery would present special risks
• If a prior birth was Cesarean

Note that Cesarean delivery is not necessarily required for subsequent births, nor is it necessary in all cases of breech birth.

The rate of Cesarean births varies widely from one area of the country to another and from one physician to another. In choosing your obstetrician, you may wish to discuss and take into consideration the doctor's attitude toward Cesarean delivery.

Cesarean may be decided on in advance

• If the mother has a history of infection with herpes or certain other viruses that might be transmitted to the baby as it passes through the birth canal
• If the mother has severe toxemia, making normal delivery hazardous
• If the mother has diabetes, and fetal monitoring suggests that early delivery is wise
• If the baby is extremely large or in a particularly difficult breech position

Most Cesareans are emergency procedures when some serious problem develops during labor. Most commonly, fetal monitoring indicates that the baby is in distress, perhaps with an abnormal heart rate due to insufficient oxygen.

In the past, the incisions in the abdomen and uterus usually were made vertically, from the navel to the pubic hair. This still may be the choice in certain obstetrical emergencies, but now most incisions are made horizontal, from side to side just above the pubic hair in what is known as a bikini incision. General anesthesia used to be standard for Cesareans. Today, more physicians use epidural (spinal) anesthesia, and the mother's partner often remains in the delivery room during the procedure.

A Cesarean is major surgery, and it may produce temporary paralysis of the gastrointestinal tract. You will be fed intravenously for a day or two after the birth and will remain in the hospital for four to eight days. It will take at least four to six weeks until you feel normal again.

When birth occurs, the cervix dilates and the muscles of the uterus contract to force the baby out through the expanded vagina. An average labor may last from 8 to 24 hours. If certain problems arise during pregnancy or labor, a Cesarean birth may be necessary.

Breastfeeding

Breastfeeding is an easy and natural way to mother your baby. You are providing a perfect food for your infant and you both enjoy the comforts of a special kind of closeness. Colostrum, the first, yellowish-colored fluid in your breasts, contains important nutrients and substances that provide immunological protection for your baby. The milk itself comes between the second and sixth days after the baby's birth. Breast milk looks thin and watery compared to cow's milk, but it is ideally suited to human infants.

Nursing mothers should eat a well-balanced, nutritious diet and continue to take the prenatal vitamins and iron prescribed by the doctor. Because it takes energy to produce milk, you will be hungrier and thirstier than usual. Eat and drink more to satisfy your hunger and thirst. Do not try to diet. If you cut out sweets and eat sensibly, you will lose weight gradually while nursing.

While you are in the hospital, if your baby is in a central nursery, nurse often, perhaps once every two hours and at least once during the night. Most doctors can make this arrangement for you. If the baby is in your room, nurse on demand, not on a preset schedule. Even after you return home, give your baby short but frequent feedings for the first several weeks. This will help prevent or reduce uncomfortable fullness in your breasts, help prevent nipple soreness, and avoid the need to give the baby any supplementary feedings. Eventually, the baby will naturally establish a schedule of eating every three to four hours.

During the early months, there is no need to give your baby any formula or solid food while breastfeeding. Indeed, the easier sucking from the bottle may cause the infant to lose interest in sucking from your breast. Supply should never be a problem. The more you nurse, the more your system is stimulated and the more milk you will have. In contrast, the less you nurse your baby, the less milk you will have. This is the reason weaning should be done naturally and gradually.

Menopause

Menopause is the time when, due to a decline in production of the hormone estrogen, the monthly release of eggs by a woman's ovaries ends, menstruation ceases, and she is no longer able to conceive children. Technically, menopause occurs when a woman no longer menstruates, but the biological

---

ESTROGEN REPLACEMENT THERAPY (ERT)

ERT can considerably alleviate menopausal symptoms for women who suffer severely. It can also reduce the risk of osteoporosis and heart attack for women at risk for those disorders, although other measures are also available. Estrogen replacement may be taken by pill or skin patch, both of which have systemic effects on your whole body, or by a cream applied to the vagina.

If you have severe menopausal symptoms, ERT may be prescribed only for a year or two until your body stabilizes. If you are at high risk for osteoporosis, especially if a special X-ray called a bone scan reveals bone density problems, or if your mother, grandmother, or aunts died of a heart attack before 75, discuss longer term therapy with a gynecologist who is well informed about the latest research and whose practice includes older women rather than focusing on obstetrics. Major medical centers sometimes have menopause units that specialize in such concerns.

Although ERT began in the 1960s, it lost favor in the 1970s, when estrogen was linked with cancer of the endometrium, the membrane that lines the uterus. Research has since shown that this risk is largely eliminated when estrogen is prescribed in much lower doses and taken with another female hormone, progesterone, to protect the uterus. (If you have had a hysterectomy, progesterone is not necessary.)

However, ERT is still not advised for women with a history of uterine cancer or any other malignancy linked to estrogen. Women with gallbladder or liver disorders may have problems when oral estrogen is metabolized by the liver. In these instances, the skin patch or vaginal cream will be suggested. Women who are using corticosteroid drugs for other illnesses will need individual evaluation to determine whether they can use ERT safely.

mechanisms leading to menopause can begin years before and symptoms can continue for several years afterward. Although most women experience menopause around the age of 50, the process may begin—with menstrual flow and cycle starting to change—as early as 40 or may not occur until the mid- or late 50's. If a woman has her ovaries removed surgically, menopause occurs immediately.

The universal sign that a woman is premenopausal is that the menstrual period becomes shorter and scantier and the cycles are further apart—sometimes with whole months skipped—until they end. The body may react in other ways to the decreasing hormone supply. The two most common signs are "hot flashes" (also called flushes or sweats) and vaginal atrophy. This loss of the top layer of mucosa in the vagina and decrease in the moisture and elasticity may cause painful intercourse and related urinary infections. The flashes may be frequent or rare and may or may not disturb sleep. If sleep is disturbed, a consequent irritability and even depression may occur. As your body adjusts to its new hormone levels, the flashes go away. But vaginal dryness continues, and moisturizing lubrication may be needed.

MALE REPRODUCTIVE STRUCTURE AND FUNCTION

The **testes,** or testicles, are two oval-shaped organs that correspond to the ovaries in a woman. They manufacture the male sex hormone, testosterone, as well as **sperm,** the cells that fertilize the female's eggs. These glands hang outside the body, suspended below the penis in a pouch of skin called the **scrotum.**

Immature sperm, called **spermatocytes,** are produced in hundreds of spaghetti-like passages known as **seminiferous tubules.** The spermatocytes are stored in other tubes—collectively called the epididymis—for about 74 days until they mature. Mature sperm cells travel to the **vasa deferentia** and then into the **seminal vesicles,** where most of the seminal fluid is manufactured. Additional fluid comes from the **prostate,** a gland located just below the bladder.

The **penis** is largely composed of the **corpora cavernosa,** cylinders of tissue linked by connective fibers and located on the upper side of the penis. These "caverns" are empty when the penis is not erect. When the male is sexually stimulated, the corpora cavernosa fill with blood, doubling the size of the penis, to enable erection to occur. Another cylinder of tissue, the **corpora spongiosum,** is located on the underside of the penis. The **urethra,** a hollow tube inside the penis, carries urine and semen out of the body. The head of the penis is called the **glans.** When a male is born, the head of the penis is covered by a thin sheath of skin known as the **foreskin**. This sheath may be removed by circumcision, revealing the **corona,** a circular rim of tissue that separates the glans from the shaft of the penis.

When the male is stimulated to orgasm, sperm collect in the seminal vessels, mix with seminal fluid, and move to a bulb near the base of the urethra. When this bulb contracts, the semen is forced out of the penis in the process known as ejaculation.

When ejaculation takes place in the female vagina, and no barrier to conception is in place, the sperm are propelled forward and penetrate the cervix to reach the uterus in less than a minute. The sperm continue to move forward, by wiggling their tails, to proceed through the uterus and into the fallopian tubes. If a fertile egg is present at the time, conception may take place when one of the sperm penetrates the egg.

Although men continue to produce sperm throughout life, questions have been raised about quality of sperm in the later years. Also, there is some evidence that men experience some type of physical menopause with certain less well-defined symptoms than those of women.

HUMAN SEXUALITY

People of all ages, from infancy through old age, are sexual beings with sexual feelings and needs. Even in infancy, babies seem to experience pleasure from the stimulation of the genitals and other areas of the body that are considered erogenous zones. It is completely normal for boy infants to have frequent erections, which have even been observed during imaging while the fetus is in the uterus.

The primary source of such orgasmic experience in children is masturbation. Infants and toddlers normally investigate their own genitals and find such touching pleasant. By the age of two or three, children often examine each other's bodies, but self-exploration and manipulation are the most common forms of sex play. Fondling the penis and manual stimulation of the clitoris, as well as rubbing against beds or toys, are the most common autoerotic techniques. A child may also learn to masturbate from seeing someone else do it or from being taught by someone more experienced. Such experiences are more common among boys than among girls. Young boys frequently get together to exhibit their genitals and masturbate. Such prepubescent sex play is a sporadic but normal activity for youngsters. Only if your child seems to be focusing too much attention on his or her genitals, to the exclusion of other interests, may there be cause for concern. Discuss the matter with your pediatrician.

ADULT SEXUAL RESPONSE

Whether adults are involved in heterosexual or homosexual relationships, they also may continue to derive pleasure from masturbation throughout life.

The excitement stage of sexual response in the man leads to erection of the penis. In women, excitement causes the genital area to become somewhat swollen and the clitoris to become firm and enlarged. The vagina also produces extra fluid, which facilitates entry of the penis during intercourse.

The excitement stage of male sexual response is quite rapid. A thought or a touch may be sufficient to prompt erection. The excitement stage of female sexual response may take longer than in the man when she is having sex with a partner. During masturbation, men and women seem to require about the same amount of stimulation to reach a climax. However, recent research suggests that the time needed for arousal for either males or females seems to depend not only on physical stimulation but also on individual feelings and circumstances. Foreplay heightens arousal in both sexes. It may include manual or oral stimulation of the genitals, as well as caresses all over the body.

In heterosexual couples, sexual excitement usually leads to intercourse. The penis is inserted into the vagina and penile thrusting for several minutes or longer typically leads to male orgasmic ejaculation. The woman may have an orgasmic climax during foreplay or intercourse or as a result of continued stimulation after the male ejaculates. However, orgasm is not always necessary to achieve sexual satisfaction. Heterosexual and homosexual couples can provide each other with satisfying sexual pleasure in other ways that may include mutual oral or manual stimulation or anal intercourse.

Sexual ability and desire continue throughout life, although the general slowing down of all body processes seen in aging affects some aspects of sexual function. Men usually take longer to achieve erection and orgasm as they age. Women may need to use a lubricating cream to supplement vaginal lubrication after hormone levels drop. After menopause, some women may be more responsive than in their younger years because they no longer need fear an unplanned pregnancy.

SYMPTOMS AND SOLUTIONS

PELVIC CRAMPS AND PAIN IN WOMEN

Although cramps in the lower abdomen may be caused by digestive problems (see Chapter 6), women can usually discern the difference between such discomforts and those related to the reproductive system. The most common cause of pelvic cramps is the normal achiness that sometimes precedes menstruation or that is sometimes felt briefly midcycle during ovulation. However, many other types of cramps may signal serious illness.

If you experience cramps, pain, or abdominal pressure and minor bleeding at a time when you think or know you are pregnant, you may have an **ectopic pregnancy** or be about to have a **miscarriage** (page 163) and need emergency care. (Although such pain can also herald serious problems in nonpregnant women, as discussed in this section, it is not likely to be an emergency.)

• Call your doctor for instructions. Make it clear to whoever answers the doctor's phone that **this is an emergency.**
• If you can't reach your doctor immediately, go to a hospital emergency room.
• If your pain is too severe to travel to the hospital on your own, call an ambulance.
• While waiting for help, lie down and remain quiet.
• Take nothing to eat or drink.
• Take no medication unless it was previously prescribed and is urgently important or you are told to do so by your physician or emergency medical personnel.

Causes and Treatment of Pelvic Cramps and Pain in Women

When cramps, just before or during menstruation, are severe and prolonged, the condition is known as dysmenorrhea. Most menstrual cramps are caused by the contractions of the uterus produced by hormone-like chemicals called prostaglandins.

Moderate cramps can be eased by drugs such as aspirin or ibuprofen. Start taking the medication a day or two before you expect cramps and continue until a day or two after your period begins. Warm baths or a heating pad applied to the painful area may also help.

Severe menstrual cramps that worsen during the last few days of your flow may indicate **endometriosis** (page 158). If use of a mild painkiller and a heating pad or hot bath don't provide sufficient relief, make an appointment to see your doctor.

Sudden, sharp abdominal pain may signal that you have a **fibroid** (page 160) tumor that has become twisted and lost its blood supply. Immediate surgery to remove the fibroid may be necessary.

Pain and tenderness in the lower abdomen, especially if accompanied by a fever, vaginal discharge, irregular bleeding, or backache, may be a sign of **pelvic inflammatory disease** (page 165). Prompt antibiotic therapy is essential to prevent the spread of infection through the reproductive tract, a complication that can lead to infertility or even life-threatening problems.

Any vague discomfort, pressure, or pain in the pelvic or abdominal area that is not otherwise explained, especially if it causes abdominal swelling, may be a sign of **ovarian cancer** (page 164) or **uterine cancer** (page 169). Such symptoms should not be ignored because there may not be more severe signs of illness until the cancer has spread.

PELVIC DISCOMFORT IN MEN

Pelvic discomfort is uncommon in men, but when it does occur, it may be a sign of **testicular cancer** (page 168). The associated sensation is most often described as a dull ache in the lower abdomen or groin or a feeling of dragging or heaviness. Testicular self-examination may or may not reveal lumps or changes in tissue consistency.

If you have persistent lower abdominal discomfort, examine your testicles carefully. Then, whether or not you find any abnormalities, call your physician. Describe what is happening so that the doctor can decide whether you should be seen immediately.

ABNORMAL VAGINAL BLEEDING

Bleeding between menstrual periods, ranging from spotting to profuse, is not uncommon. Such bleeding may also reflect abnormally short or long cycles, a condition called oligomenorrhea. Although the average cycle is 28 days, a cycle as long as 20 to 40 days may be normal for you.

Causes and Treatment of Abnormal Vaginal Bleeding
Bleeding that occurs a week or so before your expected period and is accompanied by other symptoms of menstruation, such as breast tenderness, is likely to indicate a short cycle. Irregular cycles may be caused by stress or hormonal changes and are more common in puberty and as menopause

If you have even a single episode of bleeding that saturates a sanitary pad or tampon in less than an hour, or that is accompanied by pain or fever, or that occurs when you might be pregnant, you may need emergency care.

• Call your doctor for instructions. Make it clear to whoever answers the doctor's phone that **this is an emergency.**
• If you can't reach your doctor immediately, go to a hospital emergency room.
• If your pain is too severe to travel to the hospital on your own, call an ambulance.
• While waiting for help, lie down and remain quiet.
• Take nothing to eat or drink.
• Take no medication unless it was previously prescribed and is urgently important or you are told to do so by your physician or emergency medical personnel.

approaches. They are usually nothing to worry about. Call your doctor if you have abnormal bleeding that does not appear to be a short cycle or if you have repeated cycles of less than 20 days.

Some women experience a slight cramping and blood spotting at the time of ovulation, a phenomenon sometimes called "mittelschmerz." It is normal and should disappear within a few hours.

If bleeding between periods or abnormal cycles are accompanied by fever, pain, or vaginal discharge, you may have a **vaginal infection** (page 171) or **pelvic inflammatory disease** (page 165). Call your doctor for an immediate appointment. Antibiotics or other medications may be necessary to cure the infection promptly.

If unexpected bleeding occurs with severe abdominal pain and there is even the slightest possibility that you are pregnant, call your doctor immediately. You may have an **ectopic pregnancy** (page 157)—with the embryo developing outside the uterus—and need urgent surgery.

If you are using low-dose birth control pills, breakthrough bleeding between periods may mean that you require a higher dose. Call your doctor for a consultation.

If you are using an IUD and unexpected bleeding occurs, call your doctor immediately. The device may have perforated your uterus and require immediate removal.

Minor bleeding or spotting between periods in the absence of pain may also be caused by **cervical abnormalities** (page 154), such as cervical erosion or polyps. Such abnormalities should be treated to prevent further discomfort.

Abnormal bleeding between periods may also be caused by **cervical cancer** (page 156), **ovarian cancer** (page 164), or **uterine cancer** (page 169), as well as nonreproductive problems, such as diabetes or thyroid and other hormone disorders (see Chapter 8).

Although you may think that you lose considerable blood every month, the actual quantity of the menstrual period totals only a few tablespoons. Teenagers and young women tend to have a heavier flow than women in their 30's or older. If you observe a flow that is heavier than usual for you in any one month, it is likely to be a natural variation. However, if heavier than normal flows persist, make an appointment with your gynecologist. You may have minor **cervical abnormalities** (page 154), which are easily remedied by the removal of abnormal cells during an office visit. However, a complete examination is necessary to rule out **cervical cancer** (page 156).

ABSENCE OF MENSTRUATION

Amenorrhea is the complete absence of menstruation. Primary amenorrhea is failure of menstruation to begin in a young women by the age of 18. Secondary amenorrhea is the sudden absence of menstruation for several months in a woman who has previously menstruated.

If you have not had a period by age 16, or if you are not pregnant and miss periods frequently or stop menstruating for three months, see your gynecologist. This is especially important if you have other symptoms, such as vaginal discharge or pelvic pain. Describe what is happening so that the doctor can decide whether you should be seen immediately.

Causes and Treatment of Absent Menstruation

All women skip an occasional period for no known reason. Skipping several cycles may be normal for teenagers who have not yet established a regular cycle or for premenopausal women.

The most common cause of extended amenorrhea is, of course, pregnancy. Other causes include excessive or sudden weight loss or gain, stress, and minimal body fat. Amenorrhea is not uncommon in women who go on crash diets or who are long distance runners or do other rigorous exercise.

The absence of menstruation is a signal that the diet should be ended or that the runner needs to add a little body fat for normal hormonal function.

If amenorrhea is not explained by such lifestyle factors and corrected by modified behavior, it may be due to ovarian cysts or **ovarian cancer** (page 164), poorly controlled **diabetes** (page 244), or other hormonal disorders such as **hyperthyroidism** (page 248), chromosomal abnormalities, or congenital defects such as the absence of a vagina or uterus. Treatment depends on the underlying cause.

ABNORMAL VAGINAL DISCHARGE

Vaginal secretions over the course of the menstrual cycle are normal. There is usually very little secretion immediately after menstruation. Within a few days, you will notice increased wetness and a discharge that may be white or yellow, tacky or creamy. As the time of ovulation nears, the discharge tends to become clearer and less viscous. When you ovulate, the discharge again changes, becoming thicker or decreasing until you menstruate.

Abnormal vaginal discharge is the primary symptom of vaginitis, which simply means inflammation of the vagina. Vaginitis may be caused by many different problems, ranging from simple irritation, to infection by a fungus, bacterium, or virus, to more severe disorders. Sexually transmitted disease may be the cause of such infections.

If you have frequent or persistent abnormal vaginal discharge, or if you can't explain and remedy even a single episode by any of the lifestyle changes discussed in this section, call your physician. This is especially important if you also have any pelvic pain or fever or the discharge has a foul smell. Describe what is happening so that the doctor can decide whether you should be seen immediately.

Causes and Treatment of Abnormal Vaginal Discharge

Minor vaginal irritation, itching, and discharge may be caused by the chemicals in vaginal sprays, excessive douching, nylon panties, tight jeans or girdles, use of tampons, or the perfumes or other chemicals in laundry detergents. Discontinue the use of such products and the problem usually will disappear. Your symptoms can be temporarily relieved with an over-the-counter douche product containing the anti-irritant ingredient povidone-iodine. Do not use this preparation more than twice a week, and call your doctor at the end of the week if your symptoms persist.

The three most common **vaginal infections** (page 171) are yeast infections, trichomoniasis, and gardnerella, all precipitated by the overgrowth of organisms naturally present in the vagina. Sometimes prompt use of an acidic douche can halt these infections in their earliest stages. Look for over-the-counter douche products containing acetic acid, boric acid, citric acid, lactic acid, sodium borate, tartaric acid, or vinegar.

Yeast infections cause a thick, white discharge that may look like cottage cheese and smell like baking bread. If you have had yeast infections in the past and can spot the symptoms, treatment creams are available at your pharmacy without a prescription. A first yeast infection, however, should always be diagnosed by your doctor.

Trichomoniasis causes a thin, foamy discharge that is yellowish green or gray and has a foul odor. It usually requires treatment with the oral prescription drug metronidazole.

Gardnerella causes a creamy white or grayish discharge and a fishy odor. It is usually treated with such oral antibiotics as tetracycline, ampicillin, or cephalosporin, or a sulfa cream or suppository.

Other common causes of abnormal vaginal discharge are sexually transmitted diseases such as **gonorrhea** (page 274), **syphilis** (page 284), **chlamydia** (page 268), and **herpes** (pages 278 and 279). These conditions require medical treatment with prescription medication such as oral antibiotics or antiviral drugs.

Sometimes abnormal vaginal discharge may signal the presence of such **cervical abnormalities** (page 154) as cervical erosion—the presence of abnormal cells—or hyperplasia—overgrowth of normal cells. See your gynecologist so that the abnormal cells can be removed in a simple office procedure.

In rare cases, abnormal vaginal discharge, especially if the discharge is blood-tinged, may signal **cervical cancer** (page 156) or **uterine cancer** (page 169). These possibilities emphasize the importance of prompt diagnosis and treatment of any unexplained or persistent discharge.

PAINFUL INTERCOURSE IN WOMEN

Sexual intercourse is usually a pleasurable experience. Although slight pain may occur during a woman's first experience as the hymen is broken, subsequent relations should not cause discomfort.

Causes and Treatment of Painful Intercourse in Women

If you experience a friction type of pain during intercourse, it may be due to inadequate lubrication. This may occur if there has not been sufficient

> If you have repeated episodes of painful intercourse, or if you can't
> explain even a single episode by any of the lifestyle causes discussed in
> this section, call your physician. This is especially important if painful
> intercourse is followed by even light vaginal bleeding. Describe what
> is happening so that the doctor can decide whether you should be seen
> immediately.

time for arousal and the accompanying vaginal lubrication. Both you and
your partner should be aware of the natural pacing of the experience and
time yourself accordingly.

If you have passed menopause, the vaginal lining begins to thin and you
may no longer produce as much lubrication as you did in earlier years. You
may wish to try a vaginal lubricant available in your pharmacy or to discuss
estrogen replacement therapy with your physician.

If you experience sharp pain deep in your vagina with each penile thrust,
especially if you also have low back pain during menstruation or when
standing for long periods, you may have **uterine prolapse** (page 170)—that
is, your uterus may be tipped at a variant angle. Your doctor can diagnose
this problem by a routine pelvic examination. If the prolapse is mild, simply
trying different positions for intercourse may solve the problem. If it is more
severe, you may need to be fitted with a device called a pessary to support
the uterus or undergo surgery to relocate the uterus.

If you experience sharp pain deep in your vagina and also have severe
menstrual pain that is worse at the end of your period, you may have
endometriosis (page 158). Again, trying different intercourse positions may
resolve your difficulty.

If you experience sharp pain deep in your vagina and also have mild
bleeding after intercourse, you may have a **cervical abnormality** (page 154)
such as cervical polyps. Your gynecologist can remove these polyps during
an office visit and resolve the problem.

If you have pain in your pubic area during intercourse, and especially if
you also have an abnormal vaginal discharge or vaginal bleeding, you may
have **cervical cancer** (page 156). Prompt diagnosis and treatment are
essential to help prevent the spread of the disease.

BREAST LUMPS

Many women develop one or more lumps in their breasts over the course of
their lifetime. Although these lumps can cause considerable anxiety, more
than 90 percent of all lumps found by women are not cancerous.

If you have not been diagnosed with fibrocystic breast syndrome, any lump found in your breast should be reported to your doctor. If you have cystic breasts, any *new* lump should be reported immediately. Describe the lump you have found and any other breast abnormalities observed. You should be seen by a specialist as soon as possible.

Causes and Treatment of Breast Lumps

If you have one or more breast lumps of various sizes, or a "pebbly" breast consistency, and these lumps come and go in synchronization with your period, you probably have **fibrocystic breasts** (page 159). Although it is important to have your gynecologist evaluate such lumps when they are first found, you can rest more easily if the diagnosis is made. Thereafter, you should examine your breasts frequently and get to know your own pattern. Then only variations from that pattern will warrant a doctor's appointment. In other words, any *new* lump should always be examined by a physician.

Most other breast lumps are harmless, fluid-filled cysts. Again, however, any new lumps should be reported to your doctor. If fluid cannot be easily aspirated from the lumps, a more detailed examination and biopsy will be necessary to rule out **breast cancer** (page 152).

BREASTFEEDING PROBLEMS

Although breastfeeding is the most natural way to nourish your baby, it is a learned skill. Before giving birth, study the nursing process in your childbirth preparation classes, in baby-care books, or through La Leche League (call 1-800-LA LECHE).

With few exceptions, any mother who wishes to can successfully breast-feed her baby. You will need to become accustomed to the normal sensations of breastfeeding. It should not be painful. Pain always requires further investigation. If you encounter any problems not easily remedied by the techniques discussed in this section, call your obstetrician.

Causes and Treatments of Common Breastfeeding Problems

Almost all women experience a generalized soreness during the first few days of breastfeeding. Another symptom, nipple tenderness at the beginning of each feeding, usually lasts only the few seconds it takes for the nipples and breast tissue to adjust to having an infant latch on to suckle. Sore nipples, although common, are almost completely avoidable. They are not related to how long you feed your baby but rather to how the baby is positioned and removed from the breast and to general nipple care.

When the baby latches on to the nipple to feed, the jaws should compress on your breast tissue approximately one to one and one-half inches behind the nipple. When sucking begins, the nipple and part of the dark areola are drawn deep into the baby's mouth. To remove the baby from the breast, first place your finger in the corner of the infant's mouth to break the suction and avoid hurting the nipple.

Practice scrupulous nipple care. Avoid using soap, lotions, or creams on your breasts or products containing vitamin E that can be absorbed by your baby while feeding. After each feeding, rub a little breast milk into the nipple and areola. The natural fats and enzymes of the milk have soothing and healing properties. Cool tea bag compresses or a pure oil, such as olive, vegetable, or sesame, may also soothe initial soreness and lubricate nipples. After feeding, always air-dry your breasts for 10 to 15 minutes. This helps to toughen your nipples.

Avoid using commercial suction pumps on your breasts. If a pump is necessary, rent a state-of-the-art electric standard piston pump. Pump rentals are usually covered by health insurance, especially if you have a doctor's prescription.

If nipple soreness does develop, sunlight in small doses or blowing warm, not hot, air from a hair dryer on your nipples may help them toughen. Warm compresses, gentle massage, and relaxation techniques are helpful. Try more frequent but shorter feeding periods. If pain develops during a feeding, remove the baby promptly but carefully.

A heavy fullness in the breasts two or three days after birth is called engorgement and signals an increase in milk production and in the supply of blood and lymph in the breasts. For most women, engorgement usually resolves quickly or can be prevented by regular breastfeeding. To help minimize the problem, start frequent breastfeeding as soon as the baby is born. Although feeding on demand will probably become your pattern, offering your breast more often is best in the first few days to help establish your milk supply. Avoid supplementary water feedings so that the baby will be hungry enough to remove the milk from your breasts, thus relieving the pressure.

If severe engorgement develops and the breasts feel warm, tight, painful to the touch, and lumpy in some areas, prompt steps should be taken to get the milk flowing. Take a hot shower or apply moist heat packs for 10 minutes. Gently massage your breasts in a circular motion to loosen areas of milk congestion. As soon as possible, breast-feed your child and feed every one and one-half to two hours until engorgement subsides. Then you can return to demand feeding. If you are unable to breast-feed, gently express the milk with your hand or use an electric standard piston pump. Once the milk is removed, apply covered ice packs to your breasts for 10 to 15 minutes.

If discomfort continues, contact your physician. Severe engorgement can lead to a breast infection called mastitis. If you develop a fever and an achy, fatigued feeling, suspect mastitis. Your doctor is likely to recommend rest, adequate fluid intake, hot compresses, and antibiotics. Continued frequent feedings for your baby are part of your cure. The milk is not affected by the infection.

SEXUAL DYSFUNCTION

Sexual dysfunction is the inability of a person to express his or her sexuality adequately and to enjoy sexual relations. Although sexual dysfunctions can be distressing to you and your partner, almost none is hopeless. Sexual counseling and certain medical treatments can help most couples develop a satisfying relationship.

If you are having a sexual problem, consult your physician first. Certain difficulties may be caused by physical disorders or by medications you are taking. If your doctor rules out a physical disorder or corrects it and you still have problems, consult an experienced and well-recommended sex counselor for help in identifying and solving the problem.

Causes and Treatment of Sexual Dysfunction

The four most common sexual dysfunctions in women are disorder in the excitement phase leading to intercourse, disorder in the orgasm phase of intercourse, dyspareunia, and vaginismus. (Frigidity, a term once used to describe a woman totally unaroused by sex, is extremely rare.)

In excitement phase disorders, a woman may have inhibitions that prevent arousal and therefore inhibit vaginal lubrication or expansion. In orgasm phase disorders, a woman has difficulty reaching a climax or is unable to do so. In dyspareunia, sexual intercourse is painful. In vaginismus, involuntary spasm of the muscles surrounding the vaginal opening causes the vagina to close tightly.

The most common male sexual dysfunctions are impotence, premature ejaculation, and retarded ejaculation. These terms are not absolute but refer to generalized deviations from average behavior.

Impotence is the term used to describe a man's inability to develop or maintain an erection. Its occasional occurrence is normal, especially if a man is overtired, under a lot of stress, or has consumed too much alcohol. Certain medications may inhibit erection, and dosage modification may return normal function. Impotence is not normal if it occurs frequently or if the man is never able to achieve an erection.

Premature ejaculation, the most common male sexual problem, has been described as ejaculation that occurs within 30 seconds of vaginal entry, within 2 minutes of stimulation, or in less than 10 penile thrusts. A better definition may be that orgasm occurs before the man wants it to happen. Occasional premature ejaculation is normal, especially in situations where the man feels anxious about performing well.

Retarded ejaculation, the opposite problem, is also difficult to define. It refers, in general, to the inability to achieve orgasm after extended stimulation. Again, occasional ejaculation delays are normal, especially in situations similar to those that may prompt impotence, but persistent problems merit attention.

Sexual problems have many complex causes—physical illness, certain medications, stress outside the sexual relationship, or serious psychological problems. On the other hand, some may be caused more simply by lack of information and understanding. Sometimes one partner's supposed dysfunction really reflects a problem that the couple shares. For example, when a man tends to ejaculate prematurely, he may blame his partner, who, on the other hand, may unconsciously lose interest in sex in order to avoid another frustrating experience. Couples who put too much stress on sexual performance may trigger apparent dysfunction, usually in the man. In sexual therapy, both partners and the counselor talk about their relationship and their attitudes toward sexuality. Sometimes exercises may be prescribed to help the relationship.

COMMON DISORDERS OF THE REPRODUCTIVE SYSTEM

BREAST CANCER is the most common malignancy in women. About one in every nine American women will eventually develop a breast malignancy. However, your overall chances of survival are 67 percent, and

they are better when the condition is diagnosed before the cancer cells have
spread.

What are the symptoms?

The most common symptom is a small lump or thickening in the breast.
Such lumps are often discovered by women themselves during breast self-
examination. Nearly 90 percent of such lumps are not cancerous. Other
signs may include a change in breast shape or contour, dimpling or puckering of breast skin, retraction of the nipple or discharge from it, or an inflamed
reddish appearance. The most common early warning signs are certain
changes that show up on a mammogram, a special X-ray of the breast.

How did I get it?

The cause of breast cancer is unknown, but it occurs more commonly in
women whose mothers or sisters have had the disease, in women who have
never had children or had a first child after age 30, and in those who begin
to menstruate at a relatively early age and reach menopause relatively late.
There is some indication that a specific gene malformation predisposes
women to breast cancer that may be environmentally triggered. Some
research suggests that a high-fat diet may also be a factor.

How is it diagnosed?

The first step is usually a mammogram. Your doctor will also perform a
needle aspiration of any suspicious lump. A hollow needle is inserted into
the lump. If fluid can be withdrawn, it is probably a harmless cyst. If the cyst
grows back quickly, or if the lump cannot be aspirated, then a needle or
surgical biopsy is needed. Needle biopsy involves insertion of a corkscrew-
shaped needle that carves out a small part of the lump for laboratory
examination. Surgical biopsies may be done with local or general anesthesia,
depending on the size and location of the lump and your own preferences.
They may be performed in the doctor's office or as an outpatient procedure
in a hospital's ambulatory surgery department. The biopsy may be incisional,
removing only part of the lump, or excisional, removing all of the lump and
a margin of normal tissue around it.

How is it treated?

The treatment of breast cancer varies from location to location and doctor
to doctor. Thoroughly familiarize yourself with the options before you
proceed. Generally speaking, if the cancer is small and localized, it may be
advised that you have a lumpectomy, which is surgical removal only of the

lump and surrounding tissue, followed by radiation therapy and, sometimes, chemotherapy. A modified mastectomy may also be suggested. In this procedure, the breast is removed. In both cases, lymph nodes under the arm are also removed for examination. For larger tumors or where lymph nodes are involved, only modified or, in some rare cases, more extensive radical mastectomy is needed and chemotherapy will likely be advised.

Self-Care: All women over age 20 should perform breast self-examination every month, a few days after menstruation when the breasts will be at minimum fullness. Postmenopausal women should examine their breasts at the same time each month. First, stand in front of a mirror and look at your breasts while your hands are at your sides; then examine them with hands raised above your head and then with hands on your hips. Notice anything unusual. In most women, one breast may be slightly larger than the other, but you should look for differences in shape, for a flattening or bulging in one, but not the other, or for skin puckering. Unless you are pregnant or nursing, there should be no nipple discharge even upon light squeezing. Notice any reddening or other abnormality of the nipples, any hardness or asymmetry. Any sore on a nipple should be investigated. Next, lie down. Raise your right arm above your head and rest it on a pillow behind you. Use your left hand to gently explore your right breast, using the flat of the fingers. Move your hand in small circles around the breast, applying gentle pressure, until the entire breast is covered. After you check the right breast, repeat the procedure on the left side. Any thickening, lump, or other abnormality should be reported to your physician.

CERVICAL ABNORMALITIES that are not malignant include any variations in the structure of the cervix—the donut-shaped structure whose opening leads from the vagina into the uterus—or the mucous tissue called squamous epithelium that covers it. The most common abnormalities are dysplasia, erosion, hyperplasia, and growths. Cervical dysplasia is abnormal cell growth in or around the cervix. Cervical erosion is a wearing away of some of the squamous epithelium that covers the cervix. Cervical hyperplasia is an overgrowth of cervical cells. Cervical polyps and cysts are benign growths on the cervix.

What are the symptoms?
Often these abnormalities do not have symptoms. Some women with dysplasia may have heavy or painful menstrual periods. Some women with

erosion or hyperplasia may have a slight increase in vaginal discharge, a whitish discharge, or occasional bloody discharge if the erosion is irritated by intercourse. Polyps may occasionally cause painful intercourse or bleeding, particularly after intercourse.

How did I get it?

The cause of most cervical abnormalities is unknown. Cervical dysplasia occurs more often in women who take birth control pills, began having intercourse at an early age, have multiple sexual partners, have had one or more sexually transmitted disease, smoke cigarettes, have sexual partners with skin cancer, or have jobs (or have sexual partners who have jobs) where they are exposed to certain cancer-causing agents. Cervical erosion, which is very common, may sometimes occur in association with childbirth, abortion, infection, use of an IUD, or the friction of intercourse. Women whose mothers took a drug commonly known as DES (diethylstilbestrol) before birth may have an increased tendency to dysplasia and erosion. Hyperplasia may be the result of hormonal imbalance, use of birth control pills, or healing from cervical erosion.

How is it diagnosed?

Cervical dysplasia is initially diagnosed based on a Pap smear. This painless test is performed as part of a regular pelvic examination. A smear of cells shed by the cervix is collected and sent to a laboratory for examination. A closer look at the dysplasia is provided with colposcopy, a painless procedure in which the gynecologist uses a magnifying scope to look at the cervix. In some cases, a small tissue sample is taken for biopsy. Cervical erosion may be observed during a normal pelvic examination. Subsequent evaluations of erosion and hyperplasia are the same as for dysplasia. Polyps and cysts are observed during a normal pelvic examination, and a small tissue sample is taken for biopsy to ascertain whether cancer is present.

How is it treated?

Mild cervical dysplasia is simply monitored with more frequent Pap tests. If it is more severe, your doctor may recommend removal of the abnormal cells by freezing or cauterizing them in an office procedure. If the abnormal changes are significant or extend into the cervical canal, a cone biopsy may be necessary to make sure no cancerous cells are present. Some doctors do not treat cervical erosion at all; others follow procedures similar to those for dysplasia. Some types of hyperplasia require no treatment, but others must be surgically removed because they may be hiding cervical cancer. When cysts cause no problems, nothing need be done. If they become infected, they may be removed by freezing or cautery. Polyps are usually removed in the doctor's office.

Self-Care: If you modify the lifestyle factors associated with certain cervical abnormalities, as described in this section, you may be able to influence the subsequent course of the disorder. Avoiding the use of tampons, birth control pills, and IUDs may also reduce erosion.

CERVICAL CANCER is a malignancy that arises in the neck of the uterus that protrudes into the vagina, also called the cervix. It is a form of uterine cancer and is most common in women in their 30's, especially those who have had one or more children.

What are the symptoms?
Cervical cancer may have no symptoms in its early stages. When symptoms occur, they may include an abnormal vaginal discharge or bleeding or pain in the pubic area, especially during intercourse.

How did I get it?
Although the cause of cervical cancer remains unknown, it occurs more frequently in women who started having intercourse before the age of 18, have had multiple sexual partners, have had genital warts, have used oral contraceptives, or have a history of cervical dysplasia or some other cervical abnormality.

How is it diagnosed?
Cervical cancer can be detected at its earliest, most curable stages by a simple examination known as the Pap test. If the Pap test is abnormal, the cervix may be examined more closely with a colposcope and a small sample of tissue removed for further examination. (Pap tests and colposcopy are described in **cervical abnormalities,** page 154). If cervical cancer is confirmed, other blood tests and X-rays will be performed to determine if the cancer has spread to other parts of the body.

How is it treated?
Treatment depends on the extent of the cancer. For early cancer, simple removal of part or all of the cervix may be sufficient. In other cases, hysterectomy to remove the uterus may be necessary. If the cancer has

spread, radiation and/or chemotherapy may be required to destroy malignant cells elsewhere in the body.

Self-Care: All women age 20 and over—and even younger women who are sexually active—should have a Pap test at least every three years, after two initial negative tests a year apart. A pelvic examination is recommended every three years for women between the ages of 20 and 40 and every year for women over 40, including women who have passed menopause.

ECTOPIC PREGNANCY, also called tubal pregnancy, occurs when a fertilized egg does not implant in the wall of the uterus but grows elsewhere, most commonly in one of the fallopian tubes but occasionally on an ovary or elsewhere in the pelvis.

What are the symptoms?
Even slight vaginal bleeding and cramps during the early weeks of pregnancy may signal an ectopic. Instead of pain, some women feel only a sense of pressure in the abdomen. If nothing is done, tubal rupture may occur, causing extensive internal bleeding, severe pain, shock, and death.

How did it happen?
Sometimes an ectopic pregnancy occurs for no apparent reason. However, in about half of all cases, the cause appears to be pelvic inflammatory disease that has scarred the fallopian tubes and obstructed the passage of the fertilized egg. Women who have used an IUD may also be at greater risk. Older women may be slightly more likely to have ectopic pregnancies. Chlamydia, a sexually transmitted disease, is the most common forerunner of ectopic pregnancy.

How is it diagnosed?
An ultrasound evaluation usually can confirm suspicion of an ectopic pregnancy by revealing a swollen fallopian tube or a fetus outside the uterus.

How is it treated?
Surgery is required to remove the involved fallopian tube, if that is where the egg has lodged. Sometimes the adjacent ovary must also be removed. In most cases the uterus can be saved.

Self-Care: If you have had any pelvic infection or used an IUD, be alert for symptoms of ectopic pregnancy. Ask your doctor to monitor your condition closely during the early weeks of your pregnancy.

ENDOMETRIOSIS occurs when the tissue that normally lines the uterus grows in areas outside the uterus, notably on the ovaries, fallopian tubes, bowel, or bladder. If not treated, endometriosis can damage pelvic organs and cause infertility.

What are the symptoms?
Some women have no symptoms. Other women have atypical, severe menstrual pain that worsens during the last few days of the period. Over time, the pain begins ever earlier in your cycle. Depending on the site of the abnormal tissue, pain may also occur deep in the pelvis during intercourse, during bowel movements or urination, or elsewhere in the abdomen.

How did I get it?
How endometrial tissue gets outside the uterus is unknown. It is suspected that the movement may occur through the fallopian tubes, possibly during menstruation, or through the circulation of blood or lymph in the body. It is also suspected that certain pelvic surgery may trigger the condition.

How is it diagnosed?
In addition to a complete gynecological examination, your doctor may order an ultrasound examination, which uses sound waves to provide internal images. In some cases, a laparoscopy may be necessary to confirm the diagnosis. This is a hospital procedure in which a small incision is made just below the navel and a microscopic instrument is inserted to allow the doctor to examine the pelvic area directly.

How is it treated?
Endometriosis naturally goes into remission during pregnancy and after menopause. Treatment at other times depends on your age, disease severity, and other factors. If you want to become pregnant, hormones or other drugs may be given temporarily to halt ovulation and enable the abnormal tissue to shrink. Or surgery may be performed to remove as much of the abnormal tissue as possible. Such techniques do not cure endometriosis but may provide significant relief and enable pregnancy to occur. However, the problem is likely to recur. If you have severe symptoms unresponsive to these techniques or to medication, and if you are not hoping to become pregnant,

surgical removal of the uterus and ovaries may be advised to cure the disease permanently. As with any surgery, the risks and benefits of this procedure should be carefully weighed.

> Self-Care: A heating pad or hot water bottle applied to the pelvis may help ease discomfort. If discomfort is more severe, you may try aspirin, acetaminophen, or ibuprofen.

FIBROCYSTIC BREASTS are sometimes called lumpy breasts or fibrocystic breast syndrome or disease. Actually, the latter is a misnomer because this condition is not a disease but simply an exaggeration of changes that normally occur in the breast over the course of each month. Although fibrocystic breasts do not predispose you to breast cancer, the condition may mask malignant tumors or make it difficult to distinguish new lumps.

What are the symptoms?
You may have one or more breast lumps of various sizes, or a "pebbly" breast consistency. Also, you are likely to experience breast swelling, tenderness, or pain. These symptoms ebb and flow, most commonly developing in the week or two before menstruation and disappearing after cessation of bleeding. Although some women suffer with fibrocystic symptoms throughout their menstruating years, others find that difficulty comes and goes with no particular pattern. Fibrocystic problems usually disappear after menopause.

How did I get it?
Every month, just as the uterus prepares for pregnancy by building a thicker lining, so do the breasts change in anticipation of the need for milk production. In the first half of the menstrual cycle, cells of the milk-secreting glands and surrounding fibrous tissue increase in number, and the glands swell. In the week before menstruation, extra breast fluid normally is reabsorbed and extra fibrous tissue recedes. If this does not happen fully, the extra fluid is trapped in small sacs called cysts. These cysts are one of the causes of lumpy breasts, but, as the process is repeated month after month, the sacs may become filled with fibrous tissue. The fibrous lumps are irregularly shaped benign tumors.

How is it diagnosed?
If you have not been diagnosed with fibrocystic breast syndrome, any lump found in your breast should be reported to your doctor. Whether or not you have fibrocystic breasts, any *new* lump should be reported. The first step in

diagnosis usually involves inserting a hollow needle into the lump. If fluid is easily removed, the lump is probably a harmless cyst. If no fluid is removed and the lump is solid, other diagnostic techniques will be done, such as mammography and biopsy. Laboratory analysis of a tissue sample can determine whether you have fibrocystic breasts. If you have this syndrome, your doctor will probably advise that you examine your breasts regularly to become familiar with your own pattern. Then you need consult your doctor only for regular checkups or when you feel an unusual lump not consistent with your pattern.

How is it treated?
Fibrocystic breasts normally do not require medical treatment. The problem disappears by itself in more than half of all women with the syndrome. If your breasts are very painful, your doctor may prescribe a diuretic to prevent fluid retention or daily supplements of vitamin E, which may indirectly influence hormone levels. If these remedies and self-care fail to restore your comfort, hormonal drugs may be prescribed.

Self-Care: Some women find that reducing their intake of methylxanthines eases monthly breast tenderness. Methylxanthines are contained in coffee, chocolate, tea, colas and certain other soft drinks, and over-the-counter medications such as wake-up pills and some aspirin combinations that contain caffeine. More importantly, become familiar with your pattern of lumps through regular breast self-examination. Check your breasts daily for several months, keeping a chart of lumpiness and how changes may parallel your menstrual cycle. Any deviations from your regular pattern should prompt a call to your physician. Women with fibrocystic breasts also should have professional breast examinations regularly, preferably by the same physician so the doctor can develop a familiarity with your breast lumps. Your doctor can also advise you on the recommended frequency for mammography, because fibrocystic breasts may mask malignant tumors.

FIBROIDS are benign tumors of the uterus. They are the most common tumors affecting the female reproductive organs, occurring in about 20 percent of women over the age of 30. They range in size from microscopic to the diameter of grapefruits and usually grow in clusters. They grow more rapidly during pregnancy or when you take birth control pills or postmenopausal hormone replacement, all sources of extra estrogen.

What are the symptoms?
Most women have no symptoms. Some have heavy menstrual periods, leading to iron deficiency. Depending on the size and placement of the tumor, you may experience painful menstrual periods or a feeling of pressure. Sometimes a fibroid attached to the uterine wall becomes twisted and loses its blood supply, causing sudden, sharp abdominal pain. It is uncommon, but a fibroid sometimes grows rapidly during pregnancy and may cause pain, miscarriage, or obstruction during delivery.

How did I get it?
The cause of fibroids is unknown, but the problem seems to run in families.

How is it diagnosed?
Fibroids are usually found during a normal pelvic examination. Their size and location can be confirmed by ultrasound, a painless examination that uses sound waves to image internal structures.

How is it treated?
Because most fibroids remain small and grow very slowly, they cause few or no symptoms and require no treatment. If you are having heavy menstrual periods, iron supplements may be recommended to prevent anemia. For overly heavy menstrual flow or severe pain, surgery may be performed to remove large fibroids, or they may be destroyed by laser surgery performed through the vagina. In the most serious cases, hysterectomy may be the only way to remove fibroids effectively. If a fibroid is being strangulated and causing sudden pain, an emergency operation may be required to remove it. If a fibroid causes obstruction during delivery, a Cesarean section is usually necessary.

> Self-Care: If you know you have fibroids, avoid the use of birth control pills and do not take estrogen replacement after menopause. Do not take iron supplements unless your doctor recommends it based on a blood test.

INFERTILITY is experienced by at least 15 percent of all married couples. However, few are completely infertile—that is, sterile with a total lack of reproductive ability. Rather, most have low fertility for one or more reasons. About 35 percent of infertility derives from female problems alone, another 35 percent from male problems alone, and 25 percent from problems in both spouses. Less than 5 percent of infertility is unexplained.

What are the symptoms?
Infertility is defined as the inability of a couple to achieve conception after a year of unprotected intercourse or the inability to carry repeated pregnancies to a live birth.

How did I get it?
The most common causes in women are cervical fluids that impair sperm movement or survival; failure to ovulate; blockage or spasm of fallopian tubes; hormonal imbalance that prevents a fertilized egg from implantation in the uterine wall; abnormalities in the shape or position of the cervix or uterus; and other disorders of the reproductive organs, such as infections or growths that impair their function.

The most common causes in men are varicocele, a varicose enlargement of the spermatic cord veins; abnormalities in the location, size, or shape of the reproductive organs; and abnormalities in the size, shape, motility, or number of sperm caused by injury, stress, infection, toxic chemicals, or use of drugs, alcohol, or tobacco.

How is it diagnosed?
Both spouses must be evaluated, including a medical history, a review of sexual development and practices, a general physical, a detailed assessment of the reproductive organs, and blood tests to assess hormonal profiles. Laboratory studies include a Pap test and a culture of cervical secretions for women, and a culture of the urethral opening for men. Subsequently, the woman is likely to have a postcoital test, in which cervical mucus is evaluated after normal intercourse, and the man is asked to collect his sperm in a special container for evaluation. The woman may also undergo endometrial biopsy and other internal examinations to evaluate the functioning of the reproductive organs.

How is it treated?
More than half of infertile couples can be treated successfully and become parents. Sometimes all that is required is a simple lifestyle change, such as altering the frequency or timing of intercourse. The man may be advised to stop wearing tight underwear that may raise testicular temperature and impair sperm production. Douching with special solutions before intercourse may make the cervical mucus more receptive to sperm. If cervical fluids cause severe problems, artificial insemination with the husband's sperm (depositing it directly into the uterus) may facilitate pregnancy. Drugs useful in treating infertility include antibiotics to cure interfering infections

and hormones to promote ovulation in the female or stimulate sperm production in the male. Surgery may be required to open blocked fallopian tubes in the female or remove varicose veins in the male penis. If fallopian tubes cannot be repaired, in vitro fertilization may be the solution. This involves removing ripe eggs from a woman's ovary surgically, fertilizing them in the laboratory with the man's sperm, and then reinserting them into the uterus through the cervix.

Self-Care: Before seeking medical help, the couple should make sure that they are having intercourse daily during the woman's fertile period. Self-test kits, available without a prescription in pharmacies, can help you identify when you are ovulating. Do not douche during this time unless directed to do so by a physician.

MISCARRIAGE, also called spontaneous abortion, is the end of a pregnancy before the fetus is able to live independently outside the uterus. About one of five pregnancies ends this way, usually in four weeks to three months after conception.

What are the symptoms?
The most common symptoms are bleeding or brownish discharge from the vagina, which may or may not be accompanied by cramps or pain in the lower abdomen or back. Many women have some vaginal bleeding during the early months of pregnancy. This does not always signal the beginning of a miscarriage, but it should always be called to the attention of a doctor.

How did it happen?
In most cases, miscarriage is caused by some problem in the way the baby is developing. It may be that the mother's egg was fertilized too late in the cycle. If fertilization occurs toward the end of the 24-hour period after ovulation, the egg may be "stale" and the pregnancy won't develop properly. Many doctors believe that this is the major cause of miscarriage. Other causes include improper attachment of the placenta to the uterus; a structural defect in the uterus; hormonal imbalance in the mother; maternal infection; and complications of other diseases, such as diabetes. In many miscarriages, the cause is never discovered.

How is it diagnosed?
If bleeding is heavy and solid and blood tissue is expelled from the uterus, it is presumed that a miscarriage has taken place.

How is it treated?

In many cases, when there is bleeding but no pain, you may be told to restrict your activity, avoiding sexual intercourse and strenuous exercise. If the bleeding does not become heavier than normal menstrual flow and if there is no pain, the pregnancy may develop properly. If the uterus continues to grow normally, it means the baby is probably developing normally. However, when a true early miscarriage has begun, there is little that can be done to prevent it. A miscarriage is often nature's way of preventing a baby with serious health problems from being born. If the miscarriage is not complete, your doctor may have to suction the uterus to remove remaining fetal and placental material. If a treatable cause for the miscarriage is diagnosed afterward, your doctor can sometimes take steps to prevent future miscarriages, correcting a hormonal imbalance, for example, or stitching a weak cervix closed.

> Self-Care: The fact that you had one miscarriage does not mean that your next pregnancy will end that way. There is no reason to avoid another pregnancy. For most women, a miscarriage will only happen once. If you miscarry more than once, get a complete evaluation from a specialist before considering a third pregnancy.

OVARIAN CANCER, also known as ovarian carcinoma, accounts for less than 20 percent of all malignancies in the reproductive organs of women. However, because the disease is difficult to detect in its early stages, it contributes to a much larger share of fatalities. Although it can occur at any age, it is more frequent after menopause.

What are the symptoms?

Ovarian cancer causes no symptoms in its earliest stages. As the malignancy grows, you may experience recurrent abdominal discomfort, such as aching or gas. Rarely does ovarian cancer cause vaginal bleeding. When the disease is more advanced, abdominal swelling, pain, and weight loss occur.

How did I get it?

The cause of ovarian cancer is unknown. It is suspected that hereditary factors may be involved, because it occurs most commonly in women in North America and northern Europe. However, it also develops more frequently in women who have never had children, as well as those who have had cancer of the colon, rectum, uterus, or breast.

How is it diagnosed?
In many cases, the only clue to the presence of ovarian cancer is detection of slight enlargement of the ovary during a pelvic examination. In such cases, an ultrasound examination can use sound waves to detect structural change in the pelvis. Your doctor will also take samples of your vaginal secretions to look for abnormal cells. In many cases, laparoscopy is needed to confirm the diagnosis. In this procedure, a small microscopic tool is inserted into a small incision just beneath the navel to enable your doctor to examine the abdominal area directly.

How is it treated?
In young women with only one ovary involved and cancer still localized in the ovary, only that ovary may be surgically removed. However, because the cancer has often spread by the time it is diagnosed, complete removal of both ovaries, uterus, fallopian tubes, and adjacent lymph glands is usually advised. After surgery, you are likely to be given radiation and/or chemo-therapy to destroy any remaining cancer cells or to slow the spread of the disease.

Self-Care: Women over age 40 should have a thorough pelvic exami-nation every year or two. If you are found to have ovarian cysts, more frequent examinations are advisable.

PELVIC INFLAMMATORY DISEASE, or PID, is the term used to describe any extensive infection of the organs in the female pelvis, such as the uterus, fallopian tubes, ovaries, and surrounding tissues. For example, PID may include parametritis (infection of the uterus), salpingitis (infection of the fallopian tubes), or salpingo-oophoritis (infection of both the tubes and the ovaries). If untreated, these infections can be very serious and even life threatening.

What are the symptoms?
Pelvic infections may cause pain and tenderness in the lower abdomen, painful intercourse, heavy vaginal discharge, early or heavy menstrual periods, and/or irregular bleeding between periods. Acute infections may also cause fever, and chronic infections may prompt backaches. If not treated, the infection may spread throughout the reproductive tract. The infection may cause swelling and closure of the fallopian tubes, leading to sterility, or abscesses can form in the tubes or ovaries, which may require

surgery. Sometimes PID becomes a recurrent problem. Rarely, a rapidly spreading infection may cause life-threatening peritonitis or blood poisoning.

How did I get it?

PID often begins with a simple vaginal infection that is not treated and therefore spreads into the reproductive tract. Such infections can be contracted during sexual intercourse, after insertion of an intrauterine device for contraception, or after a miscarriage, abortion, or childbirth. The original infection may be from a bacterium, such as streptococcus or staphylococcus. PID is most often caused by chlamydia, a sexually transmitted disease. As a result of the dramatic increase in chlamydia infections in the population, there is currently an epidemic of ectopic pregnancies.

How is it diagnosed?

Sometimes the diagnosis is made based on symptoms, but laparoscopy may be required for confirmation. In this procedure, also known as pelvic endoscopy, a tiny incision is made just below the navel. Carbon dioxide gas is then pumped into the abdomen to provide a better view. A small, rigid laparoscope is inserted through the incision, enabling the doctor to examine structures inside the pelvis. If necessary, tissue samples can be extracted through the laparoscope for laboratory examination. About half of all PID cases are not diagnosed until a woman has become infertile as a result of the scarring that has destroyed the fallopian tubes. Sometimes PID is not spotted until rampant infection requires a hysterectomy or other gynecological surgery.

How is it treated?

Pelvic infections are best treated at the first signs of infection. Therapy usually includes a 10-day course of antibiotics. Sometimes aspirin or other painkiller may be prescribed as well, to reduce inflammation. Bed rest and avoidance of sexual intercourse also are advised during the treatment period. Severe cases may require hospitalization for more extensive evaluation and treatment.

Self-Care: Careful selection of sexual partners and the use of condoms to help prevent transmission of infection can reduce your risk of pelvic infection. If any abnormal symptoms occur, see your doctor immediately to ensure prompt treatment and the avoidance of complications.

PREMENSTRUAL SYNDROME, or PMS, is the general term used to describe the various discomforts experienced by more than half of all women during the week to 10 days before their menstrual period. Historically, women were told that their problems were psychological. However, recent medical research has demonstrated that real problems with physical causes trouble many women.

What are the symptoms?
The physical symptoms of PMS are diverse. Most common is water retention, which may involve noticeable weight gain or an uncomfortable bloated feeling. Breasts may be swollen and tender. You may experience backaches or dull aches in the ankles or muscles generally. You may have food cravings, particularly for sweets. Other chronic health problems, such as headaches, asthma, or depression, may be aggravated. The psychological symptoms of PMS include irritability, depression, general anxiety, and lethargy. You may just want to crawl into bed and cry.

How did I get it?
All the causes of PMS are not clear, but most doctors now believe that the condition results in part from an imbalance of the hormones estrogen and progesterone. Women who suffer from PMS often have high levels of estrogen in relation to progesterone in their blood during the latter half of their menstrual cycles. Estrogen causes the body to retain water. Water buildup in various parts of the body can lead to pelvic congestion, as well as brain tissue swelling and subsequent mood changes. This hormonal imbalance could account for other symptoms of PMS as well.

How is it diagnosed?
If you suffer with PMS symptoms that do not respond to self-care, see your gynecologist for a complete examination. If no other cause of your symptoms is identified, PMS is the presumed diagnosis.

How is it treated?
Many premenstrual problems can be cured, either by the lifestyle changes described here or with medical treatment. Aspirin, long the mainstay of self-help, works for PMS because it is a very mild antiprostaglandin drug. Another such drug, also available without a prescription, is ibuprofen. If self-care and over-the-counter medication do not significantly relieve your symptoms, your physician can prescribe drugs that help minimize water retention, or more potent anti-inflammatory drugs that help slow down the production of prostaglandins.

Self-Care: Reduce your salt intake sharply in the two weeks prior to your period. Eat nutritionally balanced meals to get all your vitamins and minerals, especially calcium, which tends to decline premenstrually and may aggravate PMS. Have small, high-protein snacks every few hours and cut back on high-carbohydrate foods. Cut back on coffee, tea, and colas, which contain a type of caffeine that can worsen the hormonal imbalance. Regular exercise increases circulation and helps carry off excess body fluids in the form of perspiration. Exercise also stimulates the brain to release endorphins, the body's own natural painkillers. Finally, hot baths or heating pads often help, especially if muscle stiffness and tension are symptoms.

TESTICULAR CANCER is one of the most common cancers in young men in their teens, 20's, and 30's; it rarely occurs in men past the age of 40. This does not mean that testicular cancer itself is common. Rather, it accounts for only 2 percent of all male cancers.

What are the symptoms?
Testicular cancer rarely causes pain in its earliest stages. So monthly testicular self-examination is important. Early changes may include a lump or nodule, a slight enlargement of one of the testes, or a change in its consistency. There may be a dull ache in the lower abdomen and groin, together with a sensation of dragging and heaviness.

How did I get it?
The causes of testicular cancer are still unknown. However, men with undescended or partially descended testes, and those whose mothers took the drug DES during pregnancy to prevent miscarriage, are at greater risk.

How is it diagnosed?
If you have a lump that is suspicious, your doctor will probably have it removed for laboratory examination. If cancer is detected, X-rays and blood tests will be done to determine whether it has spread beyond the testicle.

How is it treated?
When detected early, testicular cancer can be treated effectively. Treatment usually requires surgical removal of the affected testicle. Such surgery does not impair sexual functioning, because the other testicle still produces hormones and semen. If the cancer already has spread, you will probably also receive radiation and/or chemotherapy. When cancer is detected early,

about 75 percent of all patients now survive at least five years. For certain types of testicular cancer, the five-year survival rate is almost 100 percent, if detected early.

Self-Care: Testicular self-examination should be performed monthly. The best time is after a warm bath or shower when the scrotal skin is most relaxed. Rub each testicle gently between the thumb and fingers of both hands. You are looking for any hard lumps or nodules or any change in the size or consistence of your testes. It may take a few months to get to know your body. You need to learn what your testes normally look and feel like. If you notice any abnormalities, see your doctor promptly.

UTERINE CANCER can occur in either of two areas of the womb. When it occurs in the neck of the uterus, also known as the cervix, it is called **cervical cancer** (page 156). What is generally called uterine cancer starts in the upper part, or body of the uterus, also known as the corpus. Uterine cancer most commonly develops in the endometrium, the membrane lining the uterus, and is sometimes called endometrial cancer. However, a small fraction of uterine cancer arises from the myometrium, the muscular tissue that forms the walls of the womb.

What are the symptoms?
Uterine cancer may have no symptoms in its early stages. When symptoms do occur, they may include an abnormal vaginal discharge or bleeding, pain or pressure in the pelvic area, or abdominal swelling.

How did I get it?
Although the cause of uterine cancer is unknown, hormonal factors are believed to be involved. It may occur more frequently after menopause and especially among women who entered puberty late and who have not had children.

How is it diagnosed?
Although the Pap test is very good at detecting cervical cancer at the neck of the uterus, it is not quite as good for detecting cancer of the body of the uterus. If uterine cancer is suspected, your doctor will probably recommend an ultrasound examination, which uses painless sound waves to provide images of internal structures. A D&C may also be performed—dilation of the cervix in order to scrape out a sample of the endometrium.

How is it treated?
The usual treatment for uterine cancer is hysterectomy, the surgical removal of the uterus and cervix. In many cases, the fallopian tubes and ovaries are also removed. If the cancer has spread into the upper vagina, part of it also may be removed. Following surgery, you are usually given radiation and/or chemotherapy to destroy any cancer cells not surgically removed.

> Self-Care: All women age 20 and over—and even younger women who are sexually active—should have a Pap test at least every three years, after two initial negative tests a year apart. A pelvic examination is recommended every three years for women between 20 and 40 and every year for women over 40, including those past menopause. An endometrial tissue sample should be examined for those at high risk of uterine cancer.

UTERINE PROLAPSE, also called a tipped uterus, refers to an abnormal positioning of the uterus that occurs in about 20 percent of all women. Normally, the uterus is in a slightly upward tilted position. When prolapse is present, it tilts slightly downward so that it lies against the rectal canal.

What are the symptoms?
Uterine prolapse usually causes no symptoms. However, some women experience pain during sexual intercourse, if penile penetration is deep, or low back pain, especially during menstruation or when standing for a long period of time.

How did I get it?
Most women who have a tipped uterus were born with the condition, for unknown reasons. In others, the tilt develops after childbirth or due to scar tissue from endometriosis or a pelvic infection.

How is it diagnosed?
Uterine prolapse is easily identified during a routine pelvic examination.

How is it treated?
If uterine prolapse causes no problems, nothing need be done. If you experience severe symptoms, your doctor may prescribe a pessary, a soft rubber ring, similar to the outer ring of a diaphragm, that you insert into the vagina and around your cervix to help position the uterus properly. If this does not relieve your symptoms, or if prolapse is so severe that the uterus

protrudes into your vagina, surgery may be performed to establish a normal position for the uterus.

Self-Care: Undertake self-care only if a gynecologist has diagnosed your symptoms as caused by a tipped uterus. If you experience pain during intercourse, experiment with different positions that avoid deep penetration. If you have discomfort at other times, try a mild painkiller such as aspirin or acetaminophen. If you are fitted with a pessary, make sure to visit your doctor regularly for cleaning and replacement.

VAGINAL INFECTIONS are among the most common health concerns of women. The vagina normally cleans itself constantly with secretions that wash away microorganisms and other debris. Microorganisms naturally living in the vaginal flora include cocci, coliforms, anaerobes, fungi, lactobacilli, micrococci, and trichomonas. Some of these microorganisms play important roles in self-cleansing. For example, lactic acid secretions from lactobacilli help maintain the normal vaginal acidity that protects against overgrowth of yeast, fungi, and bacteria, as well as from outside organisms that may invade the vagina. The three most common vaginal infections are yeast infections, trichomoniasis, and gardnerella.

What are the symptoms?
The primary symptoms are abnormal discharge from the vagina and mild to severe itching or burning sensations around the vagina or vulva. You also experience redness and swelling of the vagina or vulva; chafing of your thighs; and pain, stinging, or itching during intercourse.

How did I get it?
When infections occur, the vagina's normal self-cleansing process has broken down. Yeast infections, trichomoniasis, and gardnerella are all precipitated by the overgrowth of organisms naturally present in the vagina. Other common causes are the infectious agents that precipitate gonorrhea, syphilis, chlamydia, and herpes.

How is it diagnosed?
Your gynecologist may be able to diagnose a vaginal infection simply by examining your vagina and vulva, as well as smelling and observing the discharge. For example, yeast infections cause a thick, white discharge that may look like cottage cheese and smell like baking bread, and trichomoni-

asis causes a thin, foamy discharge that is yellowish green or gray and has a foul odor. In other cases, a smear of the discharge may need to be sent to a laboratory for examination.

How is it treated?
Yeast infections are treated with a seven- to ten-day course of a vaginal cream or suppository containing clotrimazole, miconazole nitrate, or nystatin. If the infection is not completely cured, your doctor may apply a stronger medication directly to the vagina and vulva, or oral nystatin may be prescribed. Trichomoniasis is usually treated with an oral drug called metronidazole. Gardnerella is treated with such oral antibiotics as tetracycline, ampicillin, or cephalosporin, or a sulfa cream or suppository. All vaginal infections should be treated promptly. If allowed to spread, they may cause pelvic inflammatory disease and infertility.

> Self-Care: If you have had a yeast infection before and know for sure that the symptoms are the same, you can self-treat by purchasing an over-the-counter yeast-killing cream or vaginal insert. Look for products containing clotrimazole or miconazole nitrate, and follow package directions carefully. Although you will probably feel better within a few days, be sure to complete the full course of treatment. If your symptoms don't ease within a few days, call your doctor.

6

Digestive Disorders

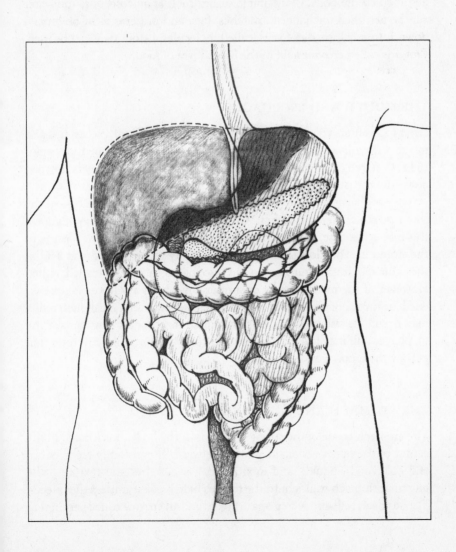

HOW THE DIGESTIVE SYSTEM WORKS

The digestive system largely consists of the gastrointestinal tract, a long hollow tube running from the mouth to the anus. In between are the esophagus, stomach, and intestines. At various sites in this tube, nutrients are extracted from the food you eat, broken down into usable form, and delivered into the bloodstream, which carries them to other organs for their use. Waste products are then eliminated from the body. Also important in the digestive process are the liver, gallbladder, and pancreas.

The term **digestion** refers to the overall process by which food is broken down mechanically and chemically and converted to forms that can be absorbed by the body. Only simple sugars, such as glucose, salt, and water can be absorbed unchanged. Starches, fats, and proteins must be broken down into much smaller forms, called molecules, before they can be used. Proteins called **enzymes** aid in the breakdown of food.

THE MOUTH AND ESOPHAGUS

After food enters your mouth, chewing breaks it into small pieces. It is also mixed with saliva, which contains ptyalin, a digestive enzyme that begins to break starch down into simple sugars. Your tongue then directs the food down the throat to the **esophagus,** also known as the **gullet.**

The esophagus is a firm muscular tube that extends from the base of the throat to the center of the chest. Gravity helps draw food and liquids down this tube to its base, where a ring of muscles relaxes to open the passage to the stomach. The closing of this ring normally prevents food and acid in the stomach from returning to the esophagus, a process called reflux. However, if the muscular ring or surrounding structures have been weakened, or if you are obese, or if you recline too soon after a meal, such reflux may occur. Persistent reflux of powerful stomach acids can damage the esophagus and may lead to more serious complications, like strictures that narrow the esophagus or even cancer.

THE STOMACH AND DUODENUM

The **stomach** is one of the strongest organs in the body. It is located in the center of the upper abdomen, above the waist. It constantly receives hot and cold foods, liquids, and mixtures of various sizes and textures. The muscular stomach walls churn the food to help break it into smaller pieces. The stomach wall also secretes gastric acid and an enzyme called pepsin that breaks down protein. Special cells within the stomach normally prevent it from digesting its own tissues with these strong digestive juices. As a result of the mechanical churning and biochemical activity, food is converted to a semifluid called chyme.

At the base of the stomach, food, or chyme, then passes through another muscular ring called the **pyloric sphincter.** This sphincter controls entry of food into the **duodenum,** the first few inches of the small intestine. The duodenal walls secrete sodium bicarbonate, which you may know as baking soda and may use as an antacid. The sodium bicarbonate neutralizes some of the stomach acids to prepare the chyme to enter the small intestine for further digestion.

THE LIVER, GALLBLADDER, AND PANCREAS

Digestive action in the small intestine gets some help from three organs. The **liver,** one of the most important organs in the body, is located just under the lower rib cage on the right side. It is a large, soft organ and is intimately concerned with various metabolic and digestive functions of the body. It synthesizes many products, such as some of the factors necessary for proper blood clotting. It also has an important function in the digestion of fats, proteins, and carbohydrates. Perhaps the best known activity of the liver is the formation and storage of bile, a green fluid that helps digest fats.

After its manufacture in the liver, bile passes into the **gallbladder** for concentration and storage. The gallbladder is a small pear-shaped organ located directly beneath the liver. It releases bile into the duodenum through the bile duct.

The **pancreas** is located directly beneath the stomach. It produces the hormones insulin and glucagon to help the body metabolize sugar (see Chapter 8). Pancreatic enzymes also enter the duodenum through the bile duct. At this point in the digestive process, the pancreas and the duodenal walls work together to secrete three more enzymes: Amylase further converts starch into simple sugars, trypsin breaks down protein into polypeptides and amino acids, and lipase breaks down fats into fatty acids.

THE SMALL AND LARGE INTESTINES AND APPENDIX

Taking up considerable space in the body below the waist are the intestines, muscular tubes that move food along by rhythmic contractions called peristalsis.

It is in the **small intestine** that the breakdown of food is finished and nutrients begin to be absorbed through the intestinal walls for use by the body. The small intestine of an adult is about 20 feet long. Its walls are lined with millions of hair-like projections called **villi.** Villi have special surface membranes that allow nutrients to pass through them and into attached tiny blood vessels. As nutrients are absorbed through the villi, protein in the form of amino acids and sugar in the form of glucose are absorbed directly into the bloodstream; some are immediately transported to cells throughout the body, and others go to the liver for further breakdown or storage. As smaller fat molecules also go directly into the blood, larger ones enter the lymph system. Undigested chyme is then moved into the large intestine.

Depending on the contents of your meal and your individual metabolic rate, it usually takes two to six hours for food to be converted to chyme, moved out of the stomach, and absorbed by the body. Simple sugars are broken down rapidly and may enter the bloodstream within minutes of eating. Starches require an hour or longer. Proteins need two to three hours for digestion and absorption. Fat takes the longest time, from four to six hours. That's why protein and fat satisfy hunger for far longer periods than sugars and carbohydrates.

The **appendix** is a worm-shaped appendage located at the junction of the small and large intestines in the right lower abdomen. It serves no useful purpose in the bodies of human beings, and most people are not even aware that they have an appendix unless it becomes swollen and painful. Most waste matter from the bowel flows past the appendix, but material can enter it. Normally, the appendix keeps itself clean, but sometimes waste can block it and lead to infection and inflammation, causing appendicitis.

The **large intestine,** also called the colon, is about five feet long in an adult. It is here that water needed by the body is absorbed from the chyme through the intestinal walls. Then the waste products of digestion are formed into a semi-solid stool. The walls of the large intestine are lined with mucous glands whose secretions facilitate the movement of the stool through the colon. Stools enter the final segment of the large intestine, called the rectum, and are then eliminated from the body through the anus as bowel movements.

SYMPTOMS AND SOLUTIONS

The digestive system has a relatively small repertoire of symptoms: Pain, bloating, cramping, diarrhea, constipation, and flatulence are all common symptoms. They may be completely normal or may be associated with some

WHAT IS A "NORMAL" BOWEL MOVEMENT?

Many people spend too much time worrying about whether their bowel movements are "normal" and "regular." Such concern often comes from erroneous information in advertisements for laxatives. There is no such thing as a bowel pattern that is normal for all people. Rather, your own pattern is normal for you. Some people have bowel action after every meal. Some have it as rarely as once a week. Most have it once a day. In each case, the bowel action may be perfectly normal.

Not having a daily bowel movement is not dangerous. It does not harm your health in any way. Your bowel will move when it is ready to do so. You can maintain good bowel habits by eating raw fruits and vegetables and bran and other high-fiber foods that provide bulk and by drinking a reasonable amount of water. Such a diet should provide a reasonably soft but well-formed stool that will move painlessly and at its own speed through your bowel. Some nutritionists describe self-care for bowel irregularity as "hard in, soft out and soft in, hard out." This means that minor changes in bowel habits may be attributable to, and correctable by, your eating choices. Eating some "hard" fiber foods such as salads, raw vegetables, and bran helps contribute to a softer stool. Eating "soft" foods, such as bananas or rice pudding, can help firm a stool.

Laxatives should not be used except in special circumstances when directed by a doctor. Some people who have trouble with a hard, dry, painful stool but who cannot eat a high-fiber diet find that they get relief using a special softening and lubricating medicine available without prescription. It is much better to use these products than the violent laxatives or cathartics that can be habit forming.

Possible medical problems are signaled not by a lifetime pattern that you think may vary from some artificial norm but by sudden changes in bowel habits that persist. If you have been having stools twice a week for years and suddenly find that you are having bowel action twice a day, you should be concerned. If your normal pattern is a once-a-day schedule and this routine changes so that several days pass without a bowel movement, this, too, indicates a possible problem. In both examples it is the change in your normal pattern that indicates something may be wrong and warrants medical attention.

factor in your lifestyle, such as diet or the stresses of everyday living. Excitement, disappointment, fear, anxiety, and other strong emotions can cause some upset in your digestive system and should not be of concern if they are transient. However, because the digestive system has a limited set of symptoms for expressing distress, such symptoms also may be caused by very serious problems, ranging from ulcers to cancer. Therefore, any persistent symptoms that do not respond to dietary change or efforts at stress management should cause concern and prompt a call to your physician.

ABDOMINAL PAIN OR CRAMPS

Pain is your body's distress call. Pain in the upper abdomen or chest may be due to simple indigestion, reflux, or an ulcer. However, symptoms of a heart attack, including indigestion, heartburn, nausea, and vomiting, can easily be misinterpreted as a problem in the upper gastrointestinal tract. Gastrointestinal discomfort in the lower abdomen is more likely to be experienced as cramps rather than pain, unless appendicitis or another very serious illness is under way.

Causes and Treatment of Abdominal Pain or Cramps

Ulcers (page 209) are one of the most well-known causes of pain in the center of the chest. The pain—usually worse when the stomach is empty (except before breakfast) and better after eating or taking an antacid—may range from a gnawing or burning to a severe searing sensation. Other symptoms may include heartburn, burping, bloating, and gas. Many people try to self-treat ulcers by taking antacids after meals and at bedtime—which may be just what your doctor will first prescribe—and that may be an appropriate, temporary course of action until you can get an appointment with your doctor. However, because your pain may signal a far more serious condition, it is wise to avoid self-diagnosis and see your doctor promptly.

Reflux is the return of some stomach contents upward into the esophagus. The stomach acids in the fluid cause a burning sensation in the esophagus. Occasional reflux is not uncommon. It may be caused by too large a meal, especially if it included fatty foods and alcohol and ended with coffee, chocolate mints, and/or a cigarette—all substances that weaken the muscular sphincter at the base of the esophagus. Reflux may also occur if you recline within an hour after eating, losing the aid of gravity in the downward movement of food. Avoiding such practices should alleviate your reflux. Obesity can cause a weakening of the sphincter, and weight loss should ease the problem.

If there is even the suspicion that upper abdominal pain may be signaling a heart attack or that lower abdominal pain is caused by appendicitis, get emergency care immediately. This is especially urgent if you are over 35 years of age and experience chest pain that lasts for more than two minutes, or if you have lower abdominal pain in conjunction with nausea, vomiting, and fever.

• Call your doctor for instructions. Make it clear to whoever answers the doctor's phone that **this is an emergency.**
• If you can't reach your doctor immediately, call an ambulance. Again, make it clear that **this is an emergency.**
• If someone can get you to a hospital faster by car or taxi, get going. Don't try to go by yourself. You may collapse on the way.
• While waiting for help, remain quiet.
• Sit up rather than lie down.
• Take nothing to eat or drink.
• Do not take a laxative, even if you are constipated.
• Take no medication unless it was previously prescribed and is urgently important or you are told to do so by your physician or emergency medical personnel.

Most abdominal pain is far less severe. However, if you have persistent pain, or if you can't explain a single episode of moderate to severe pain by lifestyle factors, call your physician. Describe what is happening so that the doctor can decide whether you should be seen and when.

Persistent reflux could be a sign of **hiatal hernia** (page 201), a condition in which the opening in the diaphragm where the esophagus meets the stomach has widened, allowing part of the stomach to protrude upward. Again, your doctor is first likely to recommend lifestyle changes, as well as medications to reduce or neutralize stomach acids. If such conservative measures fail, surgery may be needed to return the stomach to its proper position.

Upper abdominal pain that is associated with alcohol consumption, gallstones, or certain medications and that worsens with movement or breathing but lessens when you sit up or bend at the waist is the hallmark of **pancreatitis** (page 205), an inflammation of the pancreas. Acute pancreatitis, where pain escalates quickly and is accompanied by nausea, can be a medical emergency that requires hospitalization for effective treatment. Delay can cause pancreatic rupture that may require surgery. Chronic pancreatitis develops more slowly, is often accompanied by diarrhea and weight loss due to inadequate food absorption, and is aggravated by eating or drinking alcohol. Again, serious problems can occur if medical care is not prompt.

Sudden, severe pain on the upper right side of the abdomen may signal an attack of **gallstones** (page 197). Sometimes the pain is felt in the back under the right shoulder blade. Pain usually begins after a meal and may be accompanied by fever, chills, and vomiting. The pain usually lasts for several hours until the stone passes through the bile duct and into the intestines. Nonetheless, call your doctor right away at the first sign of such pain because some stones can rupture the gallbladder, causing life-threatening problems. Surgical removal of the gallbladder is usually recommended for those who have frequent attacks.

Moderate discomfort in the right upper part of the abdomen may signal a problem with your liver. If you have experienced a general deterioration of health, including loss of weight and appetite, weakness, fatigue, and easy skin bruising, **cirrhosis** (page 191) of the liver may be suspected. In the earliest stages, elimination of the underlying cause of the cirrhosis—often, excessive alcohol consumption—may halt the damage. People with cirrhosis need prompt medical care and special nutrition to help slow progression of the disease. If liver failure occurs, a transplant may be able to save your life.

Lower abdominal pain that comes on suddenly and is accompanied by nausea, vomiting, and fever often signals **appendicitis** (page 189). The pain may begin high in the center of the abdomen and then migrate to the lower right side or, less commonly, to the lower left. It should be reported to your doctor as a medical emergency. If you can't reach your doctor immediately, go to a hospital emergency room. Even if you are constipated, do not take a laxative or enema if you have these symptoms. It may worsen your problem and cause the appendix to rupture.

Intermittent lower abdominal pain, cramps, and diarrhea can be signs of a series of digestive disorders, including lactose intolerance, Crohn's disease, irritable bowel syndrome, diverticulosis, colorectal cancer, and ulcerative colitis. When and where the pain occurs, and accompanying symptoms, can aid in the diagnosis.

If the symptoms only occur a few hours after consuming milk or milk products, and you also develop excessive flatulence, it could be **lactose**

intolerance (page 204). Many people, particularly women, lose their ability to digest milk products in early or late adulthood. If that's your problem, eliminating all milk products for a few days should eliminate your symptoms—and they won't recur unless you consume milk products again. Some infants are lactose intolerant from birth. Oral enzyme supplements are available that can help those with this problem to tolerate dairy products.

Blood in your stool might be caused by gastrointestinal bleeding due to an **ulcer** (page 209) or **gastritis** (page 198). Or it might be **Crohn's disease** (page 195), a chronic inflammatory disease that usually affects the lower part of the small intestine and/or the large intestine. Although Crohn's disease has no cure, your doctor can prescribe medications to reduce the inflammation and alleviate the cramps and diarrhea. As a last resort in the worst cases, surgery to remove part of the bowel may be necessary.

Intermittent symptoms only after eating, together with bloating, nausea, and alternating bouts of diarrhea and constipation, may signal **irritable bowel syndrome** (page 203). Although there is no cure, your doctor can prescribe drugs and suggest lifestyle patterns that can ease your symptoms and discomfort, such as a diet high in fiber.

If you have severe lower abdominal pain with diarrhea and fever, it may signal **diverticulitis** (page 196). This won't be a surprise if you have already been diagnosed with a common condition in those over age 60 called **diverticulosis,** small outpouchings protruding from the intestinal wall that can cause abdominal cramps, gas, and diarrhea alternating with constipation. In most people diverticulosis causes no symptoms. However, an infection in the pouches can lead to the sudden pain caused by diverticulitis. The primary treatment of diverticulosis is a high-fiber diet that helps keep the intestines clean and reduces risk of infection. To treat diverticulitis, a clear liquid diet is prescribed at first and then a bland diet. Antibiotics and other medications also may be used. In the worst cases of diverticulitis, hospitalization and surgery to remove the infected areas are necessary.

If you have pain or bloating in your lower abdomen, a change in the typical size or shape of your stool, and persistent or intermittent diarrhea or constipation, it could be **colorectal cancer** (page 193). Prompt surgery to remove the diseased portion of the colon often provides a complete cure.

If you have intermittent attacks of abdominal pain, bloating, cramping, and bloody diarrhea, you may have **ulcerative colitis** (page 208). Attacks last from one to several days and alternate with intervals without symptoms. Your doctor can prescribe steroid drugs to reduce the inflammation and alleviate symptoms. You will also have to follow a bland, low-fiber diet to reduce intestinal irritation. If infection is suspected, you will need antibiotics therapy as well. In the worst cases, only surgery to remove inflamed parts of the intestine can help.

Both ulcerative colitis and Crohn's disease are categorized as inflammatory bowel disease and may increase your risk for colorectal cancer. So regular medical checkups and bowel exams are important.

Rarely, very large **colon polyps** (page 192) may cause pain in the lower abdomen. However, before this occurs, you probably will have noticed other abnormalities in your normal bowel function, such as changes in the size and shape of your stools or bloody stools.

RECTAL BLEEDING OR BLACKISH STOOLS

A very occasional few drops of bright red blood on your toilet tissue after a difficult bowel movement most likely signals hemorrhoids, although it could be a sign of far more serious illness. When blood is mixed with a bowel movement there may be no red appearance. Rather, the stool will have a very dark, blackish appearance known as a tarry stool, technically called melena.

Bleeding from the rectum or tarry stools is never normal. If you have such symptoms, call your physician. Describe what is happening so that the doctor can decide whether you should be seen immediately.

Causes and Treatment of Rectal Bleeding or Blackish Stools

Hemorrhoids (page 199) are the most common cause of rectal bleeding. You also may experience rectal pain and itching, soiled underwear due to mucous discharge, or a sensation of incomplete evacuation after a bowel movement. Discomfort can be eased by sitting in a warm bath, applying witch hazel compresses, or using stool softeners to prevent constipation. However, there is no point in suffering with persistent hemorrhoid symptoms when sophisticated treatments, often available in your doctor's office without hospitalization for surgery, can eliminate the problem.

Depending on other symptoms, rectal bleeding can also be a sign of much more serious disorders, such as **colorectal cancer, colon polyps, Crohn's disease,** or **ulcerative colitis.** Because these disorders usually cause abdominal pain as well, they are discussed more fully in the section on abdominal pain or cramps.

INDIGESTION

Indigestion, also called dyspepsia, is a vague term referring to a cluster of seemingly minor digestive problems. They include a sense of upper abdominal discomfort or stomachache, fullness or bloating, and perhaps minor twinges of pain, slight nausea, and burping or flatulence—all occurring after meals.

> Persistent indigestion is not normal. If you have daily or even intermittent but frequent indigestion that you can't explain and remedy with lifestyle changes, call your physician. Describe what is happening so that the doctor can decide whether you should be seen and when.

Causes and Treatment of Indigestion

Most episodes of indigestion are caused by eating too much or too fast, especially if you talk while eating and thus swallow air. Such habits can be provoked by stress, which may also interfere with proper digestion. Take time to enjoy your meals slowly. If you eat more slowly, you give your "appestat" time to learn that food has been received and to signal satiety, which usually occurs about 20 minutes after you start eating. Then you are more likely not to overeat.

In addition, some foods seem to prompt indigestion in many individuals. Onions, beans, and cabbage are frequent offenders. Keep a food diary to help you identify and eliminate your own personal problem foods.

Indigestion is the hallmark symptom of **gastritis** (page 198), which is the medical term for an upset stomach triggered by inflammation of the stomach lining. Gastritis is most commonly caused by frequent use of irritating drugs, such as aspirin, other nonsteroidal anti-inflammatory medications, steroids, and alcohol. You can reduce the risk of stomach irritation by taking such products with food or an antacid. Gastritis also can be caused by infectious organisms and require antibiotic therapy. Although antacids provide immediate relief, people with chronic gastritis should see a physician, as the same symptoms can be caused by more serious problems. Further, frequent gastritis may increase your risk of developing ulcers.

Unfortunately, persistent indigestion is also the most common symptom of **stomach cancer** (page 207). In addition to indigestion, you may experience occasional nausea and vomiting and loss of appetite and weight. The earlier stomach cancer is diagnosed, the better. Although effective treatment requires surgical removal of part or all of the stomach, you can still live normally and eat a fairly regular diet.

Indigestion may also be a symptom of **lactose intolerance** (page 204), especially if accompanied by considerable cramps, flatulence, or diarrhea. Symptoms may arise within a half hour after eating, will disappear if you avoid all milk products for several days, and will not return as long as you continue to avoid such products. If eliminating milk products from your diet does not resolve the problem, call your doctor.

CONSTIPATION

Constipation is any condition in which the bowels move less often than usual and with difficulty.

> Occasional constipation is normal. However, if your normal bowel pattern changes, with movements suddenly and persistently becoming less frequent and difficult to pass, call your physician. Describe what is happening so that the doctor can decide whether you should be seen immediately.

Causes and Treatment of Constipation

Eating habits, physical activity, emotions, and time—all can affect bowel frequency. Eating the wrong things or eating too little can cause constipation. The residue of food you eat is easier to eliminate if it contains liquid from water, juice, or other nonalcoholic beverages and roughage in the form of fibers. Whole-grain breads and cereals, such as barley, brown rice, oats, wheat, and bran, and green leafy vegetables are good sources of roughage. Ensuring that your diet contains these elements should be your first step toward self-care for constipation.

Exercise is also important. A sedentary lifestyle and inadequate exercise can trigger constipation. If your job requires you to sit a lot, start a regular exercise regimen, even if it is just a half-hour walk before dinner every evening.

If you are feeling very anxious or stressed—uptight—don't be surprised if your bowels tighten up too. Try to practice relaxation and stress management skills to ease the strain on your body.

The time you choose to move your bowels may also be a factor. After food is digested in the stomach and intestines, the residue is passed along in watery material. The water is absorbed in the colon. If feces remain there too long, they may become hard and difficult to pass. Because most people eat their main meal in the evening, the following morning may be when the remains of that meal have accumulated in the lower bowel. However, your digestive system may operate at a different pace. Try to cultivate regular elimination habits, but don't worry about it if you don't develop a daily morning habit.

Occasionally, constipation may be an adverse side effect of some medication. If you have recently begun using a new drug, call your doctor for advice.

If persistent constipation does not respond to lifestyle changes, it could be due to a serious problem. Digestive disorders that can cause constipation include **diverticulosis, diverticulitis, irritable bowel syndrome, colorectal cancer,** and **ulcerative colitis.** Because these problems also cause abdominal pain, they are discussed in greater detail in the section on abdominal pain or cramps.

Beyond the digestive system, constipation may be a symptom of **hypothyroidism** (page 250). Symptoms may include feelings of lethargy, aching muscles, heightened sensitivity to cold, and weight gain despite a decreased appetite. The most common cause of hypothyroidism is an autoimmune disorder that is treated by taking daily pills of thyroid hormone.

Never take a laxative without the recommendation of your physician. If a laxative is suggested, you should know the different types:

Psyllium hydrophilic compound, although technically a laxative, is really a seed that provides the bulk and roughage the colon needs to function. It can be taken without any danger or harmful effects.

Stool softeners, such as Colace, enable the stool to hold water, so that the stools become softer and bulkier. Although not as effective as a bulk provider, stool softeners frequently work well with them. Stool softeners can be taken for prolonged periods with no serious side effects.

Saline cathartics, such as milk of magnesia or phosphor soda, cause the intestine to produce a large amount of fluid. They generally should not be used for chronic constipation.

Stimulant or irritant laxatives, such as Senna, Dulcolax, and Ex-Lax, should be avoided unless specifically prescribed by a physician, a rare occurrence. These laxatives irritate the nerves of the colon, stimulating it to contract. Over long periods, they damage the nerves within the colon wall, sometimes permanently. Many "natural" over-the-counter laxatives contain these drugs and should be avoided. They are likely to cause dependence on them for bowel function.

DIARRHEA

Diarrhea is the frequent passage of loose or watery bowel movements. Not a disease in itself but, rather, an indicator of some disorder, diarrhea can lead to dehydration—a loss of important fluids from body tissues—and the loss of large amounts of salts (sodium, potassium, and chlorides) essential for normal body functions. This can be very serious. If vomiting occurs with diarrhea, the water and salts lost are more difficult to replace and could lead to death if left untreated for an extended period. The person may need to be hospitalized for intravenous replacement of water and salts. Depending on the severity of the problem and the condition of the individual, it usually takes a week or more for such a crisis to arise in an adult. However, diarrhea is more serious in children, especially infants, who can become very dehydrated in less than a day if diarrhea becomes severe. They may require oral rehydration with balanced solutions such as Pediolyte or Gatorade.

Occasional mild diarrhea can usually be managed at home. However, if diarrhea lasts for more than two days or worsens during that time (or one day if the victim is a child under two), if there is blood, mucus, or worms in the bowel movement, if there is severe abdominal pain, or if diarrhea is accompanied by vomiting or fever, call your physician. Describe what is happening so that the doctor can decide whether you should be seen immediately.

Causes and Treatment of Diarrhea

Although diarrhea can be a sign of a serious malady that warrants medical attention, most episodes are minor and temporary and can be managed with dietary modification.

Diarrhea is often brought on by stress or other emotional problems or an excess of certain foods, such as prunes. Learning to cope with stress more effectively or modifying your diet can usually resolve these problems.

Diarrhea may also accompany some other illnesses, ranging from some varieties of flu, to so-called "traveler's diarrhea," to food poisoning. Call your doctor to describe your symptoms. Self-care at home may be sufficient in some cases, but more severe illness may warrant medication or even hospitalization. If self-care is recommended, the first step usually requires avoidance of solid food. Rather, drink small amounts of warm fluids, such as flat sodas (cola or ginger ale allowed to stand and fizz out), tea, or broth or other clear soup. If you can keep these down, add binding foods, such as bananas, toast, rice, rice cereals, or chicken/rice soup. As the diarrhea eases, add baked potatoes and other bland, low-fat foods to the diet. Avoid salads and fruits until your bowels are back to normal.

Doctors vary in their opinions on the use of over-the-counter diarrheal products, such as Pepto-Bismol, Kaopectate, and Imodium AD. Some think they are fine for nonspecific diarrhea or that related to minor illness. Others feel that it is best to let your system expel whatever is bothering you in order to ensure more rapid healing. Do not use such products for more than a day or two without consulting your physician.

Some medications cause diarrhea. For example, excessive use of antacids that contain magnesium can precipitate the problem. Switching to a different brand may resolve it. Sometimes antibiotics kill so many normal bacteria in the intestines—while they are killing bad bacteria elsewhere in the body—that an overgrowth of a toxin-secreting bacteria called *Clostridium difficile* triggers diarrhea. Eating yogurt with live cultures may repopulate the colon with bacteria that will compete with *C. difficile* and avert antibiotic-associated diarrhea. If diarrhea occurs while you are taking any medication, inform your doctor.

Diarrhea is also the primary symptom of **celiac disease** (page 190), a disorder in which you are unable to properly digest gluten, a cereal protein found in wheat, rye, barley, and oats. Although it most commonly causes symptoms in infants when they start to eat cereal, yielding particularly malodorous diarrhea, mild cases occasionally arise in adults. If you have unexplained diarrhea and also experience skin disorders and weight loss, this could be your problem. Consult your physician to rule out other possible causes of your symptoms. If celiac disease is diagnosed, dietary modification to avoid certain grains should be able to eliminate your discomfort.

Diarrhea also can be caused by other serious digestive problems, including **colorectal cancer, Crohn's disease, diverticulosis, diverticulitis, irritable bowel syndrome,** and **ulcerative colitis.** Because these disorders also cause abdominal pain, they are discussed more fully in the section on abdominal pain or cramps.

WARNING: Alternating bouts of constipation and diarrhea, interspersed with periods of normal bowel function, may be caused by irritable bowel syndrome or colorectal cancer, as well as by stress. Such symptoms should not be allowed to persist for more than a few weeks without medical evaluation.

FLATULENCE

Flatulence is gas in the intestinal tract that passes out of the body through the rectum. This natural body process occurs in normal, healthy people. Individuals may produce from six ounces to two quarts daily of intestinal gas. Most flatus is produced during the digestion of food in the large intestine. As complex sugars are broken down, carbon dioxide, hydrogen, and methane are produced. Swallowed air adds oxygen and nitrogen to the flatus. Fatty acids, ammonia, and other substances also are part of flatus.

In most cases, flatulence is normal and can be controlled by lifestyle change. However, if you have what seems to be excessive flatulence as well as any other digestive symptoms discussed earlier, especially abdominal pain or diarrhea, call your physician. Describe what is happening so that the doctor can decide whether you should be seen immediately.

Cause and Treatment of Flatulence

Flatulence cannot be totally eliminated because flatus is a normal body product, not a medical problem. When the rectal muscles relax, flatus may escape and cause embarrassment. This can sometimes be controlled through diet and by intentionally expelling gas in privacy.

The odor of flatus depends on the type of food eaten. For example, the digestion of fats contributes in large part to the odor of intestinal gas. Though fat is essential to the human diet and cannot be eliminated, the amount eaten can be controlled. Eating large amounts of fat increases the potential for malodorous flatus. In addition, there is a hereditary component; some people are more likely to make methane, which contributes to the bad odor.

The quantity of flatus often depends on diet as well. Some foods are associated with an increase in the body's production of gas. For example, the habitual bean eater will produce several times the amount of gas daily than the non–bean eater. Other foods associated with increased gas production are cabbage, spinach, cauliflower, broccoli, brussels sprouts, eggplant, and fibrous foods such as bran and fruit. In some people dairy products cause excess flatus.

You can control your gas production to some extent by adjusting your diet. Different foods have a different impact on people. Only by trial and error can you find the ones that get your own intestinal tract into an uproar.

In addition to those already listed, some people are bothered by onions, celery, carrots, raisins, pastries, apricots, wheat germ, and prune juice. Once you find the foods that offend your intestinal tract, you can at least reduce their amount in your diet, if not eliminate them totally. Also, make sure that you eat calmly, not rushing and not talking with your mouth full, which tends to increase air swallowing. Eating too much at one time or eating while under stress also can inhibit normal digestive processes and lead to excessive gas production.

Occasionally, flatulence is caused by a digestive disorder. If you develop flatulence and bloating, as well as abdominal cramps or diarrhea, only a few hours after consuming milk or milk products, it could be **lactose intolerance** (page 204). Some people lose their ability to digest milk products in early or late adulthood. If that's your problem, eliminating all milk products for a few days should eliminate your symptoms—and they won't return as long as you avoid such products.

Far less commonly, flatulence may be caused by **celiac disease** (page 190), a disorder in which you are unable to properly digest gluten, a cereal protein found in wheat, rye, barley, and oats. Although it most commonly causes symptoms in infants, mild cases occasionally arise in adults, causing flatulence, diarrhea, skin disorders, and weight loss. Consult your physician to rule out other possible causes of your symptoms. If celiac disease is diagnosed, dietary modification should be able to eliminate your discomfort.

COMMON DISORDERS OF THE DIGESTIVE SYSTEM

APPENDICITIS is inflammation of the appendix, a small pouch that extends from the beginning of the large intestine, in the lower right side of the abdomen. The swollen appendix sometimes ruptures or perforates, permitting pus to enter the abdominal cavity or the peritoneum. The resulting contamination and inflammation is called peritonitis. Appendicitis and peritonitis are more likely to be problems in children and in elderly people. In both groups the early warning signs may not be fully recognized.

What are the symptoms?
Abdominal pain is the primary symptom. The pain comes on suddenly and may be accompanied by nausea, vomiting, a mild fever, and constipation. The pain may start high in the center of the abdomen and then migrate to the right lower side or, less commonly, the lower left side.

How did I get it?
Although waste matter in the bowel normally flows past the appendix, it can sometimes enter the appendix. It can become blocked by its own twisting or if the appendix then fails to clean itself properly. When this happens, the blood vessels in the appendix are shut off, pus begins to form, and the appendix swells.

How is it diagnosed?
Your doctor will diagnose appendicitis based on a complete history and physical exam, in conjunction with blood tests to determine whether infection is present.

How is it treated?
Appendicitis is treated with surgery to remove the appendix. You are usually in the hospital less than a week and back to your normal routine within three weeks. This procedure offers little risk and should not be delayed for more than a few hours due to the serious risk of peritonitis. If the appendix has already ruptured, surgery is more complex and infected tissue must also be removed.

Self-Care: If your symptoms suggest appendicitis, call your doctor immediately. If you can't reach your doctor, go to a hospital emergency room. Laxatives, which are used commonly by older people, may worsen appendicitis and cause perforation. Never use a laxative or enema in the presence of abdominal pain unless told to do so by your physician.

CELIAC DISEASE is a disorder in which you are unable to properly digest gluten, a cereal protein found in wheat, rye, barley, and oats. Also called celiac sprue or gluten enteropathy, it is an intestinal malabsorption problem.

What are the symptoms?
No symptoms occur until an infant starts to eat cereal. Those afflicted then develop pale, watery bowel movements that are particularly malodorous. These infants also become irritable and do not grow normally, developing large bellies due to abdominal gas. If not diagnosed and treated promptly, infants with celiac disease become seriously malnourished and the disorder can be fatal. In very mild cases, minor bowel problems may not be noticed

and more serious concerns do not arise until adulthood. Adult problems may include weight loss, skin disorders, and anemia.

How did I get it?
Celiac disease is an inherited disorder. If there is any history of the disorder in your family, cereals should be introduced into a baby's diet with caution.

How is it diagnosed?
Your doctor will suspect celiac disease based on your report of the baby's abnormal stools, a swollen belly, and failure to thrive. Diagnosis is confirmed based on blood tests, special X-rays, and in some cases, an intestinal biopsy.

How is it treated?
The primary therapy is changing the diet to one that completely excludes all sources of gluten. If an infant is severely malnourished, hospitalization for intravenous feeding may be necessary. However, most youngsters can be treated at home with the appropriate diet and vitamin and mineral supplements. Symptoms usually disappear within a few weeks of eliminating gluten from the diet.

> Self-Care: The gluten-free diet must be continued throughout life. You can get help in planning an appropriate diet from a registered dietitian. When buying prepared foods, be sure to read package labels carefully because gluten is often used as a food additive.

CIRRHOSIS is severe, permanent scarring of the liver due to a condition in which it has become enlarged, tender, and sensitive. The liver can no longer perform the functions necessary to do its part in keeping the body healthy.

What are the symptoms?
There is a general deterioration of health, characterized by weight and appetite loss, weakness, and fatigue. As the disease progresses, you may experience discomfort in the right upper part of the abdomen, and your skin may bruise easily. As the disease worsens, your skin and the whites of your eyes may take on a yellowish cast, a condition called jaundice. In advanced cases of cirrhosis, there may be mental changes, ranging from simple forgetfulness and insomnia to stupor and coma. Veins in the esophagus and upper abdomen may enlarge and rupture, causing potentially life-threatening bleeding.

How did I get it?
There are many causes of cirrhosis, including hepatitis, infection from viruses, bile duct problems, alcoholic damage from excessive drinking, and certain medications and genetic conditions.

How is it diagnosed?
Before the liver reaches the stage of permanent damage from cirrhosis, changes taking place in the individual cells can be discovered by your doctor through a series of tests. These changes may sometimes be spotted during a checkup before you notice any symptoms. Cirrhosis is diagnosed based on a physical examination, blood tests, special imaging procedures, and a liver biopsy.

How is it treated?
In the early stages of liver damage, elimination of the underlying cause—commonly, excessive alcohol consumption—may be able to halt or even reverse the injury. Once cirrhosis has been diagnosed, the damage cannot be reversed, although elimination of the cause may be able to slow its progression. For a person with alcoholic liver disease, every drink of alcohol contributes to destruction of the liver. Treatment is usually aimed at maintaining good nutrition and preventing the life-threatening complications of advanced liver disease. You may have to control your protein and salt intake. If liver failure occurs, a liver transplant may be possible, depending on the cause of the cirrhosis. Alcoholics are transplant candidates only if they are committed to abstinence.

> Self-Care: Because the most common cause of cirrhosis is alcohol ingestion, avoid alcohol overuse throughout life. There is no form of alcohol that is incapable of producing cirrhosis of the liver. Beer, wine, vodka, gin, rum, bourbon, blended whiskey, and home brews—all produce the disease.

COLON POLYPS are small benign tumors that grow on the inside walls of the lower part of the large intestine. They range in size from a tiny grape pit to a small plum. Most adults develop such polyps at some time in life.

What are the symptoms?
Most colon polyps remain small and cause no symptoms. In some cases, they grow sufficiently large to interfere with normal bowel function, causing a change in the size and shape of stools, bloody stools, or abdominal pain.

How did I get it?
Some types are inherited, but the cause of most colon polyps is unknown.
However, they become more common after age 40.

How is it diagnosed?
You will require a special examination called a colonoscopy. In this procedure, a hollow tube is inserted into the rectum and up into the colon. A
viewing device attached to the tube enables the doctor to examine the inner
colon wall. If any polyps are observed, tools inserted through the tube can
be used to take tissue samples for laboratory examination. Small polyps can
be completely removed by this method.

How is it treated?
Small benign polyps that are not causing problems do not necessarily need
to be removed. However, many doctors recommend that all colon polyps
be removed because of the risk that they may become cancerous. Because
colon cancer is a leading cause of death, it is hoped that removal of colon
polyps can reduce the toll.

Self-Care: People over age 40 should have an annual digital rectal
examination. Those over 50 should have more extensive examination
of the lower bowel by a procedure known as sigmoidoscopy, which is
similar to but not as extensive as colonoscopy. The frequency of such
examinations should be discussed with your physician based on your
personal and family medical history.

COLORECTAL CANCER refers to any malignancy of the last few feet
of the large intestine, known as the colon, or the rectum. Such cancers are
second only to lung cancer as the greatest cause of cancer death. However,
when diagnosed early, colorectal cancer can be effectively treated. About
70 percent of patients undergoing surgery for early colorectal cancer survive
the crucial first five years after treatment.

What are the symptoms?
Early colorectal cancer may cause no symptoms for months or years. Then
you may experience persistent or intermittent diarrhea or constipation for
no apparent reason. Later symptoms include bleeding from the rectum, a
blackish stool that signals the presence of blood, a change in the typical size
or shape of the stool, or pain or bloating in the lower abdomen.

How did I get it?

The precise cause of colorectal cancer is unknown. However, there is growing indication that diet may play a key role. People who eat a diet high in beef and fat and low in fiber seem to be at greater risk. You may also be at greater risk if you have colon polyps, if you have inflammatory bowel disease, or if there is a history of the disease in the family, because genetic factors may play a major role.

How is it diagnosed?

Colorectal cancer can be detected at an early stage with several procedures. First, there is the digital rectal examination, which enables your doctor to feel the presence of abnormal growths in the first few inches of the bowel. Second, there is the stool slide test, in which a sample of your bowel movement is checked for the presence of blood. Third, there is sigmoid-oscopy, in which a lighted tube is inserted into the rectum, enabling your doctor to examine the lower colon. Finally, there is colonoscopy, which is similar to sigmoidoscopy but enables examination further up in the large intestine. During this procedure, small growths can be removed and samples of larger growths taken for laboratory examination.

How is it treated?

Colorectal cancer requires surgery to remove the cancer and part of the intestine directly above and below the tumor site. Usually, the two ends of the colon are rejoined and normal function returns. However, if the cancer is in the rectum and it must be removed, a new way for waste to exit the body must be created. This is called a colostomy. A small, permanent opening is made in the lower abdomen, and a bag is attached to collect waste. New surgical techniques, including a "pull-through" procedure, may avert the need for colostomy and should be discussed with your doctor. Depending on the type and stage of the disease, radiation or chemotherapy may be recommended after surgery.

Self-Care: To reduce the risk of colorectal cancer, or a recurrence if you already have had a tumor removed, try to eat a low-fat, high-fiber diet. Foods high in fiber include whole grains, such as bran and other whole-grain cereals and whole wheat bread, and fresh fruits and vegetables. Fruit fiber is thought to be even more effective than grain fiber.

CROHN'S DISEASE is a chronic inflammatory disease that most commonly affects the lower part of the small intestine, called the ileum, and/or the large intestine. The illness is also called regional enteritis or ileitis. Inflammation and ulceration cause permanent scarring of the intestines, which can narrow or obstruct the channel for body waste. Ashkenazic Jews may be at higher risk.

What are the symptoms?
Crohn's disease causes abdominal pain, cramping, persistent diarrhea, and blood in the stool, as well as hemorrhoids and abscesses in the anal area. You also may experience weight loss, fever, joint pains, and skin or eye irritations. When Crohn's disease strikes children, growth and sexual maturation may be delayed.

How did I get it?
The cause is unknown, although doctors think that it may be an autoimmune disorder because there seem to be familial or genetic factors involved. Although the disorder is not caused by emotional stress or dietary factors, it may be worsened by these problems.

How is it diagnosed?
Diagnosis can be difficult and usually requires blood tests, laboratory examination of the stool, special X-rays, and sigmoidoscopy (page 194), during which a tissue sample usually is taken to help confirm the diagnosis.

How is it treated?
There is no cure for Crohn's disease, and it is difficult to treat. You will be given oral medications, such as corticosteroids and sulfasalazine, to help reduce the inflammation and alleviate the cramps and diarrhea. If this therapy does not provide sufficient relief, you may be given other drugs that suppress the immune system. Discuss new approaches with your doctor. If medical therapy is not adequately successful, or if an intestinal obstruction occurs, surgery may be necessary to remove the affected areas. Surgery, however, is the treatment of last resort, because scar tissue in the bowel may cause future obstructions. Unfortunately, the disease is likely to recur later in other areas of the bowel.

Self-Care: In addition to medication, people with Crohn's disease should get plenty of rest and follow a bland, low-fiber diet to reduce intestinal irritation. Because people with Crohn's disease are at greater risk of colon cancer, discuss routine screening with your doctor.

DIVERTICULOSIS and **DIVERTICULITIS** are abnormalities of the large intestine. Diverticulosis refers to small outpouchings or sacs protruding from the intestinal wall. At least one-third of all Americans over age 45 and more than two-thirds of those over age 60 have diverticulosis. Women are at greater risk than men. When one or more of the pouches becomes infected, a more serious condition called diverticulitis may occur. About 15 percent of those with diverticulosis develop diverticulitis, whose complications may include an abscess or perforation or obstruction of the intestine.

What are the symptoms?
Most people with diverticulosis have no symptoms, although some suffer with abdominal cramps, gas, and diarrhea alternating with constipation. These symptoms may be more related to the irritable bowel syndrome that often precedes the disorder than to the diverticulosis itself. Diverticulitis usually causes severe abdominal pain, diarrhea, and fever.

How did I get it?
The sacs, called diverticula, contain the same outer and inner linings as the rest of the bowel but they are missing the middle muscular layer. The pressure of intestinal contractions causes the inner lining to push through the muscle to create the sacs. When bits of food enter the sacs, they can trigger the diverticulitis infection. Although the exact causes of diverticular problems are not known, contributing factors are believed to include aging, which causes the colon walls to weaken; regular use of laxatives, which weakens the colon; and a low-fiber diet, which can compromise colonic muscle tone.

How is it diagnosed?
Your doctor will suspect diverticulosis based on your symptoms and by listening to your intestinal sounds with a stethoscope. Blood tests and an examination of your stool will be done. Finally, you will have a sigmoidoscopy (page 194), as well as special X-rays taken after you have been given an enema containing barium, a substance that highlights the contents of the bowel.

How is it treated?
Diverticulosis cannot be reversed, but medication to help relax intestinal muscles can ease discomfort temporarily. More important, to help prevent

the development of diverticulitis, drink at least eight glasses of fluid daily and add fiber to the diet. Fiber, also called roughage, is a nonnutrient but it is essential for normal bowel function. High residue fiber goes through your intestines like a "roto-rooter," cleaning every corner. However, avoid nuts and seeds. Diverticulitis can usually be controlled with medication and a temporary diet of clear liquids only to let the bowel rest. However, sometimes hospitalization, intravenous antibiotics, and even surgery to remove infected areas of the intestine are required.

Self-Care: One way to add fiber to your diet is by eating one or two ounces of natural unprocessed bran daily. Regular bran cereals are helpful, but they contain a large percentage of sugar and are otherwise not as efficient. Fresh fruits and vegetables are also high in fiber. You may prefer them, if, like many people, you cannot tolerate the roughage of bran.

GALLSTONES are crystalline formations of cholesterol or bile salts that may form in the gallbladder. Also known as biliary calculi, they may be as small as grains of sand or as large as walnuts. If recurrent gallstone attacks are not treated, the stones can lodge in the bile duct and cause infection or inflammation of the gallbladder, liver, pancreas, or other nearby organs. Another major threat is rupture of the gallbladder, leading to peritonitis, which can be life threatening.

What are the symptoms?
About half of all people who have gallstones never know it because they have no symptoms. This is known as silent gallstones. Others suffer attacks known as cholecystitis that cause sudden severe pain in the upper abdomen, usually on the right side; sometimes the pain is felt in the back and under the right shoulder blade. Pain usually begins after a meal. In addition, fever, chills, and vomiting may occur. An attack can last for several hours, until the stone passes through the duct and into the intestines.

How did I get it?
An imbalance in the composition of bile salts in the gallbladder, such as excess cholesterol, is believed to contribute to the formation of stones. The tendency to develop gallstones may run in families. They are also more common in people who are overweight or who eat a high-fat diet. Acute attacks of gallstone pain occur when a stone that was previously floating in the fluid becomes lodged in the duct that carries bile from the gallbladder

to the intestines. Attacks may occur spontaneously but more often are triggered by a large fatty meal. In some people, attacks become progressively more severe or frequent.

How is it diagnosed?
A sonogram that uses painless ultrasound waves, special X-rays, or other imaging studies can identify the presence of gallstones.

How is it treated?
For those who have frequent painful attacks, the preferred treatment is surgical removal of the gallbladder, called cholecystectomy. You can have a completely normal life without this organ. Although medication can be prescribed to dissolve stones, its effectiveness is not certain, the dissolution can take several years, and the drug must be taken for the rest of your life to prevent further stones.

Self-Care: If you have already been diagnosed with gallstones and know the symptoms, call your doctor if you have frequent recurrences or if any attack lasts for more than three hours. Such a prolonged attack indicates that the stone is too large to be passed and may require immediate surgery. You may be able to reduce the frequency of attacks by avoiding high-fat foods, large meals, and any food that tends to give you indigestion. If you are overweight, reduce. If you are a woman, avoid oral contraceptives or any other form of estrogen therapy, which may increase stone formation.

GASTRITIS is the medical term for an upset stomach triggered by inflammation of the lining of the stomach, also known as the gastric mucosa. Acute gastritis is very common; it arises suddenly and soon disappears. In chronic gastritis, symptoms are persistent or intermittent over a long period. Frequent gastritis may increase your risk of developing stomach ulcers.

What are the symptoms?
Indigestion and abdominal pain are the primary symptoms. Some people also experience heartburn, nausea, and vomiting. Sometimes, especially in acute gastritis, you may vomit blood or have blackish stools indicating the presence of blood.

How did I get it?

Both acute and chronic gastritis may be caused by drugs, especially aspirin, other nonsteroidal anti-inflammatory medications, steroids, and alcohol, as well as by an infectious organism known as *Campylobacter pylori*. Acute gastritis often occurs in those who have undergone severe trauma, such as serious burns, other physical injuries, shock, and blood or food poisoning. Chronic gastritis is more common among people over the age of 40, those who are smokers, and those who have Crohn's disease or herpes infections.

How is it diagnosed?

Mild gastritis is diagnosed based on your description of symptoms. More severe or persistent gastritis warrants fuller evaluation, which may include blood tests, evaluation of a stool sample, and special X-rays and gastroscopy. This examination involves insertion of a flexible tube down your throat, through the esophagus, and into the stomach. It enables the doctor to observe the stomach lining directly and, if necessary, retrieve a tissue sample for laboratory examination.

How is it treated?

Treatment depends on the severity of the gastritis and whether an underlying cause is found. Mild gastritis may be treated with behavior modification as described below. Taking over-the-counter antacids one hour after meals and at bedtime can neutralize stomach acid and help heal stomach inflammation. Or your doctor may recommend prescription drugs to reduce the release of acid into the stomach. If severe stomach bleeding occurs, you may need hospital treatment and, in the worst cases, surgery to remove all or part of the stomach.

Self-Care: To alleviate gastritis, avoid aspirin and other nonsteroidal anti-inflammatory drugs, such as ibuprofen. If you must use such drugs, always take them with food to ease irritation. If you smoke, quit. Avoid alcohol, spicy foods, and any other foods that seem to trigger symptoms. Eat frequent small meals rather than fewer larger ones.

HEMORRHOIDS are normal structures in the lower rectum and anus of all adults. They contain blood vessels and other tissues. Painful hemorrhoids are usually those in which an acute change, consisting of ulceration or blood clot formation, has occurred. Hemorrhoids are also known as piles or anal varicose veins.

What are the symptoms?
Hemorrhoids can cause rectal pain, rectal bleeding, protrusion of the veins from the anus, soiled underwear due to mucous discharge, or a sensation of incomplete evacuation after a bowel movement.

How did I get it?
The most common cause of painful hemorrhoids is straining to move your bowels, which more commonly occurs in people who are constipated, obese, or pregnant. Hemorrhoids also may be a symptom of liver disease. Some external hemorrhoids may be provoked by sedentary jobs, prolonged standing, or frequent diarrhea.

How is it diagnosed?
Because hemorrhoids either protrude from the rectum or are located just inside the anus, the initial diagnosis is made by physical examination. The doctor also may insert a hollow tube into the rectum to check for internal hemorrhoids further up or to rule out other disorders.

How is it treated?
Treatment depends on the type and severity of the hemorrhoid, with some responding well to the self-care described below. Some hemorrhoids, left alone, heal themselves. Severely painful hemorrhoids can be removed. Many hemorrhoids are treated in the doctor's office by rubber band ligation, which has eliminated 95 percent of hemorrhoid surgery. A small elastic band is slipped around some internal hemorrhoids. Cut off from its blood supply, the hemorrhoid falls off in 4 to 14 days. Little or no pain is involved. Bleeding hemorrhoids are treated with rubber band ligation or with injections. Other hemorrhoids can be destroyed by freezing techniques. Yet others require surgical removal. For example, surgery is usually required for acute attacks involving hemorrhoids that are prolapsed, strangulated, and swollen, causing severe pain.

Self-Care: Home care can often ease hemorrhoid discomfort. Pain may be eased by sitting in a warm bath, applying witch hazel compresses, and using stool softeners to prevent constipation. Over-the-counter ointments and suppositories have little effect on hemorrhoids, although those containing cortisone may alleviate itching and pain. A healthy diet, including plenty of fiber and at least eight glasses of fluid daily, can also help to alleviate or prevent hemorrhoids.

HERNIA (HIATAL) is a condition in which the hiatus, the normally small opening in the muscular diaphragm where the esophagus meets the stomach, has widened. As a result, part of the stomach protrudes upward through the hiatal opening. Symptomatic hiatal hernia, if left untreated, can lead to severe and potentially life-threatening esophageal damage, including ulceration, bleeding, narrowing, and even obstruction.

What are the symptoms?
Most often, hiatal hernia causes no symptoms and no problems. However, it can cause heartburn, reflux of stomach acid into the esophagus and throat, and burping. *Because the symptoms of a heart attack can often be misinterpreted as heartburn or indigestion, any chest pain that is not eased promptly by an antacid should be reported to your doctor immediately.*

How did I get it?
Some hiatal hernias are present at birth. Others develop during life as the hiatal opening becomes stretched or weak or as pregnancy or obesity place upward pressure on the stomach. Severe coughing, vomiting, straining when moving the bowels, or sudden physical exertion may also cause injury. About half of all Americans over age 40 have a hiatal hernia, but most don't know it because they do not have any symptoms. You are at greater risk if you are overweight or if you are a woman who has had a child.

How is it diagnosed?
If you have frequent heartburn and reflux, your doctor may make an assumption of hiatal hernia and recommend treatment. Diagnostic tests, such as special X-rays and endoscopy, may be performed only if you do not respond to conservative treatment.

How is it treated?
The first line of therapy is the self-care described below. Your doctor may recommend an antacid to neutralize stomach acid, histamine$_2$ blockers like cimetidine to reduce stomach acid output, or acid pump inhibitors like omeprazole. If conservative lifestyle and medical treatment do not alleviate symptoms, surgery may be recommended to reposition the stomach below the diaphragm and narrow the hiatal opening. Such surgery, though, is rarely needed.

Self-Care: If you are overweight, lose weight to alleviate pressure on your stomach. Avoid tight belts, girdles, and other clothing that constricts your belly. Avoid large meals, taking several small meals rather than fewer big ones. Avoid reclining, stooping, or bending for at least an hour after meals. Avoid substances that can weaken the diaphragmatic muscle, such as fatty foods, alcohol, chocolate, peppermint, wine, and tobacco. Avoid foods that tend to irritate your stomach—spices, carbonated beverages, citrus juice, tomato juice, and coffee.

HERNIA (INTESTINAL or ABDOMINAL) occurs when a portion of the intestines begins to bulge through the abdominal wall, forming a soft lump. Men develop these hernias more often than women in a ratio of about 20 to 1. Hernias may be aggravated by coughing, sneezing, heavy lifting, or straining to pass bowel movements. One possible complication is strangulation, when a portion of intestine becomes caught and its blood supply is cut off. The strangulated loop can become gangrenous, a life-threatening condition if not treated immediately.

What are the symptoms?
The location of the lump, which may look like an egg under the skin, depends on the type of intestinal hernia. Inguinal hernia, the most common, occurs in the groin in men and women. The femoral hernia, on the upper thigh just below the groin, is most frequent in women. In some infants, the navel (bellybutton) protrudes. Called an umbilical hernia, it usually goes away by itself soon after birth. If not, it can be a cause of concern as adult hernias are. An umbilical hernia can also occur later in life, after the abdomen is stretched by pregnancy or weight gain.

How did I get it?
Intestinal and abdominal hernias occur when a weak spot or a tear develops in the bands of muscle tissue in the abdominal wall. They may develop gradually or bulge suddenly when you lift a heavy object or otherwise strain yourself. Once a hernia develops, it tends to worsen progressively.

How is it diagnosed?
Your doctor usually can diagnose a hernia by simple physical examination.

How is it treated?
The best treatment is surgical repair of the muscle tear or weakness. This is a relatively minor operation that may be done as an outpatient procedure or with only a day or two of hospitalization. The use of trusses, an old-fashioned approach to hernias, may worsen the problem by enlarging the weak

spot and squashing or strangulating the intestine. Even a well-fitted truss does not avert the danger of a strangulated hernia.

Self-Care: If you have a hernia that suddenly gets larger or becomes painful, and the lump does not go away when you lie down, see your physician immediately or go to a hospital emergency room. You may have a strangulated hernia.

IRRITABLE BOWEL SYNDROME (IBS) is a disorder of movement within the intestines. Instead of the rhythmic muscle contractions that normally move waste through the system, irregular contractions cause abnormalities that include too little or too much fluid in the bowel. Women are affected three times as often as men.

What are the symptoms?
IBS symptoms can vary markedly from one person to another. In one type, painless but urgent diarrhea is the primary symptom. It usually occurs upon awakening or during or immediately after a meal and may lead to incontinence. In the type called spastic colon, alternating bouts of diarrhea and constipation occur, with abdominal pain, cramps, bloating, and nausea, particularly after eating. Non-bowel symptoms may include fatigue, anxiety, headache, depression, and difficulty in concentrating.

How did I get it?
No underlying cause of IBS has been identified. Although it is not caused by stress, emotional conflict, or dietary factors, it may be worsened by these problems.

How is it diagnosed?
Because there is no organic disease to identify, IBS is diagnosed by excluding all other possible causes of your symptoms, such as Crohn's disease, ulcerative colitis, and colorectal cancer. Diagnosis usually requires blood tests, laboratory examination of your stool, special X-rays, and sigmoidoscopy (page 194), during which a tissue sample also may be taken.

How is it treated?
The self-care described below is the most common treatment. In some cases your doctor may prescribe anticholinergic drugs or tranquilizers for short-term use to help alleviate abnormal muscle contractions. Other drugs may be prescribed if diarrhea or depression are severe.

Self-Care: Keep a diary of foods eaten and other lifestyle factors to help you identify what may trigger attacks. Avoid any foods that cause problems. If constipation is more severe than diarrhea, follow a high-fiber diet with plenty of fresh fruits and vegetables and whole grains. If diarrhea is more severe than constipation, or if a high-fiber diet worsens symptoms, switch to a bland, low-fiber diet.

LACTOSE INTOLERANCE is an inability to digest milk and milk products, such as cheese, ice cream, and sour cream. Lactose is a form of sugar present in milk and its products. It is digested in your intestines with the aid of an enzyme called lactase. If this enzyme is deficient or absent, you develop lactose intolerance. Instead of being broken down, lactose remains in the gut and has a laxative effect.

What are the symptoms?
After consuming a certain amount of milk or its products containing lactose, you develop gas expressed as flatulence and bloating, as well as abdominal cramps and/or diarrhea. The discomfort hits within a half hour after you consume milk products and disappears within a day after eliminating them from the diet. But symptoms recur whenever you consume milk products.

How did I get it?
In about two-thirds of the world's population, the enzyme lactase gradually begins to decrease after infancy, as people "outgrow" their need for—and ability to digest—milk. This common cause of lactose intolerance most frequently occurs in blacks, Indians, Jews, and Mediterranean, Asian, and Middle Eastern people. Two other problems can cause lactose intolerance: a small number of infants are born with congenital lactase deficiency, and some adults, whose small intestine lining becomes diseased, develop the deficiency. Lactose intolerance is not absolute in all sufferers. Some may have problems only when there are large amounts of milk in the diet. Such relative deficiencies may be revealed only when you start a high-lactose diet. Doctors report seeing more of this disorder in women who are drinking more milk to keep their calcium intake up.

How is it diagnosed?
Many people with lactose intolerance are never diagnosed. When they notice that eating milk products upsets their stomachs, they just stop using such products. Medical diagnosis may involve avoiding milk products for a

few days to see if symptoms disappear, or laboratory tests, one based on a blood sample and another based on the amount of hydrogen you exhale after ingesting lactose.

How is it treated?
Therapy simply involves exercising caution in your diet to avoid products containing lactose. These include whole, low-fat, skim, and evaporated milk (fluid or dry), cheese, ice cream, and many commercial cakes, frozen foods, cookies, prepared soups, and cereals. Those who are not highly sensitive can have products whose lactose levels have been reduced by bacterial cultures that partly predigest it; these include yogurt with live cultures, buttermilk, sour cream, and acidophilus milk.

Self-Care: People who are highly sensitive to lactose but who still want to ingest milk can add the enzyme lactase to fluid at home. Lactase, in tablet or liquid form, is sold in many health food stores and pharmacies. The use of lactase supplements may be problematic and depends on the amount of acid in the stomach at any particular time. Therefore, lactase tablets or liquid may not always work. Another alternative is lactose-free soy milk or milk with the lactase enzyme already added. People who avoid milk products should take calcium supplements.

PANCREATITIS is inflammation of the pancreas, an organ that produces enzymes and hormones important in digestion. The condition may be acute, with severe symptoms developing suddenly, or chronic, with milder symptoms appearing gradually over a period of years.

What are the symptoms?
Abdominal pain that worsens with movement or breathing and lessens when you sit up or bend at the waist is a hallmark of pancreatitis. In acute pancreatitis, severe abdominal pain may radiate from the upper abdomen to back; pain reaches a peak within minutes to hours and remains severe for days or weeks. You also may experience nausea and vomiting, as well as signs of developing shock, such as clammy skin and a fast, weak pulse. In chronic pancreatitis, moderate to severe pain is centered in the abdomen and aggravated after eating or drinking alcohol. You also may experience diarrhea, weight loss, and jaundice, as well as suffer with indigestion between attacks.

How did I get it?

The inflammation is caused by a buildup of digestive enzymes in the pancreas. More than 80 percent of acute pancreatitis cases are caused by alcohol ingestion or gallstones. It also may be caused by infections such as mumps, high levels of blood fats, structural abnormalities in the pancreatic or common bile duct, vascular disease, hereditary pancreatitis, or pancreatic injury. Chronic pancreatitis is almost always caused by alcoholism. Less commonly, it may be caused by hyperparathyroidism, hereditary pancreatic pancreatitis, repeated bouts of acute pancreatitis, diabetes, malabsorption disorders, or obstruction of the pancreatic duct by narrowing, stones, or cancer. In addition, women who take oral contraceptives may be at greater risk.

How is it diagnosed?

If your doctor suspects pancreatitis, you will need to have blood tests and special X-rays to confirm the diagnosis. Stool samples may also be taken for laboratory evaluation of fat absorption.

How is it treated?

Therapy is designed to reduce pancreatic enzymes and stem inflammation. Acute attacks require hospitalization; you cannot eat but must receive nutrition intravenously. Stomach secretions may be removed via a tube inserted through your nose. Anticholinergic drugs are given to reduce pancreatic secretions. Major painkillers, such as meperidine, are often needed. If the pancreas ruptures, internal bleeding can be severe and potentially life threatening. If an underlying disorder, such as gallstones, can be identified and treated, no further attacks may occur. If the acute attack was due to alcoholism and you do not permanently abstain from alcohol, the problem is likely to recur. Chronic pancreatitis must be treated by lifestyle measures, as well as medication to reduce pancreatic enzymes, including antacids. Severe problems may require surgery to remove part of the damaged pancreas.

Self-Care: Those with chronic pancreatitis must abstain from alcohol and follow a careful dietary regimen, reducing intake of fat and protein. Eat several small meals rather than fewer larger ones. You also may have to undertake periodic brief fasts to rest the pancreas. Some people with pancreatitis also develop diabetes, warranting further dietary precautions.

STOMACH CANCER, also known as gastric carcinoma, is any malignancy that arises in the stomach. Stomach cancer was once the leading cause of cancer death in the United States, but it has decreased significantly in the past 20 years. Only about 20,000 new cases are discovered each year. For unknown reasons, it strikes more men than women, and twice as many black Americans are likely to develop stomach cancer as are whites.

What are the symptoms?
The most common symptom of stomach cancer is indigestion. This may consist of a sense of discomfort or mild pain, fullness or bloating, heartburn, slight nausea, loss of appetite, and occasionally vomiting and weight loss.

How did I get it?
Although the cause of stomach cancer is unknown, doctors believe that nutrition plays an important role. Changing American dietary habits may have contributed to the decrease in stomach cancer in recent years. In particular, our increased intake of fresh fruits and vegetables and decreased use of smoked meats, salt-cured foods, and pickled vegetables may have contributed to the decline of stomach cancer risk.

How is it diagnosed?
Your doctor will perform blood tests and ask for a sample of your stool for examination. In addition, special imaging studies will be done, and you probably will have a gastroscopy. In this procedure, a flexible tube is inserted through your mouth, down the esophagus, and into the stomach. This enables the doctor to inspect the stomach lining and extract samples of stomach fluid and any abnormal tissue observed. When this material is examined in the laboratory, the diagnosis can be made.

How is it treated?
The usual treatment for stomach cancer is surgical removal of all or part of the stomach. If the cancer has spread locally, nearby lymph nodes or even the spleen or pancreas may also have to be removed. Depending on the stage of the cancer, chemotherapy may be recommended after surgery.

Self-Care: Even if all of your stomach is removed, you can live normally and eat a fairly regular diet. However, you will have to eat smaller meals more often because the intestines take over the work of the stomach.

ULCERATIVE COLITIS is a chronic disease in which sores or ulcers form on the inner lining of the colon. Colitis is the medical term for inflammation of the large intestine or colon. The term colitis is sometimes improperly used to refer to an irritable or so-called "spastic" colon in which there is no inflammation.

What are the symptoms?
An attack of ulcerative colitis usually produces abdominal pain, bloating, cramping, and frequent bloody diarrhea. You also may experience loss of appetite and weight and have a fever. Intermittent attacks lasting from one to several days alternate with intervals without any symptoms.

How did I get it?
The cause is unknown, although doctors think that it may be an autoimmune disorder because there seem to be familial or genetic factors involved. Although the disorder is not caused by emotional stress or dietary factors, it may be worsened by these problems.

How is it diagnosed?
Diagnosis can be difficult and usually requires blood tests, laboratory examination of your stool, special X-rays, and sigmoidoscopy (page 194), during which a tissue sample also may be taken to rule out Crohn's disease, another colon disorder, which has a different pattern of findings.

How is it treated?
Corticosteroid drugs are usually prescribed initially to reduce the inflammation. These may be given daily for several weeks, either orally or by enema to avoid the side effects of systemic steroids. The drug is then tapered off slowly after symptoms subside. Some people must have continuing low doses of steroids to prevent recurrences. Antibiotics also may be given if infection is suspected. In severe cases, hospitalization may be necessary for intravenous medication, surgical removal of some parts of the intestine, and, if rectal bleeding is severe, blood transfusions. In the worst cases, toxic distention of the bowel wall can lead to rupture of the large intestine causing peritonitis, a medical emergency requiring immediate surgery.

Self-Care: In addition to medication, people with ulcerative colitis should get plenty of rest and follow a bland, low-fiber diet to reduce intestinal irritation. Because people with longstanding ulcerative colitis are at greater risk of colon cancer, discuss routine screening with your doctor.

ULCERS are small erosions in the mucosal lining of the gastrointestinal tract. They most commonly occur in the upper portion of the small intestine, known as the duodenum, where they are called peptic ulcers. Less often, ulcers occur directly in the lining of the stomach, where they may be called gastric ulcers. About 10 percent of all Americans get ulcers. The first symptoms are most apt to occur between the ages of 20 and 40. The highest prevalence is in the 40 to 55 age group. More men than women are victims.

What are the symptoms?
The primary symptom is pain in the center of the chest, ranging from gnawing or burning to severe and searing. Other symptoms include heartburn, burping, bloating, and gas. In addition, some people experience nausea and vomiting. The pain is usually worse when the stomach is empty (except before breakfast) and less after eating or taking an antacid.

How did I get it?
Doctors long thought that ulcers were caused by an imbalance in the stomach—either too much stomach acid or pepsin, the major digestive enzyme, or too little mucus protecting the stomach lining. Such an imbalance could allow the stomach acids to, in effect, turn on and begin to digest the duodenal wall or stomach lining itself. Recent research suggests that an infection by a bacterium called helicobacter may be the trigger that starts the process leading to the imbalance. Smoking, heredity, poor dietary habits, excess stress, and heavy drinking also may contribute to your risk.

How is it diagnosed?
If your doctor suspects an ulcer, special imaging studies of the intestinal tract will be necessary. In some cases, endoscopy will also be done. This involves inserting a flexible tube down your throat, through the esophagus, and into the stomach. This enables the doctor to examine gastric and duodenal tissue directly and to take tissue samples for laboratory evaluation to look for helicobacter infection and to rule out cancer.

How is it treated?
Historically, doctors have used three different types of drugs to cure ulcers. Antacids, available over the counter, help neutralize stomach acid. The

other two types are available by prescription only. Histamine$_2$ blocker drugs, such as cimetidine and ranitidine, decrease the production of gastric acid. Sucralfate turns into a thick gel in the stomach, coating the ulcer lesion and protecting it from further attack. All three types of drugs, if taken in the proper doses, can stop ulcer pain and symptoms within days and heal them completely within a few weeks. Unfortunately, recurrences are common. Your doctor may also prescribe antibiotics to eradicate underlying helicobacter infection.

Self-Care: Lifestyle modifications can help heal your ulcers and reduce the risk of recurrence. If you smoke, quit. Limit your intake of alcohol and caffeine. Have just three meals a day, with no snacking that stimulates acid production. A milk-based bland diet, once the mainstay of ulcer therapy, is no longer recommended. Although milk provides temporary relief to symptoms, research has shown that it leads to a rebound effect—an increase in acid secretion within a few hours.

7

Urinary Tract Disorders

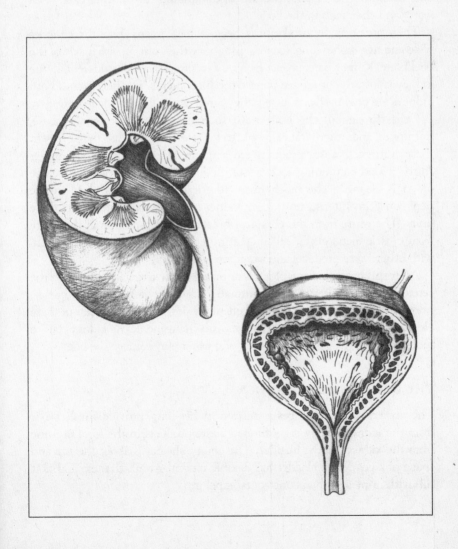

HOW THE URINARY SYSTEM WORKS

The urinary tract plays a vital role in maintaining fluid balance in the body and disposing of liquid waste. It is composed of the **kidneys, ureters, bladder,** and **urethra.** Men have an additional organ, the **prostate,** which wraps around the urethra.

THE KIDNEYS

Kidneys are vital organs that filter and clean the blood, getting rid of toxic elements, retaining important constituents of the blood, and feeding nutrients back into the system. Kidneys also maintain the delicate balance of water and chemicals in the body.

There are normally two kidneys, bean-shaped organs about three inches wide and five inches long, located just above the waist on either side of the backbone. Kidney damage can be a serious matter; but, fortunately, if one kidney is lost, the other can handle the filtering job. Further, even if both kidneys are only partly damaged, they often can still filter adequately.

Cells throughout the body need such nutrients as protein, glucose, hormones, and other vital elements to function. As cells use the energy in these nutrients, waste products are generated. The **renal artery** brings "dirty" blood containing such waste products to each kidney, where the blood is cleaned. The biochemical filtering process takes place in the **nephrons,** tiny filtering units. Each kidney has more than a million of these units. The waste from the chemical breakdown of protein and the waste from muscle metabolism, called creatinine, combine to form urea, which, with other waste products and water, creates urine.

After this process, clean blood is returned to the circulation through the **renal vein.** The filtered blood normally contains vitamins, amino acids, hormones, glucose, and other vital elements. If there is any excess of these elements, the kidneys throw them off into the urine. If the kidneys fail to function properly, excess salt, sugar, and water may damage the body.

THE URETERS AND BLADDER

The **ureters,** muscular tubes about ten inches long, provide another exit from the kidneys. They carry filtered waste products in the form of urine from the kidneys to the **bladder.** The empty bladder is about the size and shape of a pear. The bladder has flexible muscular walls that expand as it fills with urine and then contract to expel it.

The urge to urinate originates in cells in the bladder walls that respond to pressure. Although the bladder can hold about a pint of urine, these cells start signaling you to urinate when the bladder is only half full. A muscular bladder neck sphincter, not under conscious control, normally does not let urine pass out of the bladder until you consciously release a second muscular sphincter at the exit from the urethra.

THE URETHRA AND PROSTATE

When you need to urinate, urine moves out of the bladder into the **urethra,** the tube that carries it out of the body. The urethral sphincter must be released to allow urination to occur.

In women, the urethra is very short, less than two inches. It follows a straight path leading to an opening in the vulva, just in front of the vagina. In men, the urethra is much longer, about ten inches. It follows a curved path leading it behind the scrotum, then up into the penis, to an opening at its tip.

Just beneath the bladder the male urethra is surrounded for about an inch by the **prostate** gland. About the size of a chestnut, the prostate is really part of the male sex organ system. However, it is discussed here because of the pivotal role that prostate abnormalities can have in causing urinary symptoms. The fluid produced by the prostate is part of the seminal fluid that is ejaculated during male orgasm. The prostate can secrete this fluid directly into the urethra, which also serves as the passage for semen during intercourse.

SYMPTOMS AND SOLUTIONS

BLOOD IN THE URINE

Normal urine ranges from straw colored to clear. The medical term for blood in the urine is hematuria. Although you may actually see bright red blood in the urine, blood may be so dissolved that the urine has a pink, smoky, rusty, or brown coloration. Abnormal urine color may be caused by minor lifestyle changes, but blood in the urine can be a sign of very serious and possibly life-threatening illness. It should never be ignored.

Causes and Treatment of Blood in the Urine
Blood in the urine that appears suddenly and without pain is the most common sign of **bladder cancer** (page 220). Fortunately, when found early,

> Blood in the urine is never normal. If you notice any abnormal coloring of your urine that cannot be explained by the lifestyle causes discussed in this section, call your physician right away. Describe what is happening so that the doctor can decide whether you should be seen immediately.

this is one of the most easily treated cancers. Often it can be destroyed using a laser-like instrument inserted through the urethra, without open surgery.

Bloody urine may also signal **kidney cancer** (page 221). Unfortunately, kidney cancer often is not detected until serious damage has already occurred. Surgery to remove the affected kidney is almost always needed, unless the disease has already spread extensively.

Rarely, bloody urine may be a sign of **prostate cancer** (page 225) in men, especially those over the age of 50. Other more common urinary difficulties that may signal prostate cancer include a weak or interrupted urine flow, an increase or decrease in urination, or a painful or burning sensation. However, most men have few, if any, symptoms. Treatment may require surgical removal of the prostate, radiation, or hormone therapy.

Bloody urine does not always mean cancer, but there is no way you can be sure on your own. Therefore, a prompt appointment with your physician is always essential, whether or not you have pain.

If blood in the urine occurs with painful or frequent urination, it may be something as simple as a **urinary tract infection** (page 227) originating in the bladder or kidney. Antibiotics can be prescribed to cure the infection promptly.

If you have pubic, side, or lower back pain together with bloody urine, you may have a **urinary tract stone** (page 228) in your bladder, ureters, or kidney. Although the pain can be excruciating, small stones may pass on their own, or your doctor may be able to remove them during cystoscopy, which involves inserting a thin tube up the urethra. Larger stones in the kidney may need to be crushed with energy waves or surgically removed.

Blood in the urine may also be caused by chronic **nephritis** (page 223). This inflammation may be due to untreated urinary tract infections, urinary tract stones, gout, poisons, or long-term use of certain medications. Chronic nephritis can lead to kidney failure.

Abnormal urine coloration does not always signal serious illness. Eating beets, blackberries, or other red foods or foods containing artificial red dyes can cause a temporary pink to red or brown urine coloration, just as rhubarb or laxatives containing senna may turn it dark yellow to orange, or other foods may turn it green or blue. The abnormal color should disappear within a day.

Similarly, in very hot weather, your urine may become very concentrated and turn dark yellow or orange. This is a signal that you need to increase your fluid intake to at least eight to ten glasses a day.

PAINFUL URINATION

Dysuria, painful urination, is a burning or stinging sensation during urinary flow that may continue for a minute or two after the flow has ended. It normally occurs when chemicals in the urine pass over inflamed or infected tissue.

Painful urination is never normal. If you experience it, call your physician within a day. Describe what is happening so that the doctor can decide whether you should be seen immediately.

Causes and Treatment of Painful Urination

If you have painful urination together with an increased sense of urinary urgency, but have little or no flow when you try to urinate, you probably have cystitis, inflammation of the bladder. Cystitis is most commonly caused by **urinary tract infections** (page 227), which can be cured with antibiotics. Such inflammation is more common in women than men, but men who have **prostate enlargement** (page 226) are also more susceptible to cystitis.

Painful urination that occurs in men who have a thick yellow-green discharge from the penis or in woman who have a bad-smelling vaginal discharge may indicate a sexually transmitted disease such as **gonorrhea** (page 274). Again, see your doctor promptly for antibiotic treatment to prevent the infection from spreading to other parts of the body.

FREQUENT URINATION

The average adult usually urinates about six times a day, discharging about one and a half quarts of urine. However, depending on your lifestyle and fluid intake, you may urinate more or less often. Frequent urination can be described as any increase in your normal pattern of urination.

> If you notice any increase in the number of times you urinate and it cannot be explained by the lifestyle causes discussed in this section, call your physician promptly. Describe what is happening so that the doctor can decide whether you should be seen immediately.

Causes and Treatment of Frequent Urination

A first possibility a doctor often considers with a report of unexplained frequent urination is excessive fluid intake. If you are drinking more coffee, tea, colas, or alcohol, this can have a diuretic effect. Cut back on your consumption. If the problem continues, call your physician.

Anxiety may also cause frequent urination. Try to lower your stress levels and identify and deal with the cause of your anxiety.

Another common cause of frequent urination is **diabetes** (page 244). In type I, juvenile diabetes, the child or young adult may also have increased hunger and thirst. If left untreated, the disease can lead to a coma within a few days. In type II diabetes, which usually begins in middle-aged adults, there may be no further symptoms, or only some weight loss and fatigue may be noticed, and needed prompt medical attention may not be sought. Because pregnant women know that increased urination is common during the first and last trimesters, they may not realize that such frequency may also signal gestational diabetes and thus fail to seek the prompt medical attention necessary to protect their own health and that of their baby.

Although increased urination may also signal a **urinary tract infection** (page 227), greater frequency is not usually the only symptom. Such infections are also likely to cause pain or a burning sensation during urination, as discussed earlier.

In middle-aged and older men, increased urination, especially during the night, most likely signals a prostate problem. Related symptoms include a urine flow that is weak or interrupted, or difficulty in starting or stopping urination. For most men, the problem is simple **prostate enlargement** (page 226), which may be alleviated with medication or minor surgery to widen the pinched urethra. For others, the problem is **prostate cancer** (page 225).

Frequent urination sometimes arises not from the urinary tract but from increased thirst. This may be due to a disease that causes dry mucous membranes in the mouth, such as **lupus** (page 116), or to something as simple as using too much salt. If you cut back on the salt in your diet and your frequent urination still continues, call your doctor for an appointment.

With any unexplained frequent urination, you should see a doctor. If you can't get an appointment within a day or so, you can purchase test strips at your pharmacy that evaluate your urine for glucose, an indicator of diabetes, and nitrites, an indicator of infection. If you have glucose or nitrites in your urine, call your doctor back and ask for an urgent appointment.

DECREASED URINATION

The average adult usually urinates about six times a day, but lifestyle factors and fluid intake can affect the pattern. Therefore, decreased urination can be described as any decrease in your normal pattern of urination.

A less frequent urination pattern usually is not normal. If you notice any decrease in your urinary frequency that cannot be explained by the lifestyle causes discussed in this section, call your physician promptly. Describe what is happening so that the doctor can decide whether you should be seen immediately.

Causes and Treatment of Decreased Urination

If you notice decreased urination together with rapid weight gain of more than two pounds a day, it may be a sign of life-threatening acute **kidney failure** (page 222). Such failure may be caused by a local problem, such as a kidney infection, nephritis, or an obstruction, or it may be due to a major body insult, such as shock, heart attack, or other organ failure that has already put you in the hospital. Treatment of the underlying cause usually resolves the failure.

If decreased urination occurs in a middle-aged or older man, in conjunction with difficulty in urinating or in starting urination, the cause is most likely to be **prostate enlargement** (page 226) or, less commonly, **prostate cancer** (page 225).

In hot weather, if you are sweating profusely and not drinking a sufficient amount of fluid, you may have decreased urine volume. Also, your urine will be slightly darker than usual because it is concentrated. Take this as a warning to increase your fluid intake immediately to at least eight to ten glasses daily.

INCONTINENCE

Urinary incontinence is the inability to control urine flow. It can range from leakage of a few drops on occasion to constant dripping of urine from the urethra, and bedwetting. Urinary incontinence can be a very embarrassing and uncomfortable problem.

> Urinary incontinence is never normal. If you experience persistent incontinence, call your physician for an appointment. Describe what is happening so that the doctor can decide whether you should be seen immediately.

Causes and Treatment of Incontinence

Any urinary tract disorder that causes cystitis, such as **urinary tract infections** (page 227), may cause mild incontinence. Prompt treatment of the underlying problem will restore bladder control.

Although the primary indicators of a urinary tract obstruction, such as **urinary tract stones** (page 228), may be pain and a decrease in urination, the problem may also cause incontinence as urine dribbles out of the urethra before or after urination. After the stone passes or is removed, normal bladder function returns.

Bedwetting in children over age 12 is uncommon. It is believed that affected youngsters either sleep very deeply or lack the hormonal signals that will wake them to urinate. Some may have emotional problems. Try not to stigmatize the child for the problem. Instead, suggest that the youngster avoid drinking fluids for a few hours before bedtime. If the problem persists, or if any other symptoms of urinary tract disorders are present, call your child's pediatrician for an appointment.

Among men with **prostate enlargement** (page 226) and **prostate cancer** (page 225), obstruction of the urethra blocks the normal flow of urine. Then, when the bladder becomes too full, urine may leak out. Removal of urethral obstruction, by pharmaceutical shrinkage of the prostate or surgery, restores normal bladder function.

Some women experience stress incontinence, which is leakage of small amounts of urine when they sneeze, cough, or laugh. This may be more common among women who are obese or postmenopausal or whose bladder support muscles have been weakened by childbirth. You may be able to regain better bladder control by practicing Kegel exercises, tightening and releasing pelvic muscles dozens of times a day. You can learn what muscles are involved by starting and stopping your urinary stream. That gives you the feel of muscle control when you are not urinating. Practice the technique several times a day, when sitting or standing, to build local muscle strength. Tighten and release slowly, starting with 5 or 10 repetitions per session and building to 20 to 30. If this exercise does not help, make an appointment to see your doctor. Some women are helped by estrogen replacement therapy, drugs to enhance bladder muscle strength, or behavioral training. Others may need surgery to restore normal function.

Damage to nerves that participate in bladder control may cause incontinence. For example, in **multiple sclerosis** (page 64), the myelin sheath covering nerves is destroyed. In **diabetes** (page 244) and other illnesses, a condition called neuropathy can interfere with nerve messages. Similarly, those with **Parkinson's disease** (page 68) may lose bladder control. Those who have suffered **brain damage** (page 57) or spinal injuries due to **stroke** (page 71) or accidents may also become incontinent. In the later stages of **Alzheimer's disease** (page 54), the individual may lose bladder control or even awareness of urination.

In disorders that respond to treatment of the overall symptoms, the incontinence may be helped. Sometimes the precise cause of the incontinence can be identified and treated. For example, bladder relaxants can decrease contractions and thus prevent urine leakage. Or drugs that help strengthen muscle contractions at the outlet of the bladder can ensure more complete bladder emptying and help prevent later leakage. Behavioral training or surgery may also be helpful.

FATIGUE, HEADACHES, MUSCLE CRAMPS OR TWITCHES, WEIGHT LOSS

These overall "not feeling well" symptoms can be indicative of a wide variety of conditions, including urinary tract problems.

Fatigue, headaches, muscle cramps or twitches, and weight loss are a cluster of symptoms that usually suggest something seriously wrong with you. If you experience a combination of these symptoms and they are not explained by the lifestyle causes discussed in this section, call your physician right away. Describe what is happening so that the doctor can decide whether you should be seen immediately.

Causes and Treatment of Fatigue, Headaches, Muscle Problems, Weight Loss

Although you might have one or two such symptoms, it would be difficult to generate this cluster simultaneously from lifestyle factors alone. For example, if you are physically out of shape and spend a summer weekend helping a friend move—lugging furniture, sweating, straining your muscles, and getting stressed—you might be tired and have a headache and sore muscles by Sunday night. However, you should feel much better by Monday and pretty much back to normal by Tuesday—and you should not lose weight.

In contrast, the gradual development of this cluster of symptoms may indicate that you are slowly developing **chronic kidney failure** (page 222). This is more likely if you have a history of urinary tract infections, nephritis, or urinary tract stones, or if you have a chronic disease that can damage the kidneys, such as diabetes, hypertension, or lupus. If you have such a problem, you should learn to listen to your body and report any changes to your physician promptly. If not treated with dialysis or transplantation, kidney failure is potentially fatal.

COMMON DISORDERS OF THE URINARY SYSTEM

BLADDER CANCER is any malignancy in the urinary bladder. Bladder cancer occurs more commonly in men than in women, most often between ages 50 and 70.

What are the symptoms?
The most common sign is blood in the urine that appears suddenly and without pain. Depending on the amount of blood present, the color of the urine can vary from smoky or rusty to deep red. The amount of blood is not related to how far the cancer has gone.

How did I get it?
Although the exact cause is unknown, a number of environmental factors seem to be involved in bladder cancer. You are at much greater risk if you smoke or work with certain chemicals, such as aromatic amines used in aniline dyes.

How is it diagnosed?
Urinalysis is performed to seek other possible causes of your symptoms. A special X-ray called an intravenous pyelogram or a kidney or bladder sonogram may be done. Finally, your bladder is examined with a cystoscope, a flexible tube that is inserted through the urethra into the bladder to enable

the doctor to examine it directly. If any suspicious areas or growths are seen, a sample of tissue may be removed through the tube for laboratory examination. This examination, called a biopsy, is the only way of finding out for sure if cancer is present.

How is it treated?
If found early, bladder cancer is one of the most easily treated malignancies. First, surgery may be performed to remove the tumors or, sometimes, they can be destroyed by lasers that reach the bladder through the urethra without any external incision. Follow-up care may require visiting the doctor at intervals to have medications instilled directly in the bladder. This may involve chemotherapy, using drugs to kill abnormal cells, or immunotherapy, using a vaccine to stimulate the body's immune system to kill such cells. If the cancer is more extensive, radiation or chemotherapy or even complete removal of the bladder may be necessary. In some cases, a new exit for urine is created through the lower abdomen, and a bag is attached for urine collection.

Self-Care: If you smoke, quit immediately to reduce your risk of bladder cancer recurrence. If your job requires exposure to chemicals associated with bladder cancer, be sure to use all personal protective equipment available or consider changing jobs.

KIDNEY CANCER is a malignancy in the tissue that makes up the kidney. Most kidney cancers are classified as adenocarcinomas, those that start in the lining of the renal tubules. Less common are fibrosarcomas, which start in the cells of the shell that encloses the kidney, and Wilms' tumor, which occurs in children and involves cells similar to those seen in fetuses. When kidney cancer occurs, it usually affects only one of the two kidneys.

What are the symptoms?
The first symptom may be blood in urine or pain in your side or on one side of your lower back. Less commonly, a smooth, hard lump can be felt at the side of the abdomen. As kidney cancer progresses, you may experience fatigue and appetite and weight loss.

How did I get it?
Although the cause of most types of kidney cancer is unknown, there may be a familial incidence, and it can be associated with some rare disease syndromes. It may also be more common in smokers and in people whose

jobs expose them to trace metals such as cadmium. Wilms' tumor is caused by an inherited genetic defect.

How is it diagnosed?

You will require a complete examination and blood and urine tests. Various types of X-rays will be done, including a CAT scan, which provides cross-sectional views of the diseased kidney and checks on the other one as well. When cancer is diagnosed, other tests such as chest X-rays and bone scans are also performed to determine if the disease has spread to other parts of the body.

How is it treated?

The primary treatment for kidney cancer is surgical removal of the affected kidney, surrounding tissue, and nearby lymph nodes. If the cancer has already metastasized markedly, instead of surgery, chemotherapy may be given to help slow further spread.

> Self-Care: If you work in a job that involves electroplating, alloy making, or welding, take scrupulous care to protect yourself from exposure to cadmium. If you smoke, stop at once.

KIDNEY FAILURE is the cessation of normal kidney function. The organs no longer do their filtering job and fail to remove from the blood toxic wastes that are normally disposed of through the urine. Acute kidney failure comes on suddenly and is a life-threatening medical emergency. Chronic kidney failure usually develops slowly.

What are the symptoms?

In *acute* kidney failure, there is a decrease in urination and sudden weight gain of two or more pounds a day. Swollen puffiness, especially in the face, occurs and upset stomach and nausea develop. As the failure worsens, there is weakness and sleepiness, and the breath has a marked urine odor. In the early stages of *chronic* kidney failure, there may be no noticeable symptoms. As the condition worsens, fatigue, loss of mental alertness, and headaches occur. There may be muscle twitches, cramps, numbness, or pain in the arms or legs. In contrast to the weight gain of acute failure, there is weight loss, as well as loss of appetite, nausea, vomiting, and a bad taste in the mouth. The late symptoms of both acute and chronic conditions include itchy skin, confusion, convulsions, and coma.

How did I get it?
Acute kidney failure may derive from a local problem, including a kidney infection, urinary tract blockage, or obstruction of kidney blood flow. Or it may arise from a major body insult, such as shock due hemorrhaging, injury, or heart attack; failure of other organs in the body; dehydration or heatstroke; poisoning; or extensive burns. Chronic kidney failure may stem from similar problems, as well as from such underlying causes as nephritis, diabetes, atherosclerosis, or hypertension.

How is it diagnosed?
A complete physical examination is necessary, as well as urine and blood tests, X-rays, kidney scans, and, in some cases, kidney biopsy.

How is it treated?
Whatever the cause, dialysis must be performed to remove the buildup of waste products in the blood. During hemodialysis, you are connected to an artificial kidney machine that draws blood from a vein, filters it, and then returns it to the body. A hemodialysis session can take six to eight hours and must be performed several times a week. In acute failure, treatment of the underlying cause usually enables the kidneys to recuperate and return to normal function. In chronic progressive failure, dialysis must continue for life unless you have a kidney transplant.

Self-Care: If you have chronic failure, you must follow a special diet to reduce the workload of the kidney. If hypertension or diabetes is the underlying cause, control of the disorder with lifestyle modifications and drugs may slow the progression of kidney failure. If you require long-term dialysis, you can learn how to perform hemodialysis or peritoneal dialysis at home. Hemodialysis requires a machine for extended treatment, as in the hospital. Peritoneal dialysis involves pouring a special fluid into a catheter implanted in your abdomen several times a day.

NEPHRITIS, also known as pyelonephritis, is inflammation of the filtering units of kidneys, known as nephrons. Acute nephritis develops suddenly and can usually be cured completely with prompt treatment. If it is not cured, it may become chronic and lead to progressive destruction of the kidneys over a period of years.

What are the symptoms?

The most common sign of nephritis is pain in the side or at the sides of the lower back. In acute nephritis, you may experience a frequent, urgent need to urinate, as well as overall symptoms of infection, including chills, fever, nausea, and vomiting. In chronic nephritis, you may notice blood in your urine.

How did I get it?

Acute pyelonephritis usually begins when a urinary tract infection in the bladder travels upward to the kidney. This is more likely to happen in people who have a urinary tract obstruction, such as a stone, enlarged prostate, or local tumor; or in those who are taking drugs that suppress the immune system; or in women who are pregnant. Chronic nephritis may result from untreated infections or other problems that induce kidney inflammation, including kidney stones and other urinary tract obstructions, gout, poisoning, or long-term use of certain medications, such as aspirin and other nonsteroidal anti-inflammatory drugs.

How is it diagnosed?

Nephritis is diagnosed based on a complete examination, urine and blood tests, and X-rays of the kidneys. A special type of sequential X-rays is the intravenous pyelogram. Before it is performed, a contrast dye is injected into a vein to help ensure that all parts of the kidney can be seen clearly.

How is it treated?

If an infection is found, prompt treatment with antibiotics is necessary for at least 10 days and, in stubborn cases, as long as a month. Urine evaluations will be repeated to ensure that the infection has been wiped out. If chronic nephritis is caused by a treatable underlying disorder, its treatment can help relieve nephron inflammation. Corticosteroid drugs may also be prescribed to reduce inflammation. If the chronic nephritis is progressive, you will need a special diet to reduce the workload of the kidney and help slow kidney failure. When such failure occurs, you will require either a kidney transplant or weekly kidney dialysis to cleanse your blood of body wastes.

Self-Care: If you have acute nephritis, see a doctor immediately. In addition to medical therapy, you may be told to use a heating pad to ease pain and to drink at least eight glasses of fluid daily to help flush out the urinary tract. If you have chronic nephritis, ask your doctor how to monitor yourself carefully for any worsening of your condition, so that exacerbations can receive prompt treatment. In either condition, avoid all alcoholic beverages.

PROSTATE CANCER is a malignancy of the prostate gland, the chestnut-sized gland that encircles the urethra. The second most common form of cancer among men, it will afflict about 15 percent of men in their lifetimes. Prostate cancer usually does not strike until after age 40 and is more common among men over 65. Most prostate cancer is localized at the time of diagnosis. When compared with other cancers, the outlook is relatively good, especially when the cancer is detected early.

What are the symptoms?
Most men have no symptoms. When they do occur, the primary signs involve urinary difficulties, such as a weak or interrupted flow of urine, the need to urinate often, especially at night, an inability to urinate or difficulty in starting urination, blood in the urine, a flow that is not easily stopped, or painful or burning urination. Many of these problems are the same as those produced by benign prostate enlargement. In addition, some men with prostate cancer experience pain in the pelvis, lower back, or upper thighs.

How did I get it?
As with most types of cancer, the cause is unknown. However, genetic factors may be involved because the disease is much more common in men whose fathers, brothers, or uncles have had prostate cancer, and it is also more common in certain groups, such as African-Americans. High levels of fat in the diet also may play a role.

How is it diagnosed?
A digital rectal examination will be performed, in which your doctor inserts a gloved finger into your rectum to detect prostate enlargement. You will also have the PSA (prostate-specific antigen) blood test to search for a characteristic protein in the blood. Also, transrectal ultrasound is sometimes used; a probe the size of a fat cigar is inserted into the rectum and generates sound waves to provide images of the prostate. Other blood and urine tests and X-rays may also be performed. If prostate cancer is suspected, a biopsy must be performed.

How is it treated?
Treatment will depend on whether the cancer has spread to other areas, how large it is, and your age and general health. Usually, surgery is performed

to remove the prostate, or radiation therapy is given to render the malignant cells inactive. This may be followed by hormone treatment and/or chemotherapy. In some cases, hormones and chemotherapy, without surgery, may control and even shrink the cancer for long periods. Surgery, radiation, or chemotherapy for prostate cancer sometimes causes impotence, although there are surgical techniques that can spare potency.

Self-Care: All men over age 40 should have an annual digital rectal examination, which can screen them for prostate and colorectal cancer. An annual PSA test should begin at 50 or at 40, especially if other men in your family have had the disease or you are otherwise determined to be at higher risk.

PROSTATE ENLARGEMENT refers to benign enlargement of the walnut-sized gland that wraps around the male urethra. It is also called benign prostatic hyperplasia, benign prostatic hypertrophy, or BPH. Most men experience some degree of enlargement of the prostate after age 50. However, only about 10 percent will have symptoms sufficient to require treatment for the problem.

What are the symptoms?
One of the first symptoms is the need to urinate frequently and often urgently. You may also experience difficulty in starting or stopping the urinary stream and notice a decrease in the flow or caliber of the urinary stream. Symptoms range from mild to severe. Because the same symptoms may indicate a more severe problem, such as prostate cancer, any man who has these problems should see his physician promptly. Prostate enlargement also places you at greater risk for urinary tract infections and kidney problems.

How did I get it?
The cause of prostate gland enlargement is unknown, although it seems to be associated with aging.

How is it diagnosed?
Your description of symptoms plays a pivotal role. Also, the physician can feel an enlarged prostate by inserting a finger into the rectum. All men over age 50 should have such a checkup every year. If an enlargement is suspected, the physician may assess the amount of urine left in your bladder after you have finished urinating. A large amount may be a sign of severe and longstanding obstruction.

How is it treated?
Mild symptoms require no treatment. When symptoms are moderate, your doctor may recommend medication that shrinks the prostate or relaxes the sphincter over a number of months. When symptoms are severe, endoscopic or open surgery is usually required. A common procedure is called transurethral resection of the prostate, or TURP. It involves inserting a small cutting tool into the urethra and then shaving away protruding tissue.

Self-Care: Although many men worry about possible impotence after surgery, less than 1 percent of those who undergo TURP experience the problem. In the aftermath, most men acknowledge that the surgery sounds worse than it is.

URINARY TRACT INFECTIONS, also known as UTI, are those that affect the bladder or the kidneys of both men and women. If left untreated, permanent damage to the tract can occur.

What are the symptoms?
The most common symptom is frequent urination, sometimes even repeatedly during the night. The urge may be sudden and severe. Urination may be accompanied by pain or a burning sensation. If the infection is very severe, only small amounts of urine may pass and it may be bloody. There may also be a fever and achy feelings, especially in the back. Symptoms may last only a few days and then disappear, but the infection is not necessarily cured. Rather, bacteria may be doing permanent damage inside the body.

How did I get it?
UTI usually are caused by bacteria, which enter the body through the urethra—the tube that connects the bladder to the skin surface. Because the female's urethra is much shorter than the male's and because it is located so near the vagina and anus, women are much more susceptible to UTI than men.

How is it diagnosed?
Only a physician can accurately diagnose UTI, based on the results of laboratory testing of your urine. Tests reveal whether or not an infection is present and, if so, what germ is causing it—information essential to prescribing the proper drug for treatment.

How is it treated?

A ten-day course of treatment with antibiotic drugs usually cures UTI. However, if infection is severe, especially if it has been allowed to spread untreated, hospitalization for examinations to determine the cause and extent of the infection, as well as treatment, may be necessary.

Self-Care: If you have or are prone to UTI, drink at least eight glasses of fluid daily to help flush out infectious material. Due to an abnormality in the urethra, the bladder, or the kidneys, some people have repeated infections. Anyone who has recurrent UTI should be evaluated by a urologist.

URINARY TRACT STONES, also called renal calculi, occur in the bladder and kidney and are a fairly common problem, especially for men. The stones are deposits of mineral or organic substances that range in size from tiny pebbles to a "staghorn" stone, which can almost completely fill a kidney. Crystals form in urine when it is too concentrated with uric acid, calcium salts, or other substances. Tiny crystals pass out in the urine and cause no serious problems. However, larger crystals are not passed easily and are called "stones."

What are the symptoms?

"Silent" stones cause no symptoms unless, or until, they have grown sufficiently large. The most common sign is pain that can be excruciating. Bladder stones cause pain in the pubic area. Kidney stones cause pain in the kidney area that radiates across the abdomen and sometimes extends down the pelvis toward the genitals. Urinary frequency may change significantly, either more or less. Sometimes nausea, vomiting, and abdominal distension may be present.

How did I get it?

Most commonly, the cause is unknown. However, an inadequate flow of urine due to minimal fluid intake or excessive perspiration can concentrate the urine and promote stone formation. If your kidneys or bladder are infected, urine flow may be reduced, thus contributing to stone formation. Other disorders, such as gout, metabolic problems of the bowels and kidneys, and prostate enlargement, may also increase your risk.

How is it diagnosed?

To determine the cause of your pain, the doctor will do a complete physical examination, including blood and urine tests and X-rays of your pelvis and urinary tract. In some cases, a cystoscopy may be performed, insertion of a tube through your urethra to examine the bladder directly.

How is it treated?

Some stones are small and pass on their own without treatment. Sometimes the doctor may be able to remove small stones in the bladder or ureters during cystoscopy. Until recently, the only way to remove larger stones was by major surgery. However, a technique called extracorporeal shock wave lithotripsy can now help many people with kidney stones. High-energy waves are aimed at the kidney while you sit in a tub of water. The energy causes the large stone to disintegrate into sand-like grains, which then pass easily out of the body.

Self-Care: If you pass a stone at home, save it so that your doctor can have it analyzed. Knowing the content may provide guidelines for preventing new stone formation. Also, drink at least a quart of fluid daily to ensure an adequate flow of urine. In hot weather or when you sweat a lot, as after exercise, increase your fluid intake.

8

Hormone Disorders

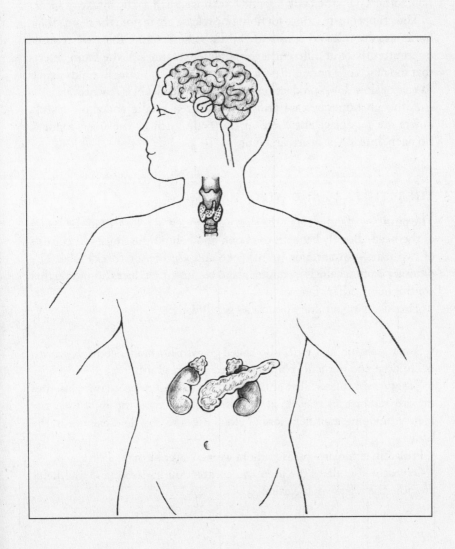

HOW THE ENDOCRINE SYSTEM WORKS

The endocrine system is a network of glands throughout the body. These glands produce **hormones,** special proteins that are secreted directly into the bloodstream and travel throughout the body to affect cell action. Hormones function as chemical messengers that may initiate, speed up, slow down, and turn off such diverse processes as growth, metabolism, and our responses to stress. They often conduct these tasks by interacting with other body substances, such as enzymes and other proteins. Some hormones, for example, those involved in blood pressure, help the body maintain a steady state; others help the body respond to change, such as the intake of sugar.

The primary instructions for hormone release come from the brain. Some hormones are released constantly at the same levels. Others are released intermittently or at different levels at different times. If the brain detects that too much of a hormone is present in the body, it normally sends signals to halt or slow down production until the needed level is reached.

Although hormones are primarily produced by the endocrine glands, others are produced elsewhere in the body, such as the liver, kidneys, stomach, intestines, heart, and lungs.

THE PITUITARY AND HYPOTHALAMUS

The **pituitary gland** is about the size of a peanut and is located in the center of the head, directly beneath the brain and behind the sinuses. It consists of two parts—an anterior (front) lobe and a posterior (back) lobe. The pituitary is often called the master gland because it produces hormones that control many other glands.

The following pituitary hormones act directly:

- Somatotrophic hormone, also called **growth hormone,** controls growth in children and normally plays a reduced role in adulthood.
- **Vasopressin,** also called antidiuretic hormone, induces contraction of smooth muscles in the blood vessels, with a secondary impact on the kidneys, helping maintain normal blood pressure and fluid balance in the body.
- **Prolactin** stimulates breast milk in women after birth.
- **Oxytocin** stimulates the uterus to contract during labor and also helps promote the release of breast milk.

In addition, the pituitary produces the following hormones that stimulate the hormone-producing activity of other glands:

- Thyrotrophic hormone, also called **thyroid-stimulating hormone (TSH),** acts on the thyroid gland.
- **Adrenocorticotrophic hormone (ACTH)** acts on the adrenal glands.
- **Follicle-stimulating hormone (FSH)** and **luteinizing hormone (LH),** also known as the gonadotropins, act on the ovaries in women and the testes in men.

The **hypothalamus** is a cluster of nerve cells at the base of the brain. It is located directly above the pituitary gland, to which it is connected by a stalk of tissue. The hypothalamus conveys messages from the brain to the pituitary and controls the release of hormones manufactured in the anterior lobe of the pituitary, that is, growth hormone, TSH, ACTH, and the gonadotropins. The release of hormones by the pituitary also may be affected by many other influences, including emotions, circadian rhythms, and seasonal changes.

THE THYROID AND PARATHYROIDS

The **thyroid,** a small gland weighing about two-thirds of an ounce, looks like a pink butterfly. It is located in the front of the neck. Its two lobes are linked by a thin strand of tissue and rest on either side of the windpipe.

The most important hormone manufactured by the thyroid is **thyroxine,** which controls the metabolic rate in your body, thus helping control weight. Those with an excess amount of thyroxine tend to be thin, and those with a short supply tend to be heavy. The thyroid also produces **calcitonin,** which plays a role in the metabolism of calcium and bone.

In order to function properly, the thyroid needs an appropriate supply of thyroid-stimulating hormone, produced by the pituitary gland and sent on its way by the hypothalamus; a regular supply of iodine with which to manufacture its main hormone; and enzymes and proteins for hormone synthesis.

When the thyroid is starved for iodine, hormone production may slow down and the gland may grow larger. It adds new cells in a desperate attempt to catch more iodine from the blood. This enlargement of the thyroid gland is called a nontoxic goiter.

Historically, this most common thyroid problem was caused by a diet low in iodine. Such problems are now rare because iodine is added to salt in the United States. However, if you are on a salt-free diet, you may need another source of iodine, such as a significant seafood intake.

The **parathyroid glands** are four pearl-sized glands. One is located at each of the four corners of the thyroid gland. They produce **parathyroid hormone,** which works together with calcitonin to control calcium levels in the body and contribute to strong teeth and bones.

THE THYMUS

The **thymus gland** is located in the upper chest, just behind the breastbone. Its two lobes consist largely of lymphoid tissue. The role of the thymus is not well understood, although it appears to produce hormones that play a role in the development of the immune system in infants and children.

THE ADRENAL GLANDS

The **adrenal glands** are two triangular-shaped glands, each about the size of a grape. They sit on top of the kidneys. Each adrenal has two main parts, the inner medulla and the outer cortex.

The medulla secretes the so-called stress hormones: **adrenaline,** also known as epinephrine; **noradrenaline,** also known as norepinephrine; and **dopamine.** These substances stimulate or calm the nervous system and play a critical role in the fight-or-flight response to stress that enables you to respond quickly to dangerous situations. For example, adrenaline increases heart activity to pump more blood, dilates the bronchi to enable you to take in more air, increases the level of glucose in the blood to provide energy, and quiets the gastrointestinal system. Noradrenaline constricts tiny arteries and veins, thus increasing blood pressure and slowing the heart. Dopamine also increases the heart's output.

Although the adrenal glands respond to directions from the pituitary, they are also highly responsive to the sympathetic nervous system and, therefore, to our emotional condition. When we are in a state of anticipation or stress, noradrenaline and adrenaline are released to prepare us for action.

The cortex of each adrenal uses cholesterol to manufacture its three groups of hormones. These include the following:

• The glucocortoids, such as **cortisol** and **cortisone,** which participate in the body's metabolism of carbohydrates, especially sugar, and act as important anti-inflammatory agents
• The mineralocorticoids, **aldosterone** and **dehydroepiandrosterone,** which participate in the body's metabolism of sodium and potassium
• The male and female sex hormones, **androgens, estrogens,** and **progestins,** which supplement hormones manufactured by the testes and ovaries and play important roles in gender and reproduction

Hormones manufactured by the medulla are also produced elsewhere in the body. However, the cortex is the body's only source of cortisone and aldosterone, which are essential for many body functions.

THE PANCREAS

The **pancreas** is a long, thin gland located horizontally behind the stomach. The pancreas manufactures **insulin** and **glucagon,** two hormones important in the body's ability to regulate its levels of glucose or blood sugar.

When you eat and digest carbohydrates, glucose is released into the blood. In response, the pancreas releases insulin to promote the absorption of glucose by cells throughout the body, providing energy for cell function, and absorption of any excess glucose by the liver for storage. Thus, insulin prevents excessive amounts of glucose in the blood.

In contrast, if your body needs energy and you have not eaten recently, the pancreas releases glucagon to promote the release of glucose by the liver, providing the energy needed.

In addition to hormone production, the pancreas manufactures enzymes important in the digestion of food.

THE GONADS

The gonads, or reproductive glands, are the **testes** in men and the **ovaries** in women. The testes are contained in a sac that hangs outside the body just behind the penis. They secrete **testosterone** and other androgens. The ovaries are located in the lower pelvis, on either side of the uterus, and secrete **estradiol, progesterone,** and **relaxin.** These glands are discussed more fully in Chapter 5.

SYMPTOMS AND SOLUTIONS

INCREASED URINATION

The average adult usually urinates about six times a day, discharging about one and a half quarts of urine. However, depending on your lifestyle and fluid intake, you may urinate more or less often. Frequent urination can be described as any increase in your normal pattern of urination.

If you notice a persistent increase in the number of times you urinate and it cannot be explained by the lifestyle causes discussed in this section, call your physician promptly. Describe what is happening so that the doctor can decide whether you should be seen immediately.

Causes and Treatment of Increased Urination

A first possibility a doctor often considers with a report of unexplained increased urination is **diabetes** (page 244), especially if it occurs in conjunction with unusual thirst, unexplained weight loss, frequent infections, or weakness and fatigue. When these symptoms occur in a child, teenager, or young adult and any drowsiness is noted, emergency medical care may be needed because the person may be headed for a diabetic coma. In middle-aged or older adults who are overweight, medical attention is less urgent, but prompt diagnosis and treatment are needed to help prevent the development of long-term complications such as heart attack, stroke, and kidney failure.

Most causes of increased urination derive from the urinary tract. See Chapter 7 for information on **urinary tract infection** (page 227) and **prostate enlargement** (page 226).

Increased urination sometimes is caused by increased thrist and fluid intake. This may be due to a disease that causes dry mucous membranes in the mouth, such as **lupus** (page 116), or to something as simple as using too much salt. If you cut back on the salt in your diet and frequent urination still continues, call your doctor for an appointment.

Other dietary modifications can also cause frequent urination. If you are drinking more coffee, tea, colas, or alcohol, this can have a diuretic effect. Again, cut back on your consumption. If the problem continues, call your doctor.

Certain medications cause frequent urination. Sometimes ridding your body of excess water is part of your medical treatment. If your doctor has not said that your medication will have such an effect, call and ask for clarification or for an appointment.

UNEXPLAINED WEIGHT CHANGE

Weight is normally determined by the net balance of how much energy you take in as food calories and how much energy you expend in daily activities and exercise. Those trying to lose or gain weight ideally do so by changing this balance. In the absence of such efforts, weight change is considered unexplained until some medical cause is identified.

> If you notice any increase or decrease in your weight without materially changing your food intake or your activity level, call your physician promptly. Describe what is happening, including the amount of weight change, the period of time, as well as any other symptoms, so that the doctor can decide whether you should be seen immediately.

Causes and Treatment of Unexplained Weight Change

Unexplained weight loss in someone who is also urinating more frequently and who has unusual thirst, fatigue, weakness, or frequent infections could signal **diabetes** (page 244). As discussed earlier, this can be a life-threatening emergency for a child, teen, or young adult when drowsiness is present. Prompt medical attention is also needed for adults.

If you experience weight gain together with decreased appetite, you may have **hypothyroidism** (page 250). Other symptoms may include fatigue, achy muscles, constipation, increased sensitivity to cold, dry skin, facial puffiness, and hair loss. Women may develop a heavier than normal menstrual flow. Hypothyroidism is most commonly caused by an autoimmune disorder that responds well to taking daily thyroxine replacement pills. Seek prompt medical care because, if allowed to progress untreated, hypothyroidism can lead to potentially life-threatening coma.

If you experience weight loss together with an increased appetite, you may have the reverse problem, **hyperthyroidism** (page 248). Other symptoms may include irritability, nervousness, increased perspiration, fatigue, insomnia, hair brittleness or loss, frequent and loose bowel movements, and mood swings. Women may have less frequent and lighter than normal menstruation. Hyperthyroidism is most commonly caused by an autoimmune disorder and can be effectively treated to reduce thyroxine production. Seek prompt medical care because, if allowed to progress untreated, hyperthyroidism can lead to a potentially life-threatening thyroid storm—a sudden explosion of symptoms that can lead to fatal cardiovascular collapse.

If unexplained weight gain occurs primarily in your face, causing a rounded appearance, and your trunk, causing a protruding abdomen, and especially if you seem to be developing a hump at the top of your back, you may have **Cushing's syndrome** (page 243). Other symptoms include loss of muscle strength, easy bruising, hair loss on your head and hair growth on your body, as well as mood swings and irritability. If you are taking a steroid medication such as prednisone for some other disorder, the development of Cushing's syndrome indicates that your dose should be reduced gradually and, if possible, eventually replaced with some other drug. If you are not taking such a medication, Cushing's syndrome symptoms may be caused by an endocrine gland tumor, most commonly affecting the pituitary or adrenal gland.

If you notice that your rings and shoes feel tight, whether or not your scale shows significant weight gain, consider whether you have any other symptoms. In some cases, these symptoms could be a sign of **heart failure** (page 21). However, if you have developed increased body hair or sweating, skin darkening, voice deepening, fatigue, headaches, or joint pain, it could be a **growth disorder** (page 246) known as acromegaly. This is more likely if you have hypertension, cardiomyopathy, or congestive heart failure, although the benign tumors that tend to trigger this disorder can arise in otherwise normal individuals. To avoid the development of severe bone overgrowth that can distort your face, hands, and feet, get prompt medical treatment.

GROWTH ABNORMALITIES

Height is normally determined by genetic factors. We tend to be about the same height as our parents, although nutrition also plays a role. Some people are naturally very tall or very short, but even short children should grow steadily, until the adolescent growth spurt. The bodies of both short and tall children should grow in proportion. Other than shape changes due to weight gain and loss, the proportions of our bodies should not change in adulthood.

Causes and Treatment of Growth Abnormalities

If growth in a child seems markedly behind that of other children, or if normal secondary sexual features do not develop around puberty—devel-

If you notice any marked abnormalities in growth in a child or adult as discussed in this section, call your physician promptly. Describe what is happening so that the doctor can decide whether you should be seen immediately.

opment of pubic hair, breasts in girls, and a deeper voice in boys—especially if such signs are accompanied by headaches and fatigue or the development of obesity, it could be a **growth disorder** (page 246) such as pituitary insufficiency. Such children need to take growth hormone replacement during their growing years.

If a child seems to be growing way ahead of peers at a time other than puberty or if growth is disproportionate at any time, causing excessively long legs and arms and possible joint and bone pain, don't assume it is a growth spurt or growing pains. It could be a growth disorder such as gigantism caused by a pituitary gland tumor. Surgery or radiation therapy can usually restore normal growth.

Abnormal growth in adults is not expressed in increased height but rather in the size of the jaw, protrusion of the brow bone, and enlargement of the nose and ears. Even before such changes occur, you may notice that rings and shoes seem tight. Other symptoms of acromegaly, an adult growth disorder, may include increased body hair, darkening of the skin, increased sweating, deepening of the voice, headaches, fatigue, and joint pain. Acromegaly is most likely to begin between the ages of 30 and 50, but the growth happens so slowly that you may not notice it for several years. Again, as in gigantism, surgery or radiation therapy is usually necessary when a pituitary gland tumor is the cause.

WEAKNESS AND FATIGUE

Healthy adults should be able to undertake a normal day of activity without feeling fatigued or weak. Although excessive tiredness can derive from a wide range of disorders, some of the more common ones have to do with the endocrine system.

Causes and Treatment of Weakness and Fatigue
When weakness and fatigue occur in conjunction with dizziness when you get up from a bed or chair, it could be **Addison's disease** (page 242). Another common symptom is the development of a suntanned appearance when you have not been out in the sun. This adrenal gland disorder, once

---

If you experience recurrent or persistent weakness and fatigue, despite eating a balanced diet and getting adequate sleep, call your physician promptly. Describe what is happening so that the doctor can decide whether you should be seen immediately.

---

life threatening, usually can be controlled with hormone replacement therapy.

When weakness and fatigue occur in conjunction with frequent urination, unusual thirst, unexplained weight loss, or frequent infections, it could be **diabetes** (page 244). When diabetes develops in a child, teenager, or young adult and any drowsiness is noted, emergency medical care may be needed. Medical attention for middle-aged or older adults is less urgent, but prompt diagnosis and treatment are important.

When weakness and fatigue occur together with episodes of sweating, shakiness, anxiety, headache, or unusual hunger, you might have **hypoglycemia** (page 249), also known as low blood sugar. This disorder most commonly occurs in people with diabetes who have taken too high a dose of insulin or who have exercised without lowering their insulin dose. However, it also may occur in those who have had too much alcohol or who are taking certain drugs. Whatever the cause, taking some easily digested sugar, such as orange juice or a soft drink, can quickly banish your symptoms. However, if none of these possible causes applies to you, make an appointment with your doctor. Rarely, hypoglycemia can be due to serious hormonal regulatory problems or liver, kidney, or pancreatic disease. However, hypoglycemia is much less common than the popular press would have us believe.

If weakness and fatigue are progressive and arise together with a decreased appetite and continued weight gain, your doctor is likely to suspect **hypothyroidism** (page 250). In most cases, treatment with a daily thyroxine pill replaces the missing hormone with no problems.

If weakness and fatigue occur in an adult who notices that facial appearance appears to be coarsening and that rings or shoes seem to be getting tight, it could be the **growth disorder** (page 246) known as acromegaly, discussed more fully earlier under growth abnormalities.

MOOD CHANGES AND IRRITABILITY

All of us have moody or irritable days now and then, most often when we are under business or social pressure, have not had enough sleep, or have not been eating properly. However, such events should be infrequent and resolve when you deal with the lifestyle cause.

If you experience persistent mood changes and irritability not accounted for by your lifestyle or other issues discussed in this section, call your physician promptly. Describe what is happening so that the doctor can decide whether you should be seen immediately.

Causes and Treatment of Mood Changes and Irritability

Mood changes and irritability can be caused by a wide range of psychological problems, including anxiety, manic depression, psychoses, and other disorders. However, only the *physical* causes of mood changes will be discussed here.

The most common cause of mood changes and irritability in women is **premenstrual syndrome** (page 167) due to the hormonal changes that occur in conjunction with menstruation. If you notice that your moodiness always develops in the week before you menstruate, that's likely to be the case. Many premenstrual problems can be cured, either by lifestyle changes, especially a reduction in salt and caffeine intake, or with medical treatment. Mood changes may also occur during pregnancy, again due to hormonal changes. If moodiness is troublesome, discuss it with your obstetrician at your next visit.

Moodiness and irritability are also common when blood sugar levels rise in poorly controlled or undiagnosed **diabetes** (page 244). If you have been diagnosed with diabetes and have problems with moodiness and irritability, ask your doctor about a home blood glucose monitor and a training program to enable you to monitor your blood glucose levels and make appropriate adjustments in your diet, exercise, and medication regimen on a daily basis.

If mood swings and irritability are accompanied by nervousness, occasional trembling and a rapid heartbeat, increased perspiration, and increased hunger despite continued weight loss, it could be **hyperthyroidism** (page 248). As discussed earlier under unexplained weight change, you need prompt treatment to reduce thyroxine production in your body.

If mood swings and irritability occur in conjunction with unexplained weight gain, especially in the face and abdomen, you may have **Cushing's syndrome** (page 243). If you are taking prednisone or other steroid drug, you probably need to have the dose gradually lowered and, ideally, another drug substituted. If you are not taking such medication, you may have an endocrine gland tumor that requires surgery or radiation treatment.

If your bouts of moodiness are episodic and always occur with such other symptoms as sweating, shakiness, weakness, or trembling, you may think you are having an anxiety attack. However, if you can't identify the source of anxiety every time, it might well be **hypoglycemia** (page 249). As discussed earlier, it most commonly occurs in people with diabetes who have overcontrolled their blood sugar, those who have had too much alcohol, or those taking certain drugs. Taking some easily digested sugar, such as orange juice or a soft drink, should quickly banish your symptoms. If that solves the problem, but none of these possible causes applies to you, make an appointment with your doctor. Hypoglycemia can also be caused by serious hormonal regulatory problems or liver, kidney, or pancreatic disease.

COMMON DISORDERS OF THE ENDOCRINE SYSTEM

ADDISON'S DISEASE is a disorder in which the adrenal glands are destroyed. Because the destruction is usually gradual, it may not be diagnosed until considerable damage has been done. It is also called adrenocortical insufficiency because you no longer have enough of the hormones produced by the adrenal glands. If the disease is not diagnosed and treated promptly, you may be at risk for potentially life-threatening adrenal crisis as a result of even minor illness or injury.

What are the symptoms?
The early symptoms are weakness, fatigue, and a sense of dizziness when you get up from bed or a chair. These problems may be worsened by physical stress. The skin may darken so that you look as if you have a suntan without sun exposure. Black freckles may develop on your face, neck, and shoulders. As the disease progresses, other symptoms may include loss of appetite and weight, decreased tolerance to cold, fainting spells, abnormal heart rhythms, and gastrointestinal problems such as nausea, vomiting, and diarrhea. With adrenal crisis, severe weakness and pain in the lower back, abdomen, or legs may occur, and the kidneys and circulatory system may fail.

How did I get it?
In most people the cause of Addison's disease is unknown, although doctors suspect it is due to an autoimmune attack, in which the body's immune

system attacks the adrenal glands as if they were foreign invaders. About one-third of those afflicted have had their adrenal gland damaged by some underlying disease, such as tuberculosis or cancer, or by certain antifungal drugs or other medications that block the body's manufacture of cortisone.

How is it diagnosed?
A complete physical examination will seek to rule out any other causes of your symptoms. The diagnostic key will be blood and urine tests that show how your body responds to an intravenous injection of corticotropin.

How is it treated?
Addison's disease can be completely controlled with twice-daily doses of hormone replacement in pill form. In the early stages of the disease, this therapy will be instituted immediately. If you are not diagnosed until a crisis occurs, you may need to be hospitalized for initial treatment.

Self-Care: Once on therapy, call your doctor if you notice any return of symptoms, such as orthostatic hypotension or dehydration, that may signal a need for a change in medication dosage. It is essential that you take your hormone replacement medication on a strict schedule. Also carry a card in your wallet that identifies you as having Addison's disease so that you can receive rapid therapy if you are in an accident.

CUSHING'S SYNDROME refers to a cluster of problems seen when your body is exposed to an excess of certain hormones, especially cortisol and cortisone. If not treated, the syndrome can lead to hypertension, osteoporosis, kidney stones, diabetes, and psychiatric problems.

What are the symptoms?
The classic symptom of Cushing's syndrome is a rounded facial appearance called a "moonface." In addition to weight gain in the face, overall weight gain occurs in the absence of increased eating; new fat is particularly distributed in the abdomen and upper back, producing a characteristic hump just below the neck. You also may lose muscle strength, develop skin bruises easily, and notice hair loss on the scalp and hair growth on the body, stretch marks on the abdomen and elsewhere, mood swings and irritability. Women experience menstrual irregularities, and children's growth may cease.

How did I get it?
The most common cause is long-term use of synthetic steroid medications, such as prednisone, to treat autoimmune diseases and other disorders. A tumor in the pituitary or adrenal glands or, less commonly, some other gland also may be responsible for Cushing's syndrome.

How is it diagnosed?
The diagnosis is based on an observation of your symptoms and on blood tests to evaluate your hormone levels.

How is it treated?
When Cushing syndrome is caused by steroid medication, it is ideally treated by gradually reducing and, if possible, eventually discontinuing use of the medication and substituting another form of therapy for the underlying problem. If a benign tumor is causing the hormone excess, surgery to remove it or radiation therapy to shrink it may solve the problem. If an entire gland must be removed, you may thereafter have to take medication to replace hormones normally produced by the gland.

> Self-Care: If you must take steroid medications, follow your doctor's directions carefully. They should be used for as short a time, and in as low a dose, as possible. Never discontinue taking steroids abruptly, because this could lead to life-threatening adrenal failure. You must be tapered off the drug gradually over a period of many weeks or months.

DIABETES is a chronic disease in which the body does not properly convert sugar, starches, and other foods into the energy needed for life. When excess glucose builds up in the blood, it damages structures throughout the body. This can cause retinopathy, which can lead to blindness, and blood vessel damage, which can lead to heart attacks, strokes, kidney failure, and other problems. High maternal blood sugar levels can jeopardize unborn babies. Research has proven that tight control of blood sugar levels can often prevent or delay these complications. The most common types of diabetes are the following:

• *Type I*, also called insulin-dependent or juvenile diabetes, is an autoimmune disease in which the islet cells in the pancreas are destroyed; therefore, you are no longer able to make insulin, a hormone essential for the metabolism of glucose.

• *Type II*, also called non–insulin-dependent or adult-onset diabetes, occurs when not enough insulin is produced to meet the body's needs, or when the cells in your body become resistant to insulin.
• *Gestational diabetes*, which occurs only in pregnant women, is similar to type II but usually disappears after the birth of the child.

What are the symptoms?

Type I may begin with frequent urination, unusual thirst, weight loss, fatigue, weakness, and uncontrollable food cravings. In type II, in addition to these symptoms, you may experience frequent infections of the skin, gums, or urinary tract; drowsiness; pain or cramps in the legs, feet, or fingers; and slow healing of cuts and bruises. Gestational diabetes may begin with increased urination and thirst or may have no early symptoms.

How did I get it?

Diabetes usually runs in families and is believed to have a genetic component. However, some environmental agent, such as a virus for type I or obesity for type II, seems to trigger the inherited predisposition. Type I, the most severe diabetes, usually starts abruptly in children or young adults who are slim. Type II usually begins slowly in people who are overweight and over 40 years of age.

How is it diagnosed?

Diabetes is diagnosed based on blood tests that measure the amount of glucose in the blood in a "fasting" state, when you have had nothing to eat or drink for eight hours, and then after you have taken a glass of sugar water.

How is it treated?

The two mainstays of diabetes treatment are a careful diet to control sugar intake, balanced with adequate exercise to use energy. Many people who have type II can be treated by diet and exercise alone, especially if they lose weight. Others may need oral medication to help their insulin function more effectively. Others may need insulin injections. All people who have type I diabetes require daily insulin injections to survive. Treatment of gestational diabetes depends on blood sugar levels.

Self-Care: People who have diabetes should test their blood sugar levels at home to monitor their blood sugar control and adjust their food-exercise-medication regimens on a daily basis. Tight control can significantly reduce your risk of the life-threatening complications of diabetes. Although you and your family will be taught the basic techniques of diabetes self-care in the immediate postdiagnostic period, that should not be the end of your educational process. People with diabetes, especially children and teenagers, need a lot of emotional support and ongoing education to accept responsibility for their own care. Joining a group for diabetics or sending a child to a diabetes camp can be a valuable step in helping the individual get over self-conscious feelings about the disease and learning self-care among peers.

THE DIABETIC DIET

A diabetic diet is not much different from the healthy diets now recommended to all Americans: get most of your calories from complex carbohydrates such as fresh vegetables, fruits, and whole grains, with lesser reliance on animal foods for protein. Avoid refined sugars, and keep your intake of cholesterol and fat very low to help reduce the risk of heart disease. When diabetes is first diagnosed, consult with a registered dietitian to develop meal plans compatible with your tastes and lifestyle, and learn to follow closely the "exchange lists" developed by the American Diabetes Association. Exchange lists provide simple formulas to ensure that you get an appropriate number of calories and other nutrients each day. Once you get comfortable with your modified style of eating, you will not need to check exchange lists as often when planning your daily meals.

GROWTH DISORDERS usually result from pituitary gland problems. These include excessive growth, called **gigantism** when it occurs in a child or teenager, and acromegaly when it occurs in an adult, or **pituitary insufficiency,** which causes the growth retardation seen in some youngsters. More severe growth abnormalities, such as dwarfism, are caused by genetic abnormalities rather than hormonal problems.

What are the symptoms?
Children should grow fairly steadily, until the adolescent growth spurt. In pituitary insufficiency, the youngster not only lags well behind peers in growth but does not develop the normal secondary sexual features around puberty—development of pubic hair, of breasts in girls, and a deeper voice

in boys. These youngsters also may complain of headaches and fatigue or become chubby in the absence of overeating. In gigantism, growth is accelerated and youngsters have disproportionately long legs and arms. In addition, they may complain of joint and bone pain. In adults, acromegaly begins very gradually. It does not affect height but causes an increase in the size of the jaw, protrusion of the brow bone, and enlargement of nose and ears. The adult may also notice that rings and shoes seem tight, body hair and sweating increase, skin darkens, and the voice deepens. Headaches, fatigue, and joint pain may also be experienced.

How did I get it?
Pituitary insufficiency may be due to a benign tumor in the pituitary gland, or to a serious head injury, a brain infection, or an abnormal swelling of brain blood vessels adjacent to the pituitary. Acromegaly and gigantism are usually caused by benign tumors in the pituitary gland, leading to excess production of growth hormone; less commonly, tumors elsewhere in the body may produce the hormone. Acromegaly is often related to other medical problems, such as hypertension, cardiomyopathy, or congestive heart failure.

How is it diagnosed?
Growth disorders are diagnosed based on a complete physical examination, a review of growth history, blood tests, X-rays, and other imaging studies to evaluate the bones and the pituitary gland itself.

How is it treated?
If a treatable cause for pituitary insufficiency can be identified and treated, no hormonal therapy may be necessary. However, such a cause cannot be found in most cases, and the youngster must take replacements for the missing growth hormone during the growing years. In acromegaly and gigantism, surgery can be performed to remove the tumor or radiation may be given to shrink it. If surgery cannot completely remove the tumor, it may be followed by radiation therapy. After treatment, until the pituitary returns to normal function, a drug called bromocriptine may be prescribed to block excessive growth hormone.

Self-Care: If a child is diagnosed with pituitary insufficiency, make sure the youngster's diet is balanced and offers adequate nutrients, especially protein, iron, and calcium.

HYPERTHYROIDISM or overactive thyroid are the terms used to describe any condition in which too much of the thyroid hormone, thyroxine, is present in the body. One of the most common types is Graves' disease. If you are alert to subtle changes in your body and see your physician promptly, hyperthyroidism can be easily treated. If not treated, it can lead to thyroid storm.

What are the symptoms?
Symptoms depend on the severity of the hormone excess and may include irritability, nervousness, increased perspiration, increased hunger and thirst but continued weight loss, fatigue, insomnia, hair brittleness or loss, rapid heartbeat, trembling, more frequent and loose bowel movements, and mood swings. Women may notice a decrease in their menstrual flow and less frequent menstruation. In Graves' disease, in addition to these symptoms, your eyes may seem larger or bulgy. As the disease progresses, you may experience muscle weakness and, if goiter occurs, a swelling in the lower front of your neck.

How did I get it?
There are many possible causes. Graves' disease, also known as diffuse toxic goiter, is caused by an autoimmune disorder that prompts generalized overactivity of the entire thyroid. Thyroiditis is an inflammation of the thyroid gland. In other types, for unknown reasons, only one or a few of the thyroid nodules become inflamed. Hyperthyroidism also may be caused by overtreatment of hypothyroidism—taking too much thyroid hormone.

How is it diagnosed?
Blood tests can determine whether you have too much thyroxine in your body and whether the problem derives from abnormal activity of the thyroid gland itself or from oversecretion of thyroid-stimulating hormone (TSH) by the pituitary gland. A thyroid scan can help differentiate the underlying cause.

How is it treated?
Several therapies are available. Treatment is based on your age, physical condition, and the cause and severity of the problem. Most commonly, beta blocker medications such as propranolol are prescribed first to lower your irritation and palpitations within hours. However, these drugs just alleviate the major symptoms and don't get at the underlying problem. For Graves' disease, radioactive iodine therapy will most commonly be prescribed. A

capsule or liquid containing radioactive iodine is swallowed, and because the thyroid needs iodine to make hormones, it absorbs the substance. Over the next few weeks, the radioactive material damages some thyroid cells and then is eliminated from the body. The damage causes the cells to shrink, reducing thyroid hormone production. Usually only one dose is necessary. However, because this treatment can't be precise, your thyroid levels will continue to be monitored for the rest of your life. Sometimes a second dose is needed. In other cases, too much tissue has been destroyed and you need thyroid hormone replacement. Children, pregnant women, and others with special problems may be unable to take radioactive iodine therapy. In these cases, antithyroid drugs may be given, or all or part of the thyroid may be surgically removed.

Self-Care: Even after treatment, you should have regular medical checkups. Subtle feelings of illness may signal a problem. Changes in your lifestyle or other factors may require modification of your medication schedule.

HYPOGLYCEMIA means low blood sugar. It is a condition in which there is an abnormally low percentage of glucose (a form of sugar) in your blood. The most common type is reactive hypoglycemia, which causes symptoms several hours after eating a high-carbohydrate meal. Such a meal contains large amounts of sugars and starches (such as fruits, cereals, breads, beans, potato, and rice), which the body converts to glucose. Less common is spontaneous, or fasting, hypoglycemia, which causes symptoms in the middle of the night or in the early morning hours before breakfast.

What are the symptoms?
Hypoglycemia is often accompanied by sweating, shakiness, weakness, trembling, anxiety, fast heart action, headache, hunger, nervousness, and irritability. More severe hypoglycemia may cause fainting, confusion, headache, and personality changes. However, the majority of people with these symptoms—many of which can simply be caused by anxiety—do not have hypoglycemia.

How did I get it?
Most commonly, hypoglycemia occurs in people with diabetes who have taken too high a dose of insulin or who have exercised without lowering their insulin dose. Occasional low blood sugar levels may also be due to drinking too much alcohol. Or the problem may be caused by certain drugs,

such as potent tranquilizers. Persistent reactive hypoglycemia in the absence of such conditions may signal that your body reacts to a high-carbohydrate load by producing too much insulin to metabolize the glucose, leading to an abnormally low glucose level. Or other hormonal regulatory systems in your body may be malfunctioning. Persistent fasting hypoglycemia may signal the presence of serious underlying liver, kidney, or pancreatic disease.

How is it diagnosed?
People with diabetes can check their blood sugar levels at home with a simple finger prick device. For others, a complete physical examination and a variety of blood tests are needed to determine whether hypoglycemia is present and to determine its cause.

How is it treated?
Diabetics can treat themselves by taking a source of easily digested sugar, such as orange juice or a soft drink. For those with reactive hypoglycemia, treatment normally is necessary only when symptoms occur on a daily basis. Usually, this only involves a change of diet: decreasing the amount of sugars and starches in any one meal to control the rise in blood sugar that leads to the rebound to low blood sugar. Rarely is medication needed. Fasting hypoglycemia is a more serious condition. If your physician diagnoses this type, you probably will need extensive medical testing, usually at a hospital. Treatment depends on the particular cause that is found.

> Self-Care: If you are diabetic, careful monitoring of your blood sugar levels and appropriate modification of your diet-exercise-medication regimen should be able to prevent hypoglycemia. If you have reactive hypoglycemia, try to lower your stress levels, which may contribute to the problem.

HYPOTHYROIDISM, myxedema, or thyroid deficiency are the terms used to describe any condition in which too little of the thyroid hormone thyroxine is present in the body. If you are alert to subtle changes in your body and see your physician promptly, hypothyroidism can be easily treated. If not treated, it can lead to myxedema coma, in which your body temperature drops markedly, your breathing is depressed, circulation to the brain is impaired, and you lose consciousness.

What are the symptoms?
Symptoms depend on the severity of the hormone excess and may include progressive fatigue and lethargy, achy muscles, constipation, increased

sensitivity to cold, decreased appetite but continued weight gain, dry skin, facial puffiness, and hair loss. Women may notice that their menstrual flow become heavier. As the disease progresses, you may experience decreased sex drive, deepened voice, impaired reflexes, numbness or tingling in your feet and hands, and psychological problems.

How did I get it?

There are many possible causes. The most common type is due to Hashimoto's thyroiditis, caused by an autoimmune disorder that leads to inflammation of the thyroid gland. It may also be caused by congenital problems, pituitary disorders, or iodine deficiency, although the latter is rare in the United States because iodine is added to most table salt. In addition, hypothyroidism may also be caused by overtreatment of hyperthyroidism.

How is it diagnosed?

Blood tests can determine whether you have too little thyroxine in your body and seek to identify the source of the problem. If no underlying disorder is identified, Hashimoto's thyroiditis will be diagnosed.

How is it treated?

Treatment usually relies on your taking daily a pill containing synthetic thyroxine. Unless a treatable underlying cause is found and corrected, you will need to take the medication for the rest of your life.

Self-Care: Even after treatment, you should have regular medical checkups. Subtle feelings of illness may signal a problem. Changes in your lifestyle or other factors may require modification of your medication schedule.

9

Infectious Diseases and Immune System Disorders

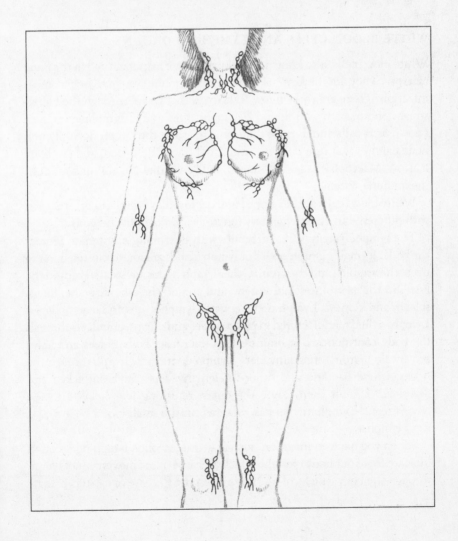

HOW THE IMMUNE SYSTEM WORKS

The immune system is a network of organs, tissues, and cells whose primary function is to defend the body from foreign invaders, such as bacteria, viruses, and parasites. Immune system malfunction can trigger a wide range of problems. If your body can't defend itself properly, you are at greater risk for many illnesses, ranging from the common cold to cancer.

The immune system works primarily by recognizing any part of the body as "self" and protecting it from anything it recognizes as "nonself." Any substance that normally triggers the immune system to start defensive action is called an **antigen.**

WHITE BLOOD CELLS AND LYMPHOID ORGANS

White blood cells, also known as **leukocytes,** are manufactured in the **bone marrow.** They are the key "soldiers" in the immune system to help combat infection. There are three types: leukocytes that travel through the blood-stream on constant patrol; and **B-lymphocytes** and **T-lymphocytes,** also known as B-cells and T-cells, that stand guard in the lymph nodes, lymph node patches that line the gastrointestinal tract, the spleen, and the bone marrow. **Macrophages** are scavenger blood cells that are also important in the immune system.

White blood cells are developed and deployed by lymphoid organs, each with different but complementary functions, throughout the body.

The **lymph system** works integrally with the immune system to protect the body. Its major **lymph nodes** or lymph glands are found clustered in the neck, the armpits, and the groin. Other lymph nodes are located behind the knee, in the gastrointestinal system, and around the elbows, spine, lungs, spleen, and kidneys. Lymph nodes contain lymphocytes and macrophages. **Lymph,** a fluid manufactured in many tissues and organs, circulates through the body continuously. It drains excess fluid from body tissues and helps protect them from foreign invaders. **Lymph ducts** carry lymph through the nodes, where bacteria and other foreign invaders can be attacked and destroyed. Lymph then leaves the ducts, returning lymphocytes to the bloodstream. **Lymphatic vessels,** channels in the small blood vessels, also carry lymph.

When you have an infection, such as a virus, swollen lymph nodes often indicate that your body is on the attack. Because of the movement of lymph through the body, the local nodes are often the first site of cancer spread.

The **thymus,** an endocrine gland (discussed more fully in Chapter 8), also plays an important part in the immune system. Stem cells from bone marrow migrate to the thymus to mature into T-lymphocytes.

DESTROYING INVADERS

Any foreign protein that enters the body, such as a bacterium, virus, or parasite, is called an **antigen.** When antigens reach the lymph nodes, they are filtered and removed from the bloodstream. In addition, lymphocytes travel in the bloodstream, patrolling for antigens throughout the body. B-cells secrete **antibodies** that attach to antigens, either neutralizing them or making them easier for the macrophages to eat and destroy. Killer T-cells destroy antigens, including tumor cells and other cells infected with viruses.

Some T-cells enhance or retard B-cell activity. For example, helper T-cells suppress antibody production when the attack has been completed. Suppressor T-cells suppress killer and helper T-cells, depending on whether the system has to be moved into higher or lower gear.

IMMUNIZATION

One of the immune system's most remarkable features is its memory. Once it has conducted a successful attack against an invader, such as the virus that causes measles, memory T-cells remember the features of that antigen. Thus, the body can respond more quickly to a second attack, often preventing a second infection with that illness and providing us with immunity.

This principle underlies the use of vaccination to prevent serious diseases. A vaccine is made from an inactivated or dead invader, such as a virus, that still retains sufficient viral features to enable the immune system to recognize it and mount an attack with lymphocytes that remember the antigen. After vaccination with polio vaccine, for example, your immune system is ready to quickly spot and destroy the real virus if you ever come in contact with it again. Other vaccines can be given that are capable of inducing immunity to toxins, such as tetanus, or to bacteria, such as pertussis, which causes whooping cough. Most vaccines provide lifetime immunization, although some require booster shots.

Such immunization works well with organisms that remain relatively stable over the course of years. Unfortunately, some viruses are constantly mutating or changing themselves slightly. A change in the properties of the protein that forms the viral coat or outer shell of the virus causes these variations. Such variations are common, for example, in the several viruses that cause influenza, commonly known as the flu. Therefore, scientists evaluate new strains of the virus every year and prepare new vaccines based on their projections of likely changes. To be immunized against influenza, you probably should have a new injection every fall, although viruses may make repeat appearances. Further, scientific forecasts of viral mutation may not necessarily yield protection against the actual virus that turns up that winter.

Another problem comes with disorders caused by many rather than one or a few viruses. The common cold, for example, may be caused by one of nearly 200 viruses, all of which mutate regularly. So far, scientists have been unable to develop a vaccine that will protect us from all of these changing viruses.

IMMUNE SYSTEM MALFUNCTION

If the immune system is deficient in one or more of its parts, you are more susceptible to disease. This condition can be inherited or can occur through exposure to environmental factors that destroy part of the immune system. For example, people with AIDS (acquired immune deficiency syndrome) have low levels of helper T-cells, putting them at greater risk of infections and cancer. A far less threatening example is allergy; hay fever and other common allergic reactions occur when the immune system responds to a false alarm, overreacting to a harmless substance like pollen.

In some people, the immune system runs amok and loses the ability to distinguish self from nonself. The result may be an autoimmune disease, in which the system attacks and destroys healthy body tissue as if it were composed of foreign antigens. Such disorders include rheumatoid arthritis, systemic lupus erythematosus, scleroderma, a type of hypothyroidism known as Hashimoto's thyroiditis, a type of hyperthyroidism known as Graves' disease, Addison's disease, the type of diabetes that most commonly starts in children and young adults, and myasthenia gravis.

The immune system can also cause trouble after organ transplantation. Although lives can be saved by the transplant of a new heart or kidney, the immune system may see the new organ as foreign and tries to reject it. Drugs given to transplant patients seek to suppress parts of the immune system in order to protect the new organ while not impairing the system's ability to protect us from foreign invaders. This is a delicate balance that is hard to achieve. A similar approach is taken in the treatment of people with autoimmune diseases.

FOCUS ON INFECTIOUS DISEASES

Because most autoimmune diseases and allergic reactions affect a particular body system, they are discussed in this book under the system affected. The balance of this chapter will deal almost exclusively with the most common infectious diseases, many of which the immune system finds it difficult to battle alone without medical help. Many of these diseases are contagious or infectious: their causative organism—whether a bacterium, virus, or other agent—is passed from one person to another or by some other physical contact. One disorder, chronic fatigue syndrome, is neither contagious nor infectious based on current scientific knowledge; it is a mysterious and debilitating disease whose cause is unknown. However, it is discussed here because its occurrence represents a failure of the immune system to protect the body.

SYMPTOMS AND SOLUTIONS

NASAL CONGESTION, SNEEZING, COUGHING

Nasal congestion, sneezing, and coughing are very common symptoms, usually caused by such self-limiting illnesses as the cold or flu that can easily be treated at home.

If you have any persistent nasal congestion, sneezing, or coughing that does not seem like the self-limiting illnesses discussed in this section, or that does not respond to the self-care measures discussed, call your physician. Describe what is happening so that the doctor can decide whether you should be seen immediately.

Causes and Treatment of Nasal Congestion, Sneezing, Coughing

A runny or stuffy nose, sneezing, and coughing most commonly signal the start of a **cold** (page 270). Cold symptoms tend to come on slowly and may also include a sore throat. If there's fever, it's usually low. Headache, if present, is mild. Colds tend to last seven to ten days.

The same nasal and throat symptoms may also signal **influenza** (page 280), commonly called the flu, although nasal congestion and sneezing tend to be less severe than in colds. Instead, headache, muscle aches, a dry cough, fatigue, and high fever are more likely. Fever may be absent in elderly people and particularly high in children. The flu starts abruptly, with severe symptoms lasting only three to five days, although feelings of weakness and fatigue may last for weeks.

Both of these upper respiratory infections are caused by viruses. When you become ill, get plenty of rest, drink lots of fluids, and take medications that are recommended by your physician for relief of symptoms. Use decongestants only as directed. If your symptoms seem worse than what is common with these illnesses, or last longer, call your doctor.

In a youngster or even an adult who has not been fully immunized, flu-like symptoms may signal one of the **vanishing childhood diseases** (page 264), such as diphtheria, mumps, polio, or whooping cough. Get a prompt diagnosis because some of these problems can be life threatening.

Nasal congestion, sneezing, and coughing also can signal **allergic rhinitis** (page 84) triggered by hay fever or some other type of allergy. The big difference from a cold or the flu is that you also are likely to experience itchiness in your nose or eyes and probably have no fever. If taking over-the-counter antihistamines and avoiding exposure to the offending allergens do not sufficiently alleviate symptoms, you may need to see an allergist.

If nasal congestion is accompanied by a severe headache or aching on one or both sides of your nose, you may have **sinusitis** (page 96). It may be caused by an underlying bacterial infection requiring antibiotics, so call your doctor.

A possible cause of coughing is **tuberculosis** (page 288). TB has increased dramatically in the United States in recent years. Particularly suspect TB if your cough produces a foul-smelling or a rust-colored sputum and if it is accompanied by fever, shortness of breath, or chest pain when you take a deep breath. You also may experience unusual fatigue, weakness, appetite loss, and unexplained weight loss. If you have any such symptoms, see your doctor right away for TB testing. If treated early in the course of infection, TB is more likely to be cured with antibiotics.

Coughing in the absence of nasal congestion and sneezing may also be caused by a variety of noninfectious lung disorders (see Chapter 3). These include asthma, bronchitis, emphysema, lung cancer, and pneumonia.

HEADACHE, FEVER, FATIGUE, MUSCLE OR JOINT SORENESS

Headache, fever, fatigue, and muscle or joint soreness are often referred to as "flu-like" symptoms, although they can occur without the presence of the other hallmarks of influenza described earlier. Fever, even if mild, is the indicator that some infectious process is underway and that you are not just overtired.

If you have persistent headache, fatigue, and muscle or joint soreness
with fever, even if all the symptoms or just the fever comes and goes,
call your physician. Describe what is happening so that the doctor can
decide whether you should be seen immediately.

Causes and Treatment of Headache, Fever, Fatigue, Muscle or Joint Soreness

This cluster of symptoms in conjunction with a sore throat, chills, and
swollen glands may signal **mononucleosis** (page 283), caused by Epstein-
Barr virus. You may also feel weak and have a poor appetite and swollen
glands. If your doctor confirms that you have mono, stay in bed and take
care of yourself until symptoms pass. Call your doctor again if discomfort
persists for more than a week or other symptoms occur that may indicate a
secondary infection or complications.

Mild and transient symptoms similar to those of mononucleosis may be
one of the first signs of infection with the human immunodeficiency virus
(HIV) that causes **AIDS** (page 265). Such symptoms may occur within a
few weeks of infection, even before blood tests can detect antibodies, but
may quickly vanish. Mono-type symptoms may not recur, or may arise as
long as ten years later, together with other problems that can signal
full-blown AIDS. Such symptoms may include night sweats, swollen lymph
glands, unexplained weight loss, diarrhea, and frequent infections. If you
suspect you may have been exposed to HIV, get tested promptly.

Headache, fever, fatigue, and muscle or joint soreness may be the first
signs of **Lyme disease** (page 282) if you live in an area where the causative
ticks are known to flourish. About half of all victims develop a rash that
expands to look like a red ring, clear in the center, that disappears within a
few weeks. Seek diagnosis and treatment before more severe arthritic,
neurological, or cardiac complications occur.

Headache, fever, fatigue, and muscle or joint soreness also may signal
hepatitis (page 276), a liver inflammation, especially if you have darker than
normal urine and lighter than normal stools. If symptoms are severe, you
may require treatment with steroid or other immunosuppressive drugs.

If these symptoms occur in conjunction with projectile vomiting and you
have a stiff neck, especially if you recently have had some other viral illness,
you may have **encephalitis** (page 271), a brain inflammation. Mild cases
may require only bed rest and self-care. Severe cases merit hospitalization
and supportive care to help prevent permanent neurological damage.

Severe fatigue, muscle or joint pain, and intermittent low fevers that tend to occur in the evening, with or without headache, may also signal **systemic lupus erythematosus** (page 116), an autoimmune disease related to rheumatoid arthritis. Symptoms may come and go over days or weeks. Other symptoms may include hair loss, increased thirst, mouth sores, depression, and a facial rash that can range from a mild blush or scaliness to severe redness and blistering in a butterfly pattern on either side of the nose. Although lupus can't be cured, a rheumatologist can prescribe medication to ease symptoms.

Particularly devastating exhaustion may signal **chronic fatigue syndrome** (page 269), a mysterious illness that also causes swollen lymph nodes, sore throat, sleep problems, and lapses of memory and reasoning. You need comprehensive testing to rule out all other possible causes of these symptoms before a diagnosis is made.

If your headache is just above your eyes, and especially if it occurs in conjunction with aching pain on both sides of your nose, you may have a sinus infection. Call your doctor promptly. If a sinus infection is treated early, it can usually be controlled, avoiding the development of chronic **sinusitis** (page 96).

If headache, fever, and pain and stiffness, especially of the jaw, and muscle spasms occur within a few weeks after any skin-penetrating injury, such as a puncture wound or burn, suspect **tetanus** (page 284). Immediate hospitalization and early treatment in an intensive care unit are essential for survival.

If sudden high fever and muscle aches occur in a menstruating woman, together with vomiting, diarrhea, and weakness, it could be **toxic shock syndrome** (page 286). Again, medical care is urgent. If you can't reach your doctor right away, go to a hospital emergency room.

SORE THROAT

Because sore throats are a common complaint, often accompanying a cold, flu, or other viral infection, you may overlook the fact that certain kinds of sore throats can be warnings of more serious illness.

Causes and Treatment of Sore Throat

Many sore throats are just due to local irritation, such as talking too much or smoking or air pollution. They are mild and will disappear in a few days with simple treatment, such as avoiding the irritant and gargling with warm salt water every few hours.

However, streptococcus bacteria often cause a severe sore throat, or strep throat as it is more commonly called. Because untreated strep can lead to **rheumatic heart disease** (page 34), prompt diagnosis and treatment with penicillin are essential. Call your doctor to arrange for a throat culture immediately. To take a throat culture, the doctor uses a cotton-tipped applicator to collect mucus from the throat. The mucus is combined with a growth medium and later examined to identify the causative organism.

If you have any sore throat not associated with a cold or flu or other illness discussed earlier under nasal congestion or headache and fever, or not attributable to local irritation and easily remedied as discussed in this section, call your physician. Describe what is happening so that the doctor can decide whether you should be seen immediately.

VOMITING

Vomiting is never normal. Although a single episode may occur due to mild stomach upset, and recurrent vomiting most commonly occurs in digestive disorders (see Chapter 6), it can also indicate infectious disease.

Causes and Treatment of Vomiting

If a single episode of vomiting occurs after excessive consumption of alcohol or rich food, or in conjunction with signs of indigestion, you are probably paying the price of dietary excess. Drink only small amounts of clear liquids and go to bed until you feel better, usually by the next morning.

If persistent vomiting occurs in conjunction with abdominal cramps and diarrhea within a few hours of eating, you might have **food poisoning** (page 272). Don't try to stop the vomiting with over-the-counter medications because your body must rid itself of the toxins. Call your doctor if symptoms become severe or don't abate within a few hours, if fever or abdominal swelling occurs, or if blood appears in the vomitus or diarrhea.

If projectile vomiting occurs in conjunction with headache, fever, fatigue, and a stiff neck, especially if you recently have had some other viral illness, you may have **encephalitis** (page 271), a brain inflammation. Mild cases may require only bed rest and self-care. But keep in touch with your doctor because severe cases merit hospitalization and supportive care to help prevent permanent neurological damage.

Vomiting also may be caused by a variety of noninfectious digestive disorders (see Chapter 6).

If you have vomiting together with abdominal cramps, diarrhea, dry mouth, fatigue, dizziness, difficulty in speaking or swallowing, blurred vision, weakness, drooping eyelids, difficulty in breathing, or any cluster of these symptoms, you could have a type of **food poisoning** (page 272) known as botulism. If the vomiting is accompanied by a high fever, diarrhea, muscle aches, weakness, decreased urination, or dizziness, and especially if a sunburn-like rash develops on your palms and soles, you could have **toxic shock syndrome** (page 286). In either case, you need emergency medical care.

• Call your doctor for instructions. Make it clear to whoever answers the doctor's phone that **this is an emergency.**
• If you can't reach your doctor immediately, call an ambulance. Again, make it clear that **this is an emergency.**
• If you can get to a hospital emergency room faster by car and have someone to drive you, do so.
• Take nothing to eat or drink.
• Take no medication unless it was previously prescribed and is urgently needed or you are told to do so by your physician or emergency medical personnel.

Most cases of vomiting are far less severe. However, if you have any persistent vomiting, especially if accompanied by other signs of illness, call your physician. Describe what is happening so that the doctor can decide whether you should be seen immediately.

BODY SORES, RASHES, OR ITCHING

Sores, rashes, and itching can occur anywhere on your body, from head to toe. When they occur in conjunction with other symptoms, they may signal an infectious disease.

Causes and Treatment of Body Sores, Rashes, or Itching
When unexplained rashes occur in a child in conjunction with fever, especially if the youngster has not been completely immunized, suspect one of the childhood infectious diseases (page 264) and call your doctor for advice. Although the illness may only be mild, some can be life threatening.

If you develop a rash that expands to look like a red ring, clear in the

> If you have any persistent sores, rashes, or itching, particularly if they occur in the presence of another symptom, call your physician. Describe what is happening so that the doctor can decide whether you should be seen immediately.

center, and you live in an area where ticks are known to flourish, suspect **Lyme disease** (page 282). Although the rash may disappear within a few weeks, you also may develop headache, fever, fatigue, and muscle or joint soreness. Seek diagnosis and treatment before more severe arthritic, neurological, or cardiac complications occur.

Development of an itchy scalp most commonly signals **seborrhea** (page 348), the mildest form of which is dandruff. But if you don't see any overt flakes, look closer. If you see tiny, silvery clumps attached to the hair shaft near the roots, you've probably got a **head lice** (page 275) infection. Immediate self-care, including checking other family members, is needed to banish the lice.

Development of one or a few painful, itchy, blistery sores on or near your mouth is probably **herpes type 1** (page 278). Try not to touch the sore and avoid touching your eyes. If the virus spreads to your eyes, you need immediate treatment to help prevent vision damage.

Development of similar sores around your genitals may signal **herpes type 2** (page 279), a potentially more serious infection that is transmitted sexually. Viral medication can help prevent recurrences and shorten attacks. If you've had oral sex, the blisters can occur around your mouth and mimic herpes type 1. A laboratory examination is needed to tell for sure which type it is.

If you develop a painless red sore that looks like a pimple anywhere around your genitals, pay attention. It could be **syphilis** (page 284), one of the most common sexually transmitted diseases. Although the sore, called a chancre, will soon disappear, the infectious organism is still spreading in your body. Within a few weeks or months, you will develop swollen lymph glands, headaches, fever, and a rash that may spread all over your body or appear only on your palms and soles. If treated with antibiotics in either of these stages, syphilis can usually be cured. If left untreated, irreversible damage to the heart and nervous system, and even death, may occur.

If itching occurs around the vagina or penis and arises in conjunction with any discharge, it may be **gonorrhea** (page 274) or **chlamydia** (page

268). Again, a laboratory examination is required. A course of treatment with antibiotics will be prescribed.

Body sores, rashes, or itching may also be caused by a variety of skin disorders (see Chapter 11).

IMMUNIZATION AND VANISHING CHILDHOOD DISEASES

Chickenpox, diphtheria, measles, mumps, polio, rubella (German measles), and whooping cough (pertussis) were once very common diseases in childhood. All are highly contagious and often occurred in local epidemics. Whereas some can be relatively mild disorders, others can be very serious and even fatal.

Except for chickenpox, *no child should ever have to suffer the threat of any of these diseases because vaccines are now available to prevent them.* (A vaccine for chickenpox is expected to be available in a few years.) Protection against these diseases should begin in infancy and involve a series of vaccinations in childhood. Ask about the schedule at your first well-baby appointment, optimally soon after your baby is born.

If your child develops a fever and a rash, but has received a full course of immunizations, it could be **chickenpox.** The rash starts out looking like lots of little mosquito bites and, within 24 hours, turns into clear blisters that break open and scab several days later. If the rash does not fit this description, and your child has not been adequately immunized, it could be **measles** or **rubella.** Any fever and rash should prompt an immediate visit to a pediatrician to ensure proper diagnosis. If chickenpox is diagnosed, antibiotics won't help because it is caused by a virus. All your child needs is acetaminophen to ease the fever and headache and calamine lotion to alleviate the rash. It also may be wise to trim the youngster's fingernails to prevent scratching, which can spread the infection and cause permanent scars. Get in touch with your doctor if any other symptoms arise, because your youngster's weakened resistance raises the risk of complications such as impetigo and pneumonia.

Other childhood diseases may start out looking like a cold or the flu, but they can be deadly. **Diphtheria** symptoms include nausea, vomiting, chills, and swollen lymph glands in the neck, underarms, and groin. **Mumps** leads to swollen glands in the neck and difficulty in swallowing; high fevers can cause seizures, and other complications may require hospitalization. **Whooping cough** leads to severe, repeated coughing attacks that end with a gasping intake of breath that produces a "whoop"; **pneumonia** is a common complication and is frequently fatal. **Polio** also causes nausea and vomiting and a stiff neck and back and can result in permanent paralysis. Call your doctor immediately if you suspect any of these illnesses.

Never give aspirin to a child if there is any possibility of chickenpox or other viral disease, such as influenza. Aspirin in these situations is associated with the subsequent development of **Reye's syndrome,** a rare but life-threatening condition that can damage the brain, liver, pancreas, heart, kidney, and spleen. Call your doctor immediately if, within a week or so after recovering from a virus, your child develops nausea, vomiting, disorientation, agitation, or seizures. If you can't reach your doctor, take your child to an emergency room and explain the sequence of events. To prevent this risk, stick to acetaminophen— not aspirin—to treat children's headaches and other discomforts.

COMMON INFECTIOUS DISEASES

AIDS is the acronym for acquired immune deficiency syndrome. "Acquired" means that you catch it from someone else and distinguishes it from disorders that arise spontaneously from within the body. It is called an "immune deficiency" because the body's natural defenses against disease are destroyed, so that even minor illnesses, such as fungal infections, can be life threatening. "Syndrome" refers to the wide range of illnesses that may afflict people with AIDS. Two of the worst ones are a rare type of pneumonia, known as *Pneumocystis carinii* pneumonia, and Kaposi's sarcoma, a form of cancer that usually involves the skin, but may affect internal organs as well. Although new treatments are under development, virtually all AIDS victims eventually die of the illness; however, with new treatments, they may live considerably longer than was the norm several years ago.

What are the symptoms?
Most people who are infected with the virus that causes AIDS notice no symptoms for a long time after infection. However, some newly infected people briefly develop a mild illness similar to mononucleosis. Symptoms include fever, swollen glands, fatigue, and possibly, a rash. Even if these symptoms occur, they usually disappear in a few weeks. From one to ten years—or sometimes even longer—after the original infection occurs,

symptoms of AIDS may begin to develop: night sweats, swollen lymph glands, unexplained weight loss, diarrhea, lethargy, headaches, intermittent fevers, frequent infections. *Pneumocystis carinii* pneumonia and Kaposi's sarcoma, which causes purplish blotches on the skin, are two classic signs of AIDS—although they do not occur in all people with AIDS and may develop in people without AIDS. As the immune system fails, you are at greater risk of opportunistic infections, including thrush, a fungal infection that causes white spots and ulcers on the tongue and mouth; chronic herpes type 1, a virus that causes blistering sores around the mouth; toxoplasmosis, a parasitic infection that can invade the brain; cryptococcosis, a fungus that attacks the nervous system, liver, bones, and skin; and cytomegalovirus, which causes pneumonia, encephalitis, and blindness. Women with AIDS also have a higher incidence of gynecological cancers.

How did I get it?

AIDS is caused by the human immunodeficiency virus (HIV). It is transmitted from one person to another by contact with bodily fluids, primarily through sexual relations or through the sharing of infected needles by drug abusers. Early in the epidemic, before tests to detect the virus in blood were available, many people contracted the virus through blood transfusions. Although homosexual men, intravenous drug abusers, and hemophiliacs have accounted for the majority of those infected to date, anyone who has not been in a mutually monogamous sexual relationship for more than ten years with someone who has no other risk factors may be at risk. In particular, women who have sexual contacts with men who have any risk factor also are at high risk. About 30 percent of infants born to HIV-infected women are infected with the virus and usually begin to have symptoms within the first year of life.

How is it diagnosed?

If you have been infected with HIV, it takes at least six weeks for your body to develop antibodies to the virus that can be detected by blood testing. In some people it can take months or, less commonly, up to a year for antibodies to develop. The test simply requires drawing a sample of blood from a vein in your arm to see if the antibody is present. Most testing centers require that you see a counselor before the test and that you return to receive your test results in person. Test results are usually confidential. A negative result means that no antibodies to HIV have been detected; depending on your risk factors, the counselor may urge that you be retested in three months. A positive result means that antibodies have been detected and that you are HIV infected; the counselor will usually refer you for psychological and medical treatment.

Another blood test measures the level of T4 helper cells in your blood to determine the extent to which HIV has damaged your immune system. The normal level is around 1,000 T4 helper cells per cubic millimeter of blood. Within five to ten years after infection with HIV, the level of these T4 cells is drastically reduced in most people. In addition to the presence of certain symptoms, the current federal Centers for Disease Control definition of AIDS includes a fall in the T4 cell count to below 200, which may not occur until five to ten years after infection. However, about 5 percent of those infected have not yet developed AIDS despite long-term infection.

How is it treated?

Some doctors do not recommend treatment of early HIV infections, whereas others prescribe AZT as soon as infection is discovered in the hope of slowing down damage to the immune system and delaying the development of AIDS. When the T4 cell count falls to 500, most doctors recommend that treatment should begin. AZT, DDI, or other antiviral drugs may be prescribed at this stage or later in the illness. These drugs can slow down the destruction of the immune system and thus protect you from potentially life-threatening opportunistic infections. However, by the time the T4 cell count falls below 200, you usually begin to have symptoms. If treatment with antiviral drugs has not been started sooner, it should certainly begin then.

Self-Care: The best approach to AIDS, if you are not already infected, is prevention. The greater the number of sexual partners, the greater the risk of coming into contact with the AIDS virus. If you have more than one partner, the risk to both of you is considerable. Whether you are homosexual or heterosexual, for any type of sexual contact, always use a latex condom lubricated with nonoxynol-9. In addition to all the other reasons to avoid drug abuse, AIDS puts the drug abuser who uses a hypodermic needle at high risk. Never share needles to inject drugs.

If you know that your past behavior patterns place you at risk of HIV infection, get an HIV test now. The sooner you learn that you have been infected, the sooner you can begin to evaluate potential treatment strategies and obtain helpful medical care. Further, if you find that you are positive, you can take steps to prevent spreading the infection to others. If you are worried about more recent exposure, or a single episode of possible exposure, wait until three months after the exposure to be tested. If the test is negative, have it repeated three months later.

CHLAMYDIA is the most common sexually transmitted (venereal) disease in the United States today. Untreated infections may be an important reason for the rising incidence of infertility due to pelvic inflammatory disease.

What are the symptoms?
Sometimes there are no early symptoms. When they do occur, men and women have different symptoms. In women, the most common signs are vaginal itching and a smelly, yellowish discharge. As the infection worsens, you may experience abdominal pain, bleeding between menstrual periods, painful or frequent urination, painful intercourse, nausea, and fever. In men, the most common signs are a discharge from the penis or burning and itching around the opening of the penis especially when urinating. If not treated promptly, symptoms may subside within a month, but the infection can then spread throughout the urinary and reproductive tracts, causing chronic bladder and urethral problems, pelvic inflammatory disease, and infertility.

How did I get it?
Chlamydia, tiny parasitic microorganisms closely related to bacteria, are usually transferred from one person to another by sexual contact. The infection also can be transferred from a pregnant woman to her baby during vaginal delivery.

How is it diagnosed?
Samples of secretions from a woman's vagina and vulva or the man's penis are taken using a cotton-tipped device. The secretions are then analyzed in a laboratory.

How is it treated?
Treatment with oral antibiotics, usually tetracycline, can cure early infections within 10 to 14 days. In some cases, infected glands may have to be drained or, rarely, surgically removed. Even after seemingly effective treatment, relapses may occur and require retreatment. Many doctors recommend retesting a month after therapy.

Self-Care: If you are sexually active with more than one partner, or if your sole partner is sexually active with others, use a latex condom during all sexual contact. Have regular medical checkups for sexually transmitted diseases. If you are diagnosed with chlamydia, avoid sexual contact until you are cured. Make sure any sexual partner is tested and, if infected, treated at the same time.

CHRONIC FATIGUE SYNDROME (CFS) is a mysterious ailment that has been called many names, such as chronic Epstein-Barr virus syndrome, herpes virus type 6 syndrome, chronic mononucleosis, neuromyasthenia, and the yuppie disease. The spectrum of illness caused by the syndrome has been reported in the medical literature for at least 100 years, but the ailment seems to have become far more prevalent in the past ten years. Women are stricken four times as often as men.

What are the symptoms?
Symptoms usually begin suddenly, and their severity varies widely from one person to another. The most common problem is devastating fatigue and exhaustion, usually severe enough to reduce daily activity by half. In addition, you may have such problems as mild fever, sore throat, painful lymph nodes, general muscle weakness, muscle aches, headaches, painful joints, and sleep problems. Neurological problems may include confusion and lapses of memory and reasoning. Some people have depression, balance disorders, heart palpitations, panic attacks, hepatitis, and pleurisy. Symptoms tend to come and go over a period of years. In about one-third of patients, the disorder disappears spontaneously in six months to two years. Another third show marked improvement. The rest seem to have constant relapses and never completely regain their health.

How did I get it?
Although the condition has been attributed to such causes as Epstein-Barr virus, low blood sugar, thyroid disorders, fungus infections, and psychosomatic problems, research has not confirmed any of these as a culprit. A predisposition to the problem may be inherited, because it often runs in families. A genetic immunological defect may be present, or the immune system may go into overdrive fighting off infection and produce substances that make the body feel sicker. Stress, environmental toxins, and virus exposure may spark the disorder or reactivate symptoms.

How is it diagnosed?
First, your doctor will do a complete examination and many tests to rule out such other disorders as diabetes, lupus, rheumatoid arthritis, tuberculosis, cancer, and AIDS. Then diagnosis is based on a certain pattern of symptoms as defined by the Centers for Disease Control.

How is it treated?
There is no cure or completely effective treatment. Drugs may be prescribed to alleviate depression, pain, or inflammation. Some research projects are studying the benefits of antiviral drugs and gammaglobulin injections. Counseling may be helpful to deal with depression. In large measure, you treat yourself at home.

> Self-Care: Your doctor will advise you to eat properly, get plenty of rest, avoid stress, and modify your lifestyle to reduce stress and unnecessary energy expenditure. A diet free of preservatives, food dyes, and caffeine and low in fats, salt, and sugar may be helpful.

COLDS, upper respiratory infections, hit millions of Americans every year. It is not uncommon for children to have half a dozen colds a winter, because they have not lived long enough to develop resistance to the viruses. Understanding how colds are transmitted may help prevent them.

What are the symptoms?
Colds usually come on slowly, with a runny or stuffy nose, sneezing, and sore throat as their most common features. If there is fever, it is usually low. Headache, if present, is mild. Coughing sometimes occurs. The typical cold lasts seven to ten days.

How did I get it?
Colds are caused by one of nearly 200 different viruses, nearly half of which are called rhinoviruses. Many people are surprised to learn that kissing is not a primary means of transmitting colds. Enzymes in our saliva may actually help destroy cold germs. Rather, germs transferred by hand, such as by shaking hands, to your nose or eyes seem to flourish best. You don't get colds from a chill; colds are more apt to flourish in winter only because we are more likely to be indoors and in closer contact with other people—facilitating germ transfer. So, to help prevent colds during the season, avoid crowds, wash your hands frequently, and keep fingers away from your nose and eyes.

How is it diagnosed?
Most people can tell when they have a cold by the symptoms, but similar symptoms can arise from an allergy attack or the flu. However, in allergy, your nose and eyes are likely to be itchy. If you have the flu, symptoms tend to be more severe and are usually accompanied by headache, muscle aches, a dry cough, fatigue, and high fever.

How is it treated?
Because antibiotics kill bacteria, not viruses, taking an antibiotic won't help to get rid of your cold. Your physician should prescribe an antibiotic only if your cold has progressed and led to pneumonia or another secondary infection, a relatively rare occurrence. Your doctor is more likely to recommend self-care and, if fever occurs, taking acetaminophen.

> Self-Care: Get plenty of bed rest to conserve energy and drink lots of fluids. Beyond these basics, select treatments specific to your symptoms. Chicken soup or other hot fluids or a cool mist humidifier will help open a stuffed nose. They can be better than decongestants, which sometimes worsen the problem if taken for more than three days. Sore throats can be eased by sucking on a hard candy or gargling with warm salt water. Try not to stifle coughs, unless they interfere with sleep, because they help you get rid of phlegm and mucus that can clog airways.

ENCEPHALITIS is a potentially life-threatening inflammation of the brain. If the spinal cord is also affected, the illness may be called encephalomyelitis. Although mild cases may never even be diagnosed, severe cases may cause permanent physical disability due to neurological damage.

What are the symptoms?
Mild cases may have few or no noticeable symptoms. The most prominent symptoms are fever, headache, stiff neck, fatigue, and projectile vomiting. You also may become restless and irritable, lose muscle strength in your arms and legs, and develop impairments in your vision, speech, and hearing. More severe cases cause seizures, varying degrees of paralysis, confusion, and coma.

How did I get it?
Encephalitis is usually caused by infection with a virus. One type, equine encephalitis, comes from an arbovirus transmitted by mosquitoes that have fed on infected horses. Infection with polio, coxsackie, or herpes viruses also

may cause brain inflammation. Encephalitis may also develop as a complication of other common viral infections, ranging from now uncommon
childhood diseases, such as measles, mumps, chickenpox, or rubella, to
influenza or even a cold. Less commonly, encephalitis may be caused by
bacterial or fungal infections.

How is it diagnosed?
Depending on your symptoms and any underlying disease, diagnosis may
involve blood tests, head X-rays, an electroencephalogram to evaluate your
brain waves, and a spinal tap to take a sample of your cerebrospinal fluid for
laboratory examination. Sometimes a sample of brain tissue is necessary to
identify the cause of the encephalitis. In severe cases, you may need physical,
occupational, or speech therapy to help you fully recuperate.

How is it treated?
No treatment is available to cure most of the viruses that cause encephalitis,
except for intravenous acyclovir illness caused by the herpes simplex virus.
If a bacterial cause is identified, antibiotics will be prescribed. Mild viral
encephalitis may require only bed rest and self-care. More severe cases
require hospitalization for supportive care that may include intravenous
nutrition, steroid drugs to reduce inflammation, and a respirator to assist
breathing. Sometimes excess fluid in the brain must be removed by needle
aspiration.

> Self-Care: Be alert for signs of encephalitis during and shortly after
> any viral infection. If you suspect a problem, go to a doctor for
> diagnosis immediately, because early treatment of certain infections
> can be lifesaving. If your doctor tells you to treat mild encephalitis at
> home, stay in bed to rest. Take acetaminophen to ease fever and
> headache. Drink plenty of fluids to avoid dehydration.

FOOD POISONING is a general term used to describe any illness caused
by eating a food that contains a toxic substance and causes illness. Although
some types of food poisoning may cause only minor, transient gastrointestinal problems, other types such as botulism are potentially fatal.

What are the symptoms?
Most types of food poisoning provoke abdominal cramps, diarrhea, and
vomiting within a few hours after eating. The severity of symptoms depends
on the type and amount of the poison eaten and the age and health of the

victim. Children, the elderly, and those with suppressed immune systems due to illness or medications are at greater risk of major problems. In botulism, symptoms don't begin for 18 to 36 hours after eating the contaminated food. In addition to gastrointestinal symptoms, botulism may cause dry mouth, fatigue, dizziness, difficulty in speaking or swallowing, blurred vision, arm and leg weakness, drooping eyelids, and difficulty in breathing. As symptoms progress, paralysis begins.

How did I get it?

Food poisoning is commonly caused by bacteria that have contaminated food that was improperly stored or prepared. These bacteria include *Clostridium botulinum*, which causes botulism due to contaminated canned foods; *Clostridium perfringens*, which can grow in foods that remain unrefrigerated for extended periods; salmonella, which contaminates undercooked animal foods such as poultry and eggs; shigella, which derives from food infected with feces; and staphylococcus, which grows in foods such as poultry stuffing, mayonnaise, and custard. Other cases of food poisoning are caused by eating a naturally poisonous item, such as certain mushrooms or fish, or a food contaminated with insecticides or other toxic substances, such as lead or mercury.

How is it diagnosed?

Your doctor usually can diagnose food poisoning based on your symptoms and your report of their onset. Identifying the specific cause of your illness often requires laboratory examination of the poisoned food.

How is it treated?

Most cases of food poisoning are self-limiting and do not require treatment. Do not try to stop the vomiting or diarrhea because your body must rid itself of the toxins. Drink frequent small amounts of clear liquids to prevent dehydration. If you think you know what food caused the poisoning, save it in the refrigerator in case more serious problems occur. Call your doctor immediately if botulism is suspected, if symptoms become severe or do not abate within a few hours, if fever or abdominal swelling occurs, or if blood appears in the vomitus or diarrhea. Severe cases of salmonellosis require antibiotic therapy. Botulism requires immediate hospitalization and antitoxin injections to help reverse the muscle paralysis.

Self-Care: When preparing foods at home, practice scrupulous hygiene to avoid food poisoning. Carefully wash any surface and utensils touched by raw meat, fish, or poultry before using them to prepare salads and other foods that will not be cooked. Cook all foods thoroughly. When canning foods, make sure they maintain a rolling boil for ten minutes before they are placed in jars. Never use food from a bulging can or any food that has a strange odor. However, do not count on your senses to warn you. Contaminated food may not look, smell, or taste unusual. Never eat any wild berry, mushroom, or other plant unless you are positive about what it is.

GONORRHEA is one of the most common sexually transmitted, or venereal, diseases. It is also called the clap or, among men, the drip. If left untreated, gonorrhea can cause serious problems. In women, the accompanying pelvic inflammatory disease can cause permanent damage to the reproductive organs, including infertility. Pregnant women can infect their baby's eyes during birth, causing serious eye problems or even blindness. In both sexes, long-term untreated gonorrhea can cause debilitating arthritis or bacteremia, a potentially life-threatening complication that damages organs throughout the body.

What are the symptoms?
Symptoms are different in men and women. Women can have the disease for months or longer without knowing it because most have no significant symptoms. Others may have a slight vaginal discharge or some burning in the vaginal area. Men usually develop symptoms within a week or two of infection. They include a thick pus-like discharge from the penis and a burning sensation during urination.

How did I get it?
Gonorrhea is caused by a bacterium that is almost invariably spread through direct sexual contact. You cannot catch gonorrhea from toilet seats.

How is it diagnosed?
A sample of the vaginal or penile discharge is taken with a cotton swab and sent to a laboratory for analysis.

How is it treated?
A two-week course of antibiotics, usually penicillin, cures most types of gonorrhea. Take the full course of the drug even if symptoms disappear sooner. Any recent sexual partners should also be tested and, if necessary,

treated to prevent reinfection. Avoid all sexual contacts until your gonor-rhea is fully cured and you have completed taking all medication.

Self-Care: Using a condom during sexual activity can reduce, but not eliminate, your risk of contracting gonorrhea. Women should never have sexual relations with a man who has a penile discharge.

HEAD LICE are tiny parasitic insects, usually less than one-eighth of an inch long and almost as wide, that survive by sucking blood from animals and humans. Although they can infect anyone, epidemics most commonly occur among children at school or at camp, who unknowingly bring the infection home. Fortunately, head lice don't carry disease and are easily banished when treated properly.

What are the symptoms?
The primary sign is intense scalp itching, frequently behind the ears and along the hairline at the back of the neck, produced by an irritant reaction to the saliva of the lice as they bite the scalp.

How did I get it?
Lice crawl from the head of a person to various objects and then to the next person. Schools are a common source of contagion because lice spread easily on hats, scarves, and jackets in coat closets. Trading headsets or haircombs and brushes can also spread lice. You can get lice from people you've never even met, through upholstered theater seats, clothing in department stores, or coat check rooms.

How is it diagnosed?
The lice themselves can be hard to spot. However, if you examine the infected person's hair and scalp closely, you can usually find their eggs (nits), which appear as tiny, silvery clumps attached to the hair shaft near the roots. Lice infestation is easy to differentiate from dandruff because the nits don't flake off; they are virtually cemented to the hair shaft.

How is it treated?
There's no need to call a doctor if you have head lice. The most effective care is given at home. Check with your doctor only if scratching has caused open sores on the scalp, if you're not sure whether lice are the cause of the

problem, if a child under two years of age is infected, or if the itching is so unbearable that extra medication is needed temporarily.

Self-Care: You can kill the adult lice with a lice-killing shampoo, available over the counter in your pharmacy. The safest ones are pyrethrin-based; follow package directions carefully. Then you need someone to use a special fine-toothed comb for the tedious task of nit-picking to remove eggs bonded to your hair shaft. Part wet hair into four sections and then carefully comb, from base to tip, a one-inch wide tuft at a time. Comb slowly, wiping nits from the comb frequently with a tissue. If hair dries during the process, wet with water again. The process can take an hour or longer if you have long, thick hair. A week to 10 days later, the entire process is repeated to catch any last nits missed on the first round. If lice have settled on the eyelashes, application of petroleum jelly three or four times a day should banish them within a week.

If one family member is infected, all others should be checked for nits and, if necessary, treated. Then you must get the lice out of your home. Adult lice die after 48 hours without a blood meal, but nits may not hatch until a month later, restarting infestation. To avoid this, all personal clothing, bed linens, and stuffed animals belonging to those infested must be either sterilized in hot water (at least 130° F), or put in a hot dryer for at least 20 minutes, or dry-cleaned. Upholstered furniture, rugs, and other objects that can't go in the machines must be thoroughly vacuumed and treated with a lice spray.

HEPATITIS is an inflammation of the liver. Although hepatitis is usually a mild and self-limiting disease, some cases can be life threatening. Although some types were frequently transmitted by blood transfusions in the past, new tests are now used to screen all donated blood for hepatitis B and C, helping to ensure the safety of our blood supply.

What are the symptoms?
Mild hepatitis may cause only flu-like symptoms, such as fatigue, weakness, fever, appetite loss, headache, and cramps, as well as darker urine, lighter stools, and a yellowish tone in your skin and the whites of your eyes called jaundice. Some people experience nausea and vomiting, hives, and joint pain. In more severe cases, almost any body system may be affected, and cirrhosis or liver failure may occur. One of the rare but worst forms of the illness is fulminating hepatitis, which may progress to a coma and be fatal,

even with the best of care. Types B and C also are more likely to develop into a chronic form of the disease.

How did I get it?

Most commonly hepatitis is caused by viruses transmitted through contaminated food (infectious hepatitis) or infected blood (serum hepatitis). The other major causes are abuse of alcohol and certain drugs. Rarely, bacterial, fungal, or parasitic infections cause liver inflammation. The three major types are named after the viruses that have been found to cause them.

• *Type A* hepatitis virus is spread primarily by contact with an infected person or their stools, or by eating food (especially shellfish) that comes from sewage-contaminated water or that has been prepared by a person with unclean hands who is infected with the disease.
• *Type B* hepatitis virus is transmitted primarily by blood transfusions, the sharing of unsterilized needles by drug abusers, and blood contact through anal sex.
• *Type C* (formerly called "non-A, non-B") may be transmitted by all of the above methods.

Carriers are people infected with hepatitis but who do not have symptoms; they can spread the disease unless they use careful sanitary measures.

How is it diagnosed?

During a physical examination, your doctor finds your liver to be enlarged and tender. Blood tests reveal inflammation of the liver; other tests identify the offending viral agent.

How is it treated?

No specific treatment can cure hepatitis. In most cases, especially of type A, all that is needed is bed rest and avoidance of alcohol and certain drugs that are metabolized in the liver; recovery takes from two to eight weeks. However, types B and C can be more severe, especially in the elderly. Severe or chronic disease may require treatment with steroids or other immuno-suppressive drugs.

Self-Care: A preventive vaccine is available only for hepatitis B; it should be given to all people at high risk for hepatitis B, such as male homosexuals, the sexual partners of hepatitis B carriers, and health care workers. Careful sanitary measures can often prevent you from contacting type A. If you have intimate contact with a person who has type A hepatitis, ask your doctor about treatment with immune serum globulin to help prevent your developing severe disease. People who have hepatitis or are carriers of hepatitis should not be involved in food preparation and should carefully wash their hands with soap and water after using the toilet; their food utensils, dishes, and glasses should be boiled after use.

HERPES TYPE 1, also called oral herpes or herpes simplex type 1, is a common viral disease that usually occurs around the mouth, where the blisters are called cold sores or fever blisters. Herpes type 1 may also affect the eyes and threaten vision if not treated promptly.

What are the symptoms?
Herpes causes painful, itchy sores that look like blisters or small bumps. In herpes type 1, they usually appear on or near the mouth, but they may also occur on the eyelid, causing it to swell. Within 24 hours of their appearance, the blisters usually break and yellowish crusts form. If herpes type 1 affects the eye itself, the cornea is usually the site, causing eye discharge, intolerance to light, and decreased vision. Less commonly, you may experience a mild fever and malaise. Sometimes herpes attacks may be preceded by a "prodrome"—tingling or burning sensations that may or may not lead to a full-blown attack. Sores eventually heal by themselves, usually within a few weeks, but the virus is still in the body. Some people never get another attack; others have repeated but milder eruptions on occasion throughout life.

How did I get it?
Oral herpes is caused by the herpes simplex type 1 virus. It is highly contagious and spread by physical contact. About 70 percent of Americans have been infected with herpes type 1 by the age of 14.

How is it diagnosed?
The sores usually can be diagnosed by their characteristic appearance. If the eye is involved, your doctor may touch the cornea itself and observe your response. Herpes-infected corneas have a reduced level of sensitivity due to nerve damage. Sometimes, samples of cells from the infected area may be sent to the laboratory for examination. This is more likely if your doctor suspects the blisters are from herpes type 2, which normally affects the genital area.

How is it treated?

There is no known cure for herpes type 1. However, most attacks are self-limiting. Attacks usually disappear within a few days. In more severe cases, a drug called acyclovir can help prevent recurrences and shorten attacks dramatically. It may be given topically or, for those with immune system problems, orally. Another drug, idoxuridine, may be prescribed for eye lesions.

Self-Care: Once you are infected with the virus, recurrences may be triggered by the onset of menstruation, as well as by stress, sunburn, or other environmental factors. If you have frequent attacks, keep track of what might have precipitated them in order to try avoidance. If you have a prodrome before outbreaks, prompt use of aspirin and ice packs sometimes forestalls the recurrence. Once the lesions appear, compresses of cold water or milk may ease discomfort. To help protect others from infection, avoid kissing anyone or sharing dishes or utensils during outbreaks.

HERPES TYPE 2, also called genital herpes, is a common viral disease that has reached near epidemic proportions in recent years. It has become one of the most common sexually transmitted diseases. If a baby gets herpes while passing through the vagina during the birth, it can suffer severe brain damage or become fatally ill.

What are the symptoms?

Herpes type 2 causes painful, itchy sores that look like blisters or small bumps. They appear inside the vagina or on the labia in women; on the penis in men; and/or in or around the anus, thighs, or buttocks in both sexes. In women, sores may also occur on the cervix, where they are not painful. Blisters may form, which can rupture into open sores. If you have had oral sex with an infected person, you may develop blisters around your mouth that can be difficult to differentiate from herpes type 1. Other possible signs are fever, enlarged lymph nodes, and flu-like symptoms. Sometimes herpes attacks may be preceded by a "prodrome"—tingling or burning sensations that may or may not lead to a full-blown attack. Sores eventually heal by themselves, usually within a few weeks, but the virus is still in the body. Some people may never get another attack; others may develop new eruptions repeatedly, every few weeks or months for years.

How did I get it?
Genital herpes is caused by the herpes simplex type 2 virus. It is usually spread by close sexual contact. When the sores are open, the virus is thought to spread very easily.

How is it diagnosed?
Accurate diagnosis of herpes is best accomplished by a microscopic examination of a smear taken from the base of one of the sores and/or a blood test for herpes antibodies. Any woman with recurrent sores in the vaginal area should suspect herpes and see a physician.

How is it treated?
There is no known cure for herpes type 2, but a drug called acyclovir can help prevent recurrences and shorten attacks dramatically. To work effectively, a five-day cycle of acyclovir must be taken as soon as the lesion appears. In addition, your physician can prescribe other medications to help ease discomfort and prevent infection of open sores. If a woman is pregnant and has active herpes that cannot be effectively treated before birth, a Cesarean section may be recommended to avoid exposing the baby to infection.

> Self-Care: Warm baths or salt water compresses can help ease inflammation. Keep the infected area clean and dry. Wash your hands after touching the sores to avoid spreading infection to other parts of your body. Because herpes type 2 is so highly contagious, those infected should never have sexual contact during an attack. Tell any prospective sexual partner that you are infected with herpes. Using a latex condom may lower, but cannot eliminate, the risk of sexual transmission.

INFLUENZA, commonly known as the flu, is a highly contagious disease. Although its symptoms are sometimes confused with those of the common cold, flu has a different cause, somewhat different symptoms, and often, a much worse course and a greater risk of complications than a cold. Indeed, flu can be fatal in infants, the aged, and people with chronic diseases.

What are the symptoms?
The primary symptoms usually start abruptly and are those of an upper respiratory infection, such as nasal congestion, sneezing, coughing, and sore throat. The flu also causes high fever, muscle ache, severe headache, and

weakness. Fever may be absent in elderly people and particularly high in children. Severe symptoms last only three to five days, although feelings of weakness and fatigue may persist for weeks.

How did I get it?

Influenza is caused by one of three types of viruses. Type A is the most common and causes the most widespread and dangerous worldwide epidemics. Type B causes milder epidemics. Type C usually causes only localized outbreaks. The virus is transmitted through the air from droplets in coughs and sneezes.

How is it diagnosed?

Diagnosis is based on the presence of the characteristic symptoms when the flu virus is circulating in your community.

How is it treated?

Most symptoms can be treated at home. Call your doctor if your symptoms persist for more than a week or seem to worsen and progress, causing a cough with dark phlegm, breathing difficulty, stiff neck, vomiting, or visual changes, or if temperature hits 103° F. If you have the flu and fall into one of the high-risk categories of people who should have been vaccinated, call your doctor right away. Although anyone can get an annual flu vaccination in the fall to prevent the disease that winter, the Centers for Disease Control urges vaccination for people at greatest risk of flu complications: those with weakened immune systems (such as those over age 65, on cancer chemotherapy, or with chronic cardiac or respiratory problems), as well as those who care for such people, including health professionals and family members. If you miss your chance at vaccination but still want to prevent the flu, an oral prescription medication called amantadine may help ward off the type A virus and ameliorate its symptoms if you are infected. You have to take it for three or four weeks, throughout the time that the influenza virus is circulating in the community.

Self-Care: Rest in bed. Drink plenty of fluids to avoid dehydration. Take acetaminophen to reduce fever and ease aches and pains. Avoid using nasal decongestant sprays for more than three days because that may cause even more severe rebound congestion. A hot shower, hot drinks, or use of a humidifier can also ease nasal congestion. Be aware that oral decongestants may cause insomnia. If you need a cough medicine, choose an expectorant that helps you bring up heavy phlegm and mucus that can clog airways. Don't block coughing with a suppressant or antitussive unless coughing keeps you awake at night.

LYME DISEASE is a tickborne infection that can cause serious illness. The disease has now been reported throughout the United States, with the highest levels of infection on the East Coast from Maine to Maryland and spreading south, as well as on the West Coast and in the upper Midwest.

What are the symptoms?
The first sign is usually a rash that develops at the site of the tick bite within days or weeks of the bite. It is often accompanied by headache, low fever, achiness, and other flu-like symptoms. The rash expands to look like a red ring, clear in the center, and then disappears within a few weeks. However, more than half of those bitten never get the rash—and most people do not remember being bitten. Weeks or months after the bite, arthritic, cardiac, and/or neurological complications may occur. Most common are joint swelling, pain, and stiffness; heart arrhythmias; meningitis; and various types of paralysis. Depression and other psychological problems may also occur. Infection in pregnant women may lead to miscarriage and other fetal problems.

How did I get it?
Named after the Connecticut town where it was first diagnosed in the mid-1970s, Lyme disease is caused by a type of bacteria known as a spirochete and is transmitted by several species of tiny ticks—no larger than the period at the end of this sentence. Although the ticks are most often found on animals, they can bite humans who come into contact with them near wooded or marshy areas, especially by walking through underbrush or even on grassy lawns.

How is it diagnosed?
Blood tests are available to check for Lyme disease, but even those infected may not test positive until months after infection. However, anyone who may have been exposed to Lyme disease and who develops unexplained symptoms similar to the disease's complications—especially arthritis—should be tested.

How is it treated?
Lyme disease usually can be cured with antibiotics, especially if treated in its earliest stages, before complications occur. Advanced cases may require hospitalization for intravenous therapy.

Self-Care: The only way to prevent Lyme disease is by avoiding tick bites. When walking in infected areas, wear long-sleeved shirts, long pants tucked into socks, closed shoes, and close-fitting hats. Use insect repellents that contain DEET. Examine yourself carefully, dressed and undressed, when you get home. When your pets come indoors, comb them carefully to remove any ticks. If you find a tick attached to your body, grasp it with a pair of tweezers as close to your skin as possible and tug gently to remove it. The sooner it is removed, the lower the risk that it will transmit infection. Place the tick in a closed jar or other container so that it can be examined. Then contact your physician promptly to obtain any medical attention that may be needed.

MONONUCLEOSIS, sometimes called "mono," is a highly contagious disease. It is often referred to by college students—a highly susceptible group—as the "kissing disease." Although mono is usually not serious, potentially life-threatening complications may occur. These include involvement of the brain and nervous system with respiratory paralysis, hemolytic anemia, obstruction of breathing by acute sore throat and swollen tonsils, or rupture of the spleen due to physical activity such as football.

What are the symptoms?
Symptoms usually start about a month or two after exposure. Initially, fatigue, headache, and chills develop, usually followed by fever, sore throat, and swollen glands, particularly in the neck. There also may be weakness, poor appetite, and sore muscles or joints. In some cases the spleen becomes swollen, the liver is involved, and jaundice may occur. Severe symptoms tend to persist for one to four weeks. However, convalescence can be extended, causing fatigue for weeks or months longer.

How did I get it?
Mono is caused by the Epstein-Barr virus (EBV). It got the nickname "kissing disease" because it is mainly transmitted by close contact with another person's saliva. However, kissing is not essential for such contact. Sharing eating utensils, toothbrushes, lipsticks—even a splashy cough— can infect you with an infected person's saliva. Most often, victims are teenagers and young adults, people who have never been exposed to Epstein-Barr virus and who, therefore, have no antibody defense to it. Mono is rare in those over age 40.

How is it diagnosed?
If your doctor suspects mononucleosis, a series of blood tests will be performed to confirm the diagnosis and rule out other possible causes of your symptoms. A negative blood test may have to be repeated for accurate results.

How is it treated?
Because there is no cure for mono, treatment is aimed at relieving the symptoms. Bed rest is important for the first one to four weeks whenever you feel tired or when symptoms are marked. Acetaminophen is recommended if needed for headaches, fever, or achiness. Antibiotics are of no value unless secondary bacterial infection occurs. No other medication is needed unless complications develop. In such cases, you may need anti-inflammatory drugs or, rarely, hospitalization for further care.

> Self-Care: Stay in bed as advised by your doctor. If your sore throat is severe, try warm salt water gargles. As you recuperate, continue to take it easy for a few weeks. Spleen problems may persist long into convalescence; in such cases, your doctor may warn you not to indulge in sports for many months.

SYPHILIS is one of the most common sexually transmitted (venereal) diseases. Although easily cured in its early stages, syphilis is difficult to treat and potentially life threatening in later stages.

What are the symptoms?
The first stage of syphilis, which commonly occurs within a month of infection, is usually a painless red sore called a chancre. It may look like a pimple at an area of sexual contact, such as the vagina, penis, rectum, or mouth. In some women, the sore may occur inside the vagina, where it is not noticed. Even if not treated, this sore soon disappears, but the infection continues to spread inside the body. Within a few weeks to a few months later, the second stage of syphilis causes new symptoms: swollen lymph glands, headaches, fever, and a rash that may spread all over your body or appear only on the palms of the hands and soles of the feet. Again, if not treated, these symptoms will disappear, but damage inside the body continues. The third stage of syphilis usually begins years later and may cause damage to the heart and nervous system, as well as blindness, insanity, or death.

How did I get it?
Syphilis is caused by a spirochete called *Treponema pallidum* that is almost invariably spread through direct sexual contact, although it may be transmitted through saliva on drinking glasses and eating utensils. You cannot catch syphilis from toilet seats. It is infectious throughout the first and second stages. Pregnant women can pass the disease to their unborn babies through the placenta.

How is it diagnosed?
In the first stage, it can be diagnosed by laboratory examination of cells from the chancre or a blood sample. In the second stage, it is diagnosed by laboratory examination of a sample of cerebrospinal fluid.

How is it treated?
In the first and second stages, syphilis usually can be cured by a full course of injections of large doses of penicillin or other antibiotics. In about 10 percent of cases, the disease recurs within a year and retreatment is necessary. Most doctors recommend regular blood tests for six months to two years after treatment to ensure that the infection has been completely eradicated. In the third stage of syphilis, hospitalization for intravenous antibiotics usually is necessary.

Self-Care: If you are sexually active with multiple partners, have annual tests for syphilis and other venereal diseases. If you are diagnosed with syphilis, make sure any recent sexual partners also receive diagnosis and, if they are infected, treatment. Avoid sexual intercourse for at least two months after treatment begins.

TETANUS, also called lockjaw, is an acute infectious disease that typically develops after the skin is broken by a wound or some other type of injury. About half of all tetanus victims die. Although the disease is relatively rare now in the United States because of immunization, you should be alert to the possibility of tetanus and take action after any skin-penetrating injury.

What are the symptoms?
Symptoms usually begin about two weeks after exposure, although they may start as soon as the day after or as long as nearly two months later. Problems start with irritability, restlessness, headache, difficulty in swallowing, difficulty in breathing, and fever, as well as pain and stiffness, especially in the jaw, abdomen, and back. Muscle pain leads to spasms and rigidity, which

may cause a severely arched back. Complications include pneumonia, irregular heartbeat, paralysis, and fatal widespread blood coagulation.

How did I get it?

Tetanus is caused by a poisonous toxin produced by *Clostridium tetani*. This bacterium is virtually ubiquitous in our environment, especially in soil, dust, and manure. Infection occurs when the bacteria enters the body through a break in the skin—for example, a deep cut while gardening, a puncture from stepping on a nail, or a dog bite. The bacteria then multiply rapidly, exuding a toxin that travels through the bloodstream and affects nerves throughout the body.

How is it diagnosed?

There are no tests for tetanus, but doctors usually can diagnose it quickly based on the classic symptoms.

How is it treated?

Immediate hospitalization and early treatment in an intensive care unit are essential for survival. You will receive tetanus antiserum injections, which can reduce the severity of the disease but cannot neutralize any toxin that has already invaded the nervous system. You also will be given muscle relaxant medication and may need a respirator to help you breathe. Surgery is sometimes necessary to open the wound and remove infected tissue. Other treatment depends on whether any complications develop.

> Self-Care: Infants should be vaccinated against tetanus as part of a series of immunizations. Adults also should have a tetanus booster about every ten years. Any skin-penetrating injury, including burns and dog bites, should be washed thoroughly with soap and water and doused with hydrogen peroxide. Because the causative bacteria cannot survive in the presence of oxygen, be concerned about any deep injury, such as a puncture wound or animal bite, in which the base of the wound would be protected from exposure to air. In such instances, discuss the possible need for an additional booster injection with your doctor.

TOXIC SHOCK SYNDROME is an infectious disease that became epidemic in 1980, causing major panic among previously healthy young women, who are its most common victims. Initial attacks are severe and potentially life threatening. About 30 percent of menstruating women who have had the disorder later have milder recurrent episodes. Less commonly, the disease strikes women who are not menstruating and men.

What are the symptoms?
The disease comes on rapidly, most often in the first day or two of menstruation. There is a sudden high fever, vomiting, diarrhea, muscle ache, and weakness. You may become disoriented or combative. Blood pressure may drop rapidly, causing shock. You may urinate less due to low blood pressure. A day or two later, a sunburn-like rash develops, especially on the soles of the feet and the palms of the hands, which then causes skin peeling. Anyone showing signs of toxic shock should call a doctor immediately; if you are unable to reach your doctor right away, go to a hospital emergency room.

How did I get it?
Toxic shock is caused by blood poisoning from a toxin produced by staphyloccal bacteria. It is believed that the 1980 epidemic in menstruating women was caused by the introduction of superabsorbent tampons, which did not need to be changed as often as regular tampons and which promoted the overgrowth of staphyloccal organisms that normally live on the skin and in the vagina and nasal passages without causing problems. When superabsorbent tampons were removed from the market, the epidemic abated. Some cases have been associated with use of a diaphragm or postsurgical infection. In others, no triggering factor can be identified.

How is it diagnosed?
Although the staph infection can be identified by blood tests, they require several days to provide results. Because the syndrome fulminates so rapidly, doctors must diagnose the disease based on symptoms and act quickly to provide treatment, even before test results are available.

How is it treated?
Hospitalization and intravenous antibiotics are needed immediately to fight the infection. Further medications and intravenous fluids are needed to restore normal blood pressure and to manage other complications, such as kidney or liver failure. If blood flow to the fingers and toes is severely impaired by shock, gangrene may occur and require amputation.

Self-Care: Menstruating women should always change their tampons at least twice a day and should switch to pads at night. Those who use diaphragms should remove them as prescribed and should not wear them continually. If you have already had toxic shock, never use tampons and ask your doctor whether it is advisable to use regular antibiotic therapy to prevent future attacks.

TUBERCULOSIS (TB) is a highly contagious disease that was one of the world's leading causes of death until the development of antibiotics. Although TB incidence in the United States declined early in the twentieth century as a result of improved sanitation and living conditions, it is now on the rise again with increasing poverty, homelessness, and drug abuse. Those at greatest risk of developing TB are health care workers, people who live with TB victims, children, the aged, and those who are malnourished or weakened by other diseases, especially AIDS. Early detection and treatment are essential, especially because of the rise of resistant strains of TB.

What are the symptoms?
The most common symptom is a chronic cough. Other lung-related symptoms include profuse and foul-smelling sputum, coughing up blood, shortness of breath, or chest pain, especially when you take a deep breath. Other symptoms are unusual fatigue and weakness and loss of appetite and weight. The bones, kidneys, and other organs can also be infected. Untreated, TB can be fatal.

How did I get it?
TB is caused by bacteria that are spread from one person to another in droplets of saliva that are expelled by coughing, sneezing, speaking, or even breathing. Although the droplets evaporate, the bacteria remain airborne and can be inhaled by other people. People who have not been treated for active TB are usually infectious and can transmit the disease; within a few weeks of beginning treatment, they are no longer considered excessively contagious, as long as reasonable sanitary precautions are taken. However, all people infected with the TB germs do not necessarily get active disease. Indeed, comparatively few "break down" with TB. Sometimes, people become ill as a result of being infected many years earlier. In the intervening period, their bodies have been able to fight the infection; lowered resistance that enabled the bacteria to multiply and spread may have been caused by illness or the subtle immune changes of aging.

How is it diagnosed?
A simple skin test can tell whether you have been infected with the TB bacteria, but it does not differentiate between active and dormant infection.

Active disease is usually determined by a culture of your sputum and chest X-rays.

How is it treated?
If TB is detected and treated early in the course of infection, it can be cured. Even if treatment is delayed, the disease can often be controlled and death prevented. Isoniazid is the drug most commonly given for TB. Because some strains of TB bacteria have become resistant to traditional antibiotics, sometimes multiple drugs must be given. People with active TB must take medication for six months to a year, depending on their doctor's prescription. Some people who are infected with TB but who have not developed active disease need extended treatment to prevent such an occurrence. Preventive treatment may also be recommended for those who live with a TB patient.

Self-Care: If you live or work with someone who has TB, you should have a skin test. If you have ever had any risk of exposure, now or years ago, discuss testing with your doctor. Although isolation in a sanitarium is no longer considered necessary, certain protective measures should be taken when active TB is present. People with the disease should not share eating or drinking utensils. They should cover their noses and mouths when sneezing or coughing. Because the bacteria that cause TB are killed by ultraviolet light, a sunny, well-ventilated environment reduces the risk of transmission.

10

Eye and Ear Disorders

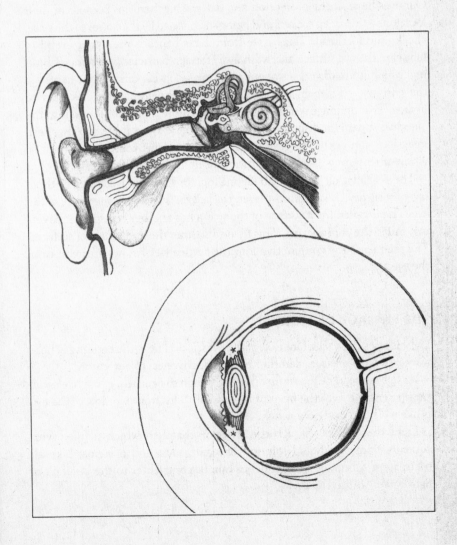

HOW THE EYES WORK

The human eye is unique among the eyes of all other creatures on earth: It can perceive color, whereas the world appears in shades of gray to other animals, and it can detect objects that are still, which most other eyes cannot. It also can perceive depth, adapt to light levels, and focus readily to accommodate changes in distance.

EYE PROTECTION

Our eyes have strong protection and defense mechanisms because of their location within deep sockets and being surrounded by the bones of the nose, cheek, and forehead. Tears issue from ducts beneath the upper eyelid to lubricate the eye surface and wash away foreign particles and germs. Blinking, which normally occurs about every six seconds, pumps tears, helps bar the entrance of foreign particles, and helps expel any particles that do invade. Tear drainage sends debris out to the nose, to be swallowed into the digestive system for disposal. When one of these systems breaks down, eye infections can occur, ranging from simple problems you can self-treat to vision-threatening disorders that warrant immediate medical care.

The eyeball itself, a sphere about one inch in diameter, is covered by three layers of tissue. The outermost layer, the **sclera,** is visible as the white of the eye. The exposed front surface of the sclera has another transparent covering, called the **conjunctiva.** This tissue also lines the eyelids' inner surfaces. The sclera and the conjunctiva join the cornea (see below) at the front of the eye.

THE PASSAGE OF LIGHT

Light is essential to the function of the eyes. Refraction, the bending of light waves, in large measure determines the effectiveness of our vision.

As light enters the eye, it first passes through the **cornea,** a tough, elastic, transparent cap over the front of the eyeball. This front window of the eye is like a clear crystal on a watch.

Light then passes through the **anterior chamber,** which is filled with **aqueous humor,** a liquid solution of water, salts, and proteins. Like all transparent substances, the aqueous humor contributes to the bending of light waves within the eye.

Behind the anterior chamber is the colored portion of the eye, the **iris,** with a small, round, black opening in the center called the **pupil.** The iris can contract to a narrow circular opening or relax to enlarge. This ability aids in focusing in different lighting conditions. The intensity of light entering the eye stimulates nerves that feed back involuntary signals to contract or relax the iris.

Light passes through the pupil and onto the crystalline, clear **lens** that bends or refracts light. Held in place by ligaments, the lens changes the focus of the eye so that you can see things at different distances. The degree of tension on the ligaments pulls on the edges of the lens, affecting its curvature and its power; lower power is used to focus on distant objects, and higher power focuses on near objects. This focusing process is called accommodation and can compensate for imbalances in the refractive powers of other parts of the eye. However, as we age, the lens stiffens and begins to lose some of its near vision accommodative ability, a condition called presbyopia, or farsightedness.

Beyond the crystalline lens is the cavity of the eyeball, which is filled with a thick fluid called the **vitreous humor.** The shape of the cavity is formed by the crystalline lens and the interior of the eyeball. This fluid also affects refraction, depending on its composition and the presence of any dissolved substances.

FOCUSING ON THE RETINA

After light from an object passes through the cornea, aqueous humor, lens, and vitreous humor, to provide clear vision it must finally be focused on the **retina,** a layer of nerve tissue that coats the inside of the back of the eyeball.

The focused image registers on millions of retinal light receptors called cones and rods. **Cones** are sensitive to individual colors and enable you to see fine detail. **Rods** distinguish only black, white, and intermediate grays and enable you to see in dim light. The **macula** is the tissue in the central portion of the retina that distinguishes fine detail at the center of the field of vision. The image produced on the retina is transmitted via the optic nerve to the brain, where the images are interpreted.

Most vision problems are caused by errors of refraction, that is, abnormalities in the bending of light in the eye. Such problems can usually be corrected with eyeglasses or contact lenses. More complex are problems resulting from damage, dysfunction, or degeneration of eye structures critical to vision, such as the lens, retina, macula, and vitreous humor.

HOW THE EARS WORK

The ear is composed of three general areas: the outer, middle, and inner ear. They work together to convert sound waves into electrical signals that the brain translates into sound. The ear also plays a critical role in maintaining balance, through the labyrinth deep within it.

THE OUTER EAR

The **outer ear,** also known as the **auricle,** gathers sound waves from the surrounding air. It is composed of the external visible ear, also called the **pinna,** and the **auditory canal,** a half-inch-long passage that leads from the external ear to the eardrum. The opening of the auditory canal is surrounded by skin containing wax-producing glands and hairs.

THE MIDDLE EAR

The **eardrum,** or **tympanic membrane,** is a thin, flexible barrier between the outer and middle ear. When sound waves reach the eardrum, it begins to vibrate and sets up a chain reaction in three small bones, collectively known as the **ossicles,** in the middle ear. Based on their respective shapes, these bones are known as the **hammer** or **malleus,** the **anvil** or **incus,** and the **stirrup** or **stapes.** The stirrup, the smallest bone in the human body, fits into the **oval window,** the opening to the inner ear. The hammer is attached to the inner lining of the eardrum. The anvil is attached to, and located between, the hammer and stirrup. Vibrations from the eardrum pass through these bones and into the fluid that fills the inner ear.

In addition to the oval window, there are other openings in the middle ear. One leads into the air spaces in the **mastoid** region of the temporal bone. This region contains all of the internal areas of the ear. Another leads to the **eustachian tube,** which extends to the cavity at the back of the nose. The eustachian tube plays an important role in maintaining normal air pressure in the middle ear. When the tube is blocked by nasal congestion, pressure can build in the ear. When the blockage clears, you may feel a popping sensation due to the sudden change in ear pressure.

THE INNER EAR

When the stirrup moves, fluid in the inner ear carries the vibrations into the canal of the **cochlea,** a delicate snail-shaped structure. More than 20,000 individual hair cells are inside the cochlea. Movement of the cochlear fluid bends these hair cells, stimulating them to generate electrical impulses. These impulses are then transported via the **auditory nerve** to the brain, where they are interpreted as sound.

Also in the inner ear is the **labyrinth,** the part of the inner ear involved in helping us maintain balance. It consists of three fluid-filled, arcing tubes located at right angles to each other, called **semicircular canals.** The auditory nerve is attached to the labyrinth, sending information on the position and movement of your head to the brain. Information from the labyrinth is combined with data from your eyes, arms and legs, and muscles to maintain balance.

Problems in the external or middle ear can impair the conduction of sound waves and may cause conductive hearing loss, disorders that are most amenable to treatment or the benefits of hearing aids. Problems in the cochlea or auditory nerve are called sensorineural hearing loss and are more difficult to solve. Some people with sensorineural problems can hear sound but may not be able to understand what they hear. Others hear no sound at all. However, new cochlear implants have been able to provide useful sound even for those who are profoundly deaf. A problem in the brain that impairs hearing is called central deafness and poses even greater challenges.

SYMPTOMS AND SOLUTIONS

BLURRINESS AND OTHER VISION ABNORMALITIES

If the images you see are not sharp but, rather, fuzzy around the edges, that is called blurred vision. It is a very vague symptom that may signal a wide variety of problems, from minor to vision threatening, depending on the circumstances and accompanying symptoms.

Causes and Treatment of Blurriness and Other Vision Abnormalities
Most cases of blurred vision are caused by errors of refraction, such as **astigmatism** (page 309) or **farsightedness** or **nearsightedness** (page 316). This explanation is most likely if the blurred vision develops slowly, is not accompanied by any symptoms other than achiness or tension around the eyes, and only affects either your distant or near vision. If your eye doctor confirms your supposition, you simply need corrective lenses.

If gradual blurred vision only affects your central vision and you can still see clearly with your side vision, it could be **macular degeneration** (page

If you have sudden blurred vision accompanied by seeing colored halos around lights, tearing, severe eye pain, and vomiting, you may have acute **glaucoma** (page 317). If blurred vision in one eye occurs suddenly, alone with vision distortion, or seeing sudden light flashes or an increase in floaters—dark spots in your visual field—it could be **retinal detachment** (page 322). In either case, you need emergency medical care.

• Call your doctor for instructions. Make it clear to whoever answers the doctor's phone that **this is an emergency.**
• If you can't reach your doctor immediately, go directly to a hospital emergency room.
• Take no medication unless it was previously prescribed and is urgently needed or you are told to do so by your physician or emergency medical personnel.

Most cases of blurred vision are far less severe. However, if you have any persistent blurring, call your physician. Describe what is happening so that the doctor can decide whether you should be seen immediately.

319), a condition more common in older people. You may have trouble reading as well as seeing distant objects. Although this is a progressive disorder, prompt laser therapy may be able to slow down central vision loss.

If you are over 60 years of age, the most common cause of gradual development of blurred vision is **cataracts** (page 310). Early cataracts may respond to corrective eyeglasses, contact lenses, or brighter light for reading. When cataracts reduce functional vision, surgery to remove the cloudy lens in the eye is recommended.

If your vision is blurred in only one eye and the eye is also bloodshot, teary, and light-sensitive, you may have a **corneal ulcer** (page 313). A corneal ulcer generally causes mild to severe eye pain and is more common in people who wear contact lenses or in the aftermath of an eye injury or infection. Get prompt medical care, which may prevent permanent corneal scarring and vision loss.

If blurred vision in one eye or both eyes is accompanied by difficulty in adjusting to seeing in the dark, you may have chronic **glaucoma** (page 317). You need prompt medical attention; special eye drops are generally prescribed to lower the pressure in your eyes.

Less commonly, blurred vision may be caused by swelling of the optic nerve due to some problem beyond the eye. For example, it may occur after a head injury and subsequent **brain damage** (page 57), or in conjunction with a **tumor** in the head (page 56), **hypertension** (page 27), or even pulmonary **emphysema** (page 89). In some cases, optic nerve swelling is caused by inflammation that may occur with a viral infection, a bee sting, or **multiple sclerosis** (page 64).

RED, ITCHY, OR PAINFUL EYES OR EYELIDS

Red, itchy, or painful eyes or eyelids are common complaints that may signal a wide variety of problems, from minor to vision threatening, depending on the circumstances and accompanying symptoms.

If you have sudden and severe eye pain accompanied by blurred vision and vomiting, you may have acute **glaucoma** (page 317). You need emergency medical care.

• Call your doctor for instructions. Make it clear to whoever answers the doctor's phone that **this is an emergency.**
• If you can't reach your doctor immediately, go directly to a hospital emergency room.
• Take no medication unless it was previously prescribed and is urgently needed or you are told to do so by your physician or emergency medical personnel.

Most cases of eye or eyelid pain or red, itchy eyes are far less severe. However, if you have any persistent eye discomfort that is not explained by the lifestyle factors discussed in this section or remedied in a day or two by the self-care guidelines described, call your physician. Describe what is happening so that the doctor can decide whether you should be seen immediately.

Causes and Treatment of Red, Itchy, or Painful Eyes or Eyelids
The most common cause of red, itchy, and achy eyes is fatigue. If you have been working long hours and not getting enough sleep, don't be surprised when many parts of your body, including your eyes, rebel and cause symp-

toms. Get a good night's sleep and your eyes will likely feel better in the morning.

Red eyes that feel gritty may also be caused by air pollution. Seek out an air-conditioned environment and rinse your eyes with cool water.

If your eyes are red and itchy, you may have allergic **conjunctivitis** (page 315). This is more likely in spring through fall if you have hay fever or other seasonal allergies. An antihistamine will help.

Many cases of red, itchy eyes are caused by **eye infections** (page 315). Conjunctivitis also causes burning eyes, a thin watery discharge, and a yellow crust that forms during sleep and causes eyelid stickiness. Sties cause a red to yellowish, itchy, painful sore that looks like a pimple at the edge of an eyelid. Some sties occur inside the lid, causing excessive tearing; you may feel as if you have a foreign object in your eye and the white part of the eye may become reddish. Blepharitis causes red, itchy, or stinging eyelid edges, a gritty sensation in the eye, a swollen eyelid, teary eyes, eye discharge, and, in the worst cases, tiny ulcers along the edge of the eyelid.

Minor eye infections should ease in a day or two with proper self-care. If yours doesn't, see an ophthalmologist, a physician who specializes in care of the eyes. Also head for professional care right away if redness and discharge are accompanied by pain, sensitivity to light, or any change in vision or reduction in the size of your pupils. You may have a **corneal ulcer** (page 313) or other more severe eye problem.

Pain that occurs only when moving the eyes may be due to inflammation of the optic nerve. This may be caused by **multiple sclerosis** (page 64), viral or bacterial infections, severe allergic reactions to bee stings, or diseases of the arteries in the brain. Prompt diagnosis and treatment of the underlying cause are essential.

DRY OR TEARY EYES

Dry eyes may cause a gritty, burning, or irritated sensation. In some cases you may not notice the dryness but, rather, teariness. When your eyes are too dry, they send signals to the brain, which increases tear production. As a result, tears may even drip out of your eyes.

If you have any persistent dry or teary eyes not explained by lifestyle factors and easily remedied, call your physician. Describe what is happening so that the doctor can decide whether you should be seen immediately.

Causes and Treatment of Dry or Teary Eyes

If you work at a computer terminal or at another job that causes you to stare for hours with minimal blinking, dry eyes are not uncommon. Try to take frequent breaks or at least stop staring and blink often. You can also ease your discomfort by using artificial tears, available at your pharmacy.

Dry eyes are often caused by an allergy to some eye medication you are using. Call your doctor to discuss the problem. A change in medication may be necessary.

Dry eyes may also be a symptom of a serious underlying illness, such as **rheumatoid arthritis** (page 121) or **systemic lupus erythematosus** (page 116). In such cases, the disorder is known as Sjögren's syndrome and is often accompanied by a less than normal amount of saliva and increased thirst. Treatment of the underlying disorder may or may not alleviate your dry eye problem. However, use of artificial tears, available at your pharmacy, can make you more comfortable.

Teary eyes may also be caused by an inflammation in the eye's tear sac due to an obstruction of the duct where tears normally leave the eyes. If teary eyes are not explained by one of these conditions, see your doctor. Minor obstructions may be resolved by applications of hot compresses. More severe ones may require a minor surgical procedure in the doctor's office to open the duct.

Although dry or teary eyes may also occur with aging in the absence of any disorder, only your eye doctor can make that determination.

CROSSED EYES

When one eye focuses properly but the other points inward, the condition is called crossed eyes. In some cases, the abnormal eye may point upward or to either side.

> Except during the first six months of life, both eyes should move in tandem. If yours or your child's do not, eye muscle dysfunction may be present. Call your physician. Describe what is happening so that the doctor can decide whether you should be seen immediately.

Causes and Treatment of Crossed Eyes

The medical term for this disorder is **strabismus** (page 323). Especially in children, it is usually due to an imbalance in muscles surrounding the eyes that can be corrected with special eyeglasses and exercises. Sometimes, if the condition does not improve, surgery may be necessary.

When abnormal eye movements occur suddenly in adults, a complete medical examination is necessary. The problem could be caused by an underlying condition, such as **diabetes** (page 244), **stroke** (page 71), **multiple sclerosis** (page 64), or **muscular dystrophy** (page 117).

LIGHT SENSITIVITY

Light sensitivity is also called photosensitivity or photophobia. If you find yourself squinting or turning away from bright light, whether from the sun or artificial light, or if you experience any eye pain when in bright light, you may have light sensitivity.

If you have sudden light sensitivity accompanied by blurred vision, severe eye pain, or vomiting, you may have acute **glaucoma** (page 317) and need emergency medical care.

• Call your doctor for instructions. Make it clear to whoever answers the doctor's phone that **this is an emergency.**
• If you can't reach your doctor immediately, go directly to a hospital emergency room.
• Take no medication unless it was previously prescribed and is urgently needed or you are told to do so by your physician or emergency medical personnel.

Most cases of light sensitivity are far less severe. However, if you have any photophobia, call your physician. Describe what is happening so that the doctor can decide whether you should be seen immediately.

Causes and Treatment of Light Sensitivity

Light sensitivity may be a symptom of **eye infection** (page 315). If an infection doesn't respond to self-care within a day or two, call your doctor. Also call your doctor right away if light sensitivity and eye infection symptoms are accompanied by pain or any change in vision or reduction in the size of your pupils. You may have a **corneal ulcer** (page 313) or other more severe eye problem.

If you currently have a cold sore, or have had such sores in the past, signs of eye infection and light sensitivity may signal a **herpes type 1** (page 278) infection that has affected your eye. You need medical care to help avoid permanent eye damage.

Rarely, light sensitivity may be caused by albinism, a rare inherited disorder that affects production of melanin, the sun-protective pigment. Albinism is likely to be diagnosed in infancy because those affected have pinkish eyes and very pale skin.

Light sensitivity accompanied by pain and redness of the eye may be caused by an inflammation called iritis that affects the inside of the eye. Although you need prompt care from an ophthalmologist, a more complete evaluation may be indicated. In about 40 percent of cases, iritis occurs in conjunction with a systemic disease, such as **ankylosing spondylitis** (page 110) or juvenile **rheumatoid arthritis** (page 121).

NIGHT BLINDNESS

Night blindness does not mean total loss of vision at night but, rather, a minor to major inability to see well in dim lighting. We all need at least a few minutes for our eyes to adjust when entering a darkened room. However, some people are relatively unable to make such vision adjustments and find it impossible, for example, to drive at night.

> If you have increasing difficulty seeing in dim lighting, call your physician. Describe what is happening so that the doctor can decide whether you should be seen immediately.

Causes and Treatment of Night Blindness

Greater difficulty seeing in dim light can be one of the early signs of **cataracts** (page 310). However, if your vision is not impaired in other situations and you do not need to drive at night, you may not need surgery.

Another cause of night blindness is a deficiency of vitamin A, which may arise from a poor diet, certain digestive disorders, or **cirrhosis** (page 191). If an underlying cause can be identified and treated with diet changes or medications, the night blindness will likely disappear.

Rarely, night blindness may be caused by certain untreatable genetic disorders, such as retinitis pigmentosa.

BLINDNESS

Blindness can occur at any time in life, from birth through old age. Because blindness most often develops slowly, regular medical eye examinations are essential to detect treatable causes of vision loss.

If you have sudden vision loss, especially after an accident that has caused head trauma, you may have **retinal detachment** (page 322) or some type of **brain damage** (page 57). If sudden vision loss is accompanied by severe eye pain, it could be acute **glaucoma** (page 317). All of these conditions need emergency medical care.

• Call your doctor for instructions. Make it clear to whoever answers the doctor's phone that **this is an emergency.**
• If you can't reach your doctor immediately, go directly to a hospital emergency room.
• Take no medication unless it was previously prescribed and is urgently needed or you are told to do so by your physician or emergency medical personnel.

Most types of vision loss start gradually. However, any noticeable vision loss should prompt a call to your physician. Describe what is happening so that the doctor can decide whether you should be seen immediately.

Causes and Treatment of Blindness

Accidents that cause eye injury are a significant cause of blindness. The most common injury is getting a foreign object in the eye. Removal of any foreign object—other than a speck of dust or other tiny material that floats in tears and is easily removed with a tissue or by tearing—should be left to a physician. If you can't reach an ophthalmologist immediately after an eye injury, go to a hospital emergency room for prompt care.

The best approach to accidents is prevention. Safety lenses of shatter-resistant glass or plastic should be used in all eyewear. Special protective lenses should be used for all sports and jobs that carry the risk of eye injuries. Children should be warned of the dangers of pointed sticks, BB guns, bows and arrows, pop-up toys, and fireworks.

Diabetes (page 244) is a leading cause of blindness. It acts primarily through a disorder called proliferative retinopathy, in which abnormal tiny blood vessels in the retina break and cause hemorrhages. Maintaining good·

control of your blood glucose levels can help prevent the development of retinopathy. When retinopathy is diagnosed early, blindness may be prevented through laser surgery.

Glaucoma (page 317), which has been called "the sneak thief of sight" because it has few warning signs, is another prevalent cause of blindness. Because chronic glaucoma is a painless eye disease, you already may have suffered permanent eye damage by the time vision loss is noticed. However, if chronic or acute glaucoma is diagnosed promptly, blindness may be prevented through daily use of eye drops or, in some cases, by surgery.

Cataracts (page 310) were once a leading cause of blindness in the elderly. However, removal of the cloudy lenses is one of the most successful surgeries performed. Intraocular implant lenses have largely replaced cataract glasses and contacts and can ensure excellent vision.

Macular degeneration (page 319) continues to be a significant cause of legal blindness among older people. Although all vision is not lost, because only central vision is damaged, your ability to read and do close work is impaired. However, you may be able to function reasonably well with side vision.

Although **eye infections** (page 315) once used to be a major cause of vision loss, most can be cured without causing permanent eye damage if diagnosed promptly. The condition is best prevented by avoiding contact with people who have a contagious eye infection. If you wear contact lenses, carefully follow professional instructions for daily lens cleaning and sterilization.

EARACHES

Any ache or pain within or around the ear may be called an earache. Earaches are especially common in babies and young children. Because children's eustachian tubes are relatively short compared with those of adults, it is easier for respiratory infections to reach the ear. Babies who are unable to talk may indicate the presence of an earache by showing irritability and by pulling or rubbing their ears.

Causes and Treatment of Earaches

The most common cause of earaches is **ear infection** (page 313). The pain of outer ear infection tends to be worsened by head movement. Infection also may provoke itching in the ear and, possibly, a yellow or greenish discharge. Middle ear infection produces severe stabbing ear pain and even temporary hearing loss; these symptoms may be accompanied by fever and,

If you develop a throbbing ear pain within a few weeks after having had a middle ear infection, you may have mastoiditis, the most severe type of **ear infection** (page 313). You need emergency medical care.

• Call your doctor for instructions. Make it clear to whoever answers the doctor's phone that **this is an emergency.**
• If you can't reach your doctor immediately, go directly to a hospital emergency room.
• Take no medication unless it was previously prescribed and is urgently needed or you are told to do so by your physician or emergency medical personnel.

Most types of earaches are far less severe. However, all earaches should prompt a call to your physician. Describe what is happening so that the doctor can decide whether you should be seen immediately.

in a baby, nausea and vomiting. Mastoiditis can occur after middle ear infection, causing throbbing pain, discharge, and hearing loss. Antibiotics are needed to cure bacterial infections, as well as to prevent secondary bacterial infections in ear problems caused by viruses.

Earaches may be caused by **allergic rhinitis** (page 84), if nasal congestion builds up and backs into the eustachian tubes. If an antihistamine does not ease the problem, you may have an ear infection.

A buildup of earwax can sometimes cause earaches. Your doctor can remove the wax with warm water and show you how to do it yourself if the problem recurs.

If your doctor finds nothing wrong with your ears, you may be urged to see your dentist, because earaches may be caused by the spread of pain from dental decay or a nerve dying in a tooth.

TINNITUS

Tinnitus is the medical name for any persistent noise heard within the head, either constant or intermittent. The sound may be described as a ringing, buzzing, roaring, or whistling in one or both ears, or it may vary in tone from a soft buzz to a high squeal. Although tinnitus is most often a minor though annoying distraction, it can be severe enough to interfere with normal activities.

If you experience any abnormal sounds in your ears, call your physician. Describe what is happening so that the doctor can decide whether you should be seen immediately.

Causes and Treatment of Tinnitus

A buildup of earwax can sometimes cause tinnitus. Your doctor can remove the wax with warm water and show you how to do it yourself if the problem recurs.

Another common cause of tinnitus can be high doses of certain drugs, especially aspirin, antibiotics in the "mycin" family, antimalarial drugs, and some tranquilizers and antihypertensive drugs. If you are taking such medications, call your doctor for advice. A change in dosage or a switch to a substitute medication will usually alleviate the problem, although some drugs can cause deafness.

Ear infections (page 313) also can cause tinnitus. Prompt treatment, usually with antibiotics, will cure the infections and should banish the sound in your ears. However, in some cases, an infection can cause permanent ear damage and leave you with untreatable tinnitus.

Less commonly, tinnitus may be caused by **otosclerosis** (page 321), the growth of spongy bone in the middle ear. Sometimes surgery can correct the problem.

If ringing in the ears is followed by dizziness, nausea, and hearing loss, you may have **Meniere's disease** (page 320). Tinnitus can be an early warning sign for you to take prescribed medications to prevent the dizziness attacks of this disorder.

A variety of non-ear disorders can also cause tinnitus. These include **allergic rhinitis** (page 84), **hypertension** (page 27), **diabetes** (page 244), **hyperthyroidism** (page 248), **brain cancer** (page 56), and **brain damage** (page 57) due to head trauma. Treatment of the underlying disease may or may not banish tinnitus.

The most common cause of tinnitus is noise trauma that damages nerves in the inner ear. This may occur slowly, over many years, due to moderate noise exposure, contributing to the higher incidence of tinnitus in older people. Many ear doctors worry that young people who attend high-volume rock concerts or who listen to music at high volume with earphones will be at greater risk of deafness as they age. Deafness may also occur suddenly due to severe noise exposure. Such damage is likely to be permanent, as is tinnitus.

Living with tinnitus may be made easier by some modest lifestyle adjustments. Most people find that the ear sounds are more noticeable when you are in a quiet room. Competing sound—a radio playing softly or a white sound machine—makes tinnitus less noticeable. Some people are helped by a special tinnitus masker, a small electronic device worn in the ear that generates a low but pleasant sound to mask tinnitus. If your tinnitus is aggravated by tension, learning relaxation techniques may help avoid or reduce the intensity of the sound. If you have impaired hearing, a hearing aid may reduce or eliminate your tinnitus.

To help prevent a worsening of tinnitus, avoid noise exposure. Wear earplugs in noisy situations. Don't wear stereo headsets. Avoid nerve stimulants such as caffeine and nicotine. Take steps to enhance your circulation through daily exercise, a healthy diet, and adequate sleep.

HEARING LOSS

Anyone at any age can suffer from total or partial hearing loss that makes it difficult or impossible to understand what people are saying or to learn speech if the loss occurs at an early age. Unfortunately, nearly 70 percent of those with hearing impairment do not get help, although a hearing aid and/or surgery or medical treatment might restore or stabilize their hearing.

If you experience any hearing loss, call your physician. Describe what is happening so that the doctor can decide whether you should be seen immediately.

Causes and Treatment of Hearing Loss

Aging is the most common cause of hearing loss, but the degree of loss varies greatly from person to person and affects men more than women. Presbycusis, a type of sensorineural hearing loss, occurs in the elderly due to deterioration of the tiny hair cells of the inner ear. These cells send electrical sound impulses to the brain, where sounds are received and processed. Excessive noise in the environment or accidents can cause similar damage.

When hearing loss occurs in infancy, it may be due to heredity or to a birth defect caused by maternal illness or medication taken by the mother during pregnancy. Such hearing damage is not reversible but, depending on the extent of the loss, may be helped by a hearing aid.

A major cause of hearing loss in children is disease, such as the complications of **childhood diseases** (page 264), including chickenpox, mumps, or measles, or **ear infections** (page 313) that are not promptly treated.

Gradual hearing loss that starts between the ages of 20 and 40 may be caused by **otosclerosis** (page 321), a degeneration of the ear bone. In some cases, surgery may be able to remedy the problem; others may be helped by a hearing aid.

If hearing problems are left untreated, particularly in children, speech, reading, behavioral, and learning problems may occur. Sometimes medical treatment or surgery can completely restore normal hearing. In other instances, a hearing aid and/or audiologic rehabilitation (including auditory training and lipreading) may be needed. If a hearing aid is necessary, it should be selected and fitted by a health professional, not a salesperson. Commercial vendors are not trained to identify the causes of hearing loss—some of which can be life threatening if ignored.

DIZZINESS

Many people think of dizziness as signaling a problem in the brain, and that may be the case sometimes. But vision, touch, hearing, and the vestibular system in the ear all contribute to helping you maintain your orientation in space, and damage to any of these senses can cause various types of dizziness.

If you experience any persistent or recurrent dizziness that is not explained by the lifestyle factors discussed in this section and easily remedied, call your physician. Describe what is happening so that the doctor can decide whether you should be seen immediately.

Causes and Treatment of Dizziness

When dizziness occurs, it is important to define clearly what you are feeling because the sensations are a critical diagnostic clue. Doctors divide dizziness into four general categories.

True vertigo involves an illusion of motion and is one of the most uncomfortable types of dizziness, often provoking nausea and vomiting. You feel as if you are spinning or that the room is spinning. Vertigo is most likely to be vestibular, coming from the inner ear, the nerve connecting it to the brain, or the brain itself.

Motion sickness can cause vertigo due to vestibular imbalance in the inner ear. You can try to override its messages with other senses. In a car, sit in the front seat and focus you eyes on a point on the horizon. Better yet, if you know you are prone to motion sickness, get prescription medication from your doctor to prevent the problem before any trip.

Labyrinthitis, an inner **ear infection** (page 313), is the classic cause of vertigo. This disorder usually develops during a cold or other upper respiratory infection. Your doctor can give you medications to ease the nausea and, if necessary, antibiotics for bacterial infections.

Less severe vertigo may occasionally be caused by **allergic rhinitis** (page 84), which causes severe nasal congestion and blocks the eustachian tubes. Decongestants should solve the problem.

A frequent cause of vertigo can be high doses of drugs toxic to the inner ear, such as aspirin, antimalarial medications, certain "mycin" antibiotics, and some tranquilizers and antihypertensive drugs. Tinnitus usually precedes the vertigo. Even modest overuse of other drugs, such as alcohol, sedatives, narcotics, or anticonvulsants, may cause vertigo. If you are taking such medications, call your doctor for advice. A change in dosage or a switch to a substitute medication will promptly alleviate the problem. If you are drinking enough to cause vertigo, you should stop.

Meniere's disease (page 320) can cause vertigo, tinnitus, and hearing loss. Attacks may last from days to weeks. Women are slightly more prone to the problem than men, and it usually begins in young adulthood. Treatment is aimed at reducing fluids in the labyrinth, which may lessen the frequency and severity of attacks. Drugs that reduce nausea are helpful.

Trauma, such as a blow to the head, can damage the inner ear or the nerve leading to the brain and cause instant vertigo that lasts for weeks until healing is complete. A relatively rare and surgically curable tumor in that nerve may also cause the problem.

More serious causes of vertigo derive from the brain and include vascular diseases that can precipitate **stroke** (page 71) and, less commonly, **multiple sclerosis** (page 64).

A second type of dizziness is a lightheadedness that makes you feel as if you might faint. Also known as near syncope, this symptom is caused by a decrease in blood pressure or some other cause of decreased blood flow to the brain.

Most people experience this type of dizziness at one time or another. One possible cause is dehydration due to excessive dieting or heavy sweating because of exercise or viral illness. Drinking fluids, especially salty ones such as soup, can restore blood volume and eliminate your dizziness.

Orthostatic **hypotension** (page 29), a drop in blood pressure upon standing up, is a classic cause of faintness. It may occur in younger people who have been confined to bed for a few days, but it should quickly vanish. The condition is more common in older people who have circulatory difficulties or who are taking antihypertensive medication. They must learn to get up from bed slowly, sitting at the side of the bed for a minute or two before standing. Such faintness can also be a warning sign of **heart valve disease** (page 22) or **arrhythmias** (page 16), which warrant immediate medical attention.

People under great stress may experience a type of fainting called vasovagal syndrome. This happens when blood is suddenly pooled somewhere in the body, decreasing the supply to the brain. People with this syndrome know they have a tendency to faint and usually feel warning signs, such as sweating or a little nausea. No medication can help. Lie down right away, before you fall down, so that blood can get back to your head. Don't put your head between your knees because, if you do faint, you could fall on your head and cause injury.

Another type of dizziness is a disequilibrium called dizziness of the feet. The unsteady feeling is comparable to the sensation experienced by people who wear reading glasses, take them off suddenly, and feel as if they might fall. The problem usually stems from a neurologic abnormality, such as a tumor or degenerative disorder. It warrants prompt medical attention. A drug such as alcohol or the anticonvulsant dilantin may also be at the root of the problem.

The last category is a poorly defined lightheadedness that people usually cannot clearly describe in any way other than to say that they are dizzy. Such dizziness often derives from anxiety or other psychological causes. It may occur in conjunction with hyperventilation, the single most common cause of dizziness. Under stress, you breathe more rapidly or deeply, taking in too much oxygen and disturbing your body's normal oxygen–carbon dioxide balance. Rebreathing into a paper bag can provide a quick solution. If you frequently have problems with this type of dizziness and your physician finds no underlying physical problems, it may be wise to consult a psychotherapist.

COMMON DISORDERS OF THE EYES AND EARS

ASTIGMATISM is an error of refraction—the bending of light inside the eye—that impairs normal vision. Although it rarely worsens with age, the development of nearsightedness, farsightedness, or other vision problems may make astigmatism more noticeable.

What are the symptoms?
The most common sign of astigmatism is blurred vision. In addition, you may have eye strain, such as achiness or tension around the eyes, and headaches, especially when you read for long periods.

How did I get it?
Astigmatism is caused by different curvatures of the cornea, the transparent membrane covering the front of the eye. As a result of these differences, light entering the eyes does not focus directly on the retina simultaneously. This improper focusing damages your ability to see sharply. The condition is most often genetic.

How is it diagnosed?
Astigmatism is diagnosed during a standard eye examination. First you read an eye chart, and then the eye doctor measures the curvature of the cornea with an instrument called a keratometer. In addition, a retinoscope is used to evaluate the degree of astigmatism and to determine the types of corrective lenses that are necessary.

How is it treated?
Astigmatism is completely correctable with lenses that properly focus light rays on the retina. Such lenses may be worn as eyeglasses or contact lenses.

Self-Care: For comfortable vision, wear your corrective lenses at all times, especially when performing tasks that require clear vision.

CATARACTS are a loss of clarity or transparency in the lens of the eye. If not treated, this loss can lead to blindness. Indeed, cataracts are one of the world's leading causes of blindness. However, surgery and lens replacement can now ensure continued clear vision for those who have cataracts.

What are the symptoms?
In the normal eye, the lens is so clear that you don't even know it is there. With age, it yellows somewhat and vision becomes slightly hazy. In some people, the changes are so severe that the lens gets cloudy, hindering the passage of light rays through it. Vision begins to fail, becoming dimmed or

blurred. Eventually, the lens may become completely opaque, causing blindness.

How did I get it?

Although aging is the most common cause of cataracts, they can occur at any time of life, even in babies. Physical injury and certain illnesses such as diabetes can promote their development. Cataracts also seem to run in some families. If you develop a cataract in one eye, you are more likely to develop it in the other eye later.

How is it diagnosed?

Cataracts can be detected by an eye doctor during a regular vision checkup using a slit lamp biomicroscope. This is a painless procedure that does not involve any contact with your eyes. The slit lamp biomicroscope simply makes eye structures appear larger for thorough examination.

How is it treated?

The size, location, and density of the cataract determine the extent of the vision loss. Cataracts usually develop slowly. Some people have such a mild cataract that they never need treatment. For others, who experience only minor blurring, a change in eyeglasses may be sufficient. In still others, surgery is essential to restore normal functional vision. Surgery to remove the cloudy lens is indicated when your vision is so impaired that corrective lenses are of no benefit and vision loss interferes with your ability to function in normal daily life. Once the lens has been surgically removed, the eye cannot focus normally. To restore normal vision, most ophthalmologists recommend the implantation of intraocular lenses as part of the surgical procedure. If for some reason you are unable to have implanted lenses, there are two other options. Cataract eyeglasses are the oldest and least expensive choice but they have rather thick lenses. They limit side vision and make objects look larger than normal. They can also cause difficulties for those who have had cataract surgery in only one eye, yielding different images in each eye. Another option is special contact lenses, which may be standard daily-wear lenses or extended-wear lenses that may be worn for a month or more without changing.

Self-Care: Cataract surgery is usually an outpatient procedure performed in an ambulatory surgical center. If you are having cataract surgery, make sure a friend is available to pick you up and take you home. Depending on the procedure and implant used, normal vision should be restored within a few weeks to two months.

COLOR BLINDNESS means that you are unable to distinguish between certain colors, sometimes only in poor light situations. The condition rarely causes a total loss of color vision. Many more men than women are affected.

What are the symptoms?
Symptoms depend on the type of color blindness. Most cases involve an inability to distinguish reds and greens in dim light, especially in their pastel tones; such people have no problem with color discernment in normal light. Some people can't distinguish these hues even in normal light. Others with color blindness can't distinguish between greens and blues.

How did I get it?
People with color blindness have a defect in the cone cells in the retina that perceive light and color. Usually, the disorder is inherited and present at birth. In some cases, however, color blindness develops in adults and may be caused by such diverse problems as some type of poisoning, glaucoma, retinal detachment, or an underlying illness such as diabetes or hypertension.

How is it diagnosed?
If the color blindness is severe, you may realize it yourself, or family members may suspect that something is wrong, for example, when you wear bizarre color combinations. Color blindness can be diagnosed by an eye doctor during a comprehensive vision checkup. The eye doctor uses pictures filled with multicolored dots; within the field of dots are numbers or pictures created with particular colors. How well you discern them will measure your ability to distinguish colors.

How is it treated?
There is no cure for color blindness, and no glasses will enable you to see the colors your cones can't perceive. If the vision problem is caused by an underlying disease, its treatment can usually halt but not reverse the damage.

Self-Care: The greatest problem is discerning the color of traffic lights when driving or crossing streets. Learn to follow other cues, such as watching traffic flow, in such situations. To avoid wearing bizarre color combinations, take a friend along when you go clothes shopping and get help lining clothes up in your closet with matching items adjacent.

CORNEAL ULCER is an opening in the transparent membrane that covers the front of the eye.

What are the symptoms?
The affected eye will be bloodshot, teary, and sensitive to bright light. In addition, you may have blurred vision and mild to severe eye pain.

How did I get it?
Most corneal ulcers are caused by eye injuries that give bacteria an opportunity to infect the eye. However, they are also common in people who wear contact lenses, especially extended-wear lenses that are not adequately cleaned. Some corneal ulcers are caused by viruses, especially herpes viruses, or fungi.

How is it diagnosed?
Your doctor can diagnose a corneal ulcer by examining the eye with a special microscope that directs a strong light beam into the eyes. In addition, a sample of tissue from the affected area or eye fluid may be taken for laboratory study to identify the infectious organism.

How is it treated?
Eye drops or ointments containing prescription medication are prescribed and may be needed for one to three weeks to cure the infection. If the condition has not been diagnosed and treated promptly, corneal scars can cause severe loss of vision. If such damage has occurred, a surgical corneal transplant may be needed.

> Self-Care: If you wear contact lenses, clean them scrupulously. If you experience any eye discomfort, remove the lenses immediately and call your ophthalmologist for an appointment. Wear protective lenses during sports or work whenever eye injury is a possibility.

EAR INFECTIONS may arise in the inner, middle, or outer ear and are called, respectively, labyrinthitis, otitis media, and otitis externa. Middle ear infections are among the most common illnesses in young children and can lead to eardrum rupture and hearing loss. Prompt diagnosis and treatment are essential. Mastoiditis—an abscess in the spongy sections of the temporal bones of the skull near the ears—is a most serious type of ear infection; if it spreads to the bloodstream, it can be fatal.

What are the symptoms?

Outer ear infections tend to cause itching in the ear; there may be a yellow or greenish discharge and ear pain that is worsened by head movement. Middle ear infections produce severe stabbing ear pain and even temporary hearing loss; they may be accompanied by fever and, in a baby, nausea and vomiting. If the eardrum ruptures due to pressure from fluid buildup, there may be a discharge of blood or pus. Inner ear infections cause severe vertigo, balance problems, nausea, vomiting, and possible temporary hearing loss. Mastoiditis causes throbbing pain that arises after a middle ear infection, as well as a discharge and hearing loss.

How did I get it?

Ears are common infection sites because they provide a moist, warm environment in which bacteria and viruses can thrive. Ear infections may be caused by cold and flu viruses that spread to the ear, by bacterial invasion such as occurs in swimmers, or less commonly, by fungi. Chronic middle ear infections may be caused by stubborn bacterial infection or problems with the eustachian tube or adenoids, lymph tissue behind the nose. Mastoiditis usually results from the spread of a bacterial middle ear infection.

How is it diagnosed?

Your doctor can diagnose ear infections based on your symptoms and ear examination with an otoscope. If a discharge is present, a sample may be sent for laboratory evaluation. When symptoms of inner ear infections occur, a complete physical examination and blood tests may also be performed to rule out other diseases that may be causing the dizziness.

How is it treated?

Viral infections usually clear up on their own. Antibiotics may be prescribed to prevent secondary bacterial infections or cure primary ones. Fungal infections are more difficult to treat and may require months of ear drops or creams. Prescription ear drops also may be given for outer ear infections, and the doctor may clean the ear canal and suction out pus. Decongestants and antihistamines may be needed to relieve the pressure from fluids in the eustachian tube for middle ear infections. In some instances, if middle ear infections have not responded to several antibiotics, the doctor may make a tiny incision in the eardrum to drain pus, a procedure called myringotomy. Inner ear infections may also require medications to alleviate nausea and, in severe cases, surgery to drain the inner ear. Severe mastoiditis may require hospitalization and intravenous antibiotics and, rarely, surgery to hollow out the spongy bone mass.

> Self-Care: Ease earaches with a heating pad or warm compresses as well as acetaminophen. Keep the ear as dry as possible by wearing a bathing cap when swimming or showering. If water gets in your ear, dry it thoroughly. For inner ear infections, remaining quietly in bed in a dim room may decrease dizziness and nausea.

EYE INFECTIONS occur when one or more of the natural defenses of the eye breaks down and the eye is infected by a foreign organism. Eye infections range from simple problems you can self-treat to vision-threatening disorders that warrant immediate medical care. The most common eye infections are conjunctivitis or pink eye, an irritation of the membrane that lines the front of the eyeball and eyelid; sties or hordeolum, infections of oil glands at the base of an eyelash; and blepharitis, inflammation of the eyelids.

What are the symptoms?
Conjunctivitis causes red eyes that may itch and burn, as well as a thin watery discharge and a yellow crust that may form during sleep and cause eyelid stickiness upon awakening. A stye is a red to yellowish, itchy, painful sore that looks like a pimple at the edge of an eyelid. Some sties occur inside the lid, causing excessive tearing; you may feel as if you have a foreign object in your eye, and the white part of the eye may become reddish. Blepharitis can cause red, itchy, or stinging eyelid edges, a gritty sensation in the eye, a swollen eyelid, teary eyes, eye discharge, and, in the worst cases, tiny ulcers along the edge of the eyelid.

How did I get it?
Conjunctivitis is most commonly caused by viruses similar to those that cause colds, although it may occasionally be due to bacteria or allergic reactions. Viral conjunctivitis is highly contagious, spreading most commonly among schoolchildren. Most sties and blepharitis are caused by staphylococcal infections. Such infections may occur for no known reason or may be prompted by oily skin or chronically dirty skin. Milder cases of blepharitis may result from allergic reactions.

How is it diagnosed?
Most minor eye infections can be self-diagnosed based on their appearance, especially if the problem has occurred before. However, infections with a thick discharge may be bacterial and warrant medical attention. Your doctor can discern bacterial problems by taking a sample of the eye discharge for laboratory examination. Internal sties or any infection that doesn't respond to a day or two of self-care warrant medical attention; other more serious conditions can look like minor infections in their early stages.

How is it treated?
Self-care usually helps improve your comfort until minor eye infections, especially viral conditions, run their course. If medical attention is needed, antibiotic eye drops or ointments may be prescribed for bacterial conditions. In severe allergic reactions, corticosteroid eye drops may be prescribed. Internal sties may require lancing and antibiotic therapy.

> Self-Care: Warm, wet compresses applied every few hours for 5 to 15 minutes usually bring improvement in minor eye infections within a day or so. They usually bring external sties to a "head" to allow them to rupture and clear up. If an infection fills your eye with "goop," irrigate it away with a sterile eyewash. Add a teaspoon of salt to a quart of water, boil it for 5 minutes and allow it to cool thoroughly. Then tilt your head over the sink and pour the water over your eye. Avoid eyecups; they tend to transfer germs from the lid into the eye. Unless advised by a doctor, avoid over-the-counter products, such as boric acid and yellow mercuric oxide; they may mask symptoms and, therefore, delay your getting professional care when you need it.

FARSIGHTEDNESS and **NEARSIGHTEDNESS** are defects in the eyes' focusing mechanism. They are errors of refraction—the way light is bent inside the eye—that impairs vision. Nearsightedness is called myopia. Farsightedness is called hyperopia when it starts early in life; in this instance, the degree of farsightedness usually remains the same until middle age. Farsightedness is called presbyopia when it begins in middle age; this type usually worsens gradually with age until a plateau is reached later in life.

What are the symptoms?
In nearsightedness, you can see near objects with ease but have problems with distant vision. Depending on the degree of nearsightedness, you may have to hold a book close to your nose to avoid blurring or you may need

to sit in the front row in movie houses to see clearly. Younger people with mild farsightedness may have no symptoms because mechanisms in the eye accommodate to resolve the problem. In older individuals with higher degrees of farsightedness, there can be blurred vision at distance as well as at near, but you may have a particular problem with blurred vision, headaches, and eyestrain when reading.

How did I get it?
Nearsightedness and farsightedness that first become apparent in childhood are usually inherited. After the age of 40, as the lens of the eye hardens due to aging, its ability to focus on close objects decreases, causing the midlife farsightedness called presbyopia.

How is it diagnosed?
People who are or become farsighted can spot the signs themselves. For example, they notice that they tend to hold a book ever further away in order for the print to be clear enough to read. In children who are nearsighted, you may see the reverse problem, with the youngster always trying to get very close to what is being looked at. Your eye doctor can diagnose far- or nearsightedness easily during a routine eye checkup according to your difficulty with the eye chart.

How is it treated?
These conditions are easily treated with corrective lenses, which may be worn as eyeglasses or contact lenses. These lenses change the angle at which light enters the eye to ensure that it focuses properly on the retina.

Self-Care: If you have presbyopia, you may be able to use reading glasses available at low cost in many stores. These are not a wise choice if there are other conditions where corrective lenses should be tailored to your specific needs. In either case, you need a thorough examination from an eye doctor to determine what your condition is and to make sure your symptoms are not caused by some more serious disorder.

GLAUCOMA is an eye disease that afflicts more than a million Americans over the age of 35. It is the second leading cause of blindness in the United States. The disease involves abnormally increased pressure inside the eye (called intraocular pressure). When a normal amount of fluid is produced but too little drains away, intraocular pressure rises. As the pressure increases, it affects the nutrition and structure of the optic nerve and causes nerve damage. The speed at which this occurs varies from person to person. Some eyes lose sight within weeks. Others may take years to become damaged, and the symptoms during that time may be so minimal as to go unnoticed. The most common type is chronic (open-angle) glaucoma. Totally painless, it produces defects in the visual field. You can have chronic glaucoma for months or years before experiencing any difficulties. Less common is acute (angle-closure) glaucoma, where pressure builds in the eye very rapidly and creates a medical emergency. If glaucoma is diagnosed and treated promptly, blindness can usually be prevented.

What are the symptoms?

The subtle symptoms of chronic glaucoma include slightly blurred or fogged vision, a feeling that your glasses should be changed, difficulty adjusting to the dark, and eventually, the beginning of significant vision loss in your visual field. The striking symptoms of acute glaucoma include severe eye pain, blurring of vision, tearing, colored halos around bright lights, and vomiting.

How did I get it?

The causative factors leading to glaucoma are not fully understood. Although glaucoma sometimes develops as a result of injury or as a complication of some other eye disease, it usually strikes people whose eyes are healthy. The disorder often runs in families, especially when certain risk factors are present. Acute glaucoma often affects farsighted people, especially in middle age. In predisposed eyes, some medications used as cold remedies may dilate the pupils and produce an acute glaucoma attack.

How is it diagnosed?

Glaucoma is diagnosed by a simple test performed by your eye doctor. Called tonometry, it measures eye pressure.

How is it treated?

Usually, glaucoma is treated effectively by the use of one of several types of drops placed in the eye every day. These prescription drops regulate eye pressure. In some situations, surgery may be necessary, although it may not provide complete relief. Although lost vision cannot be restored, treatment with eye drops can prevent further vision loss.

Self-Care: Because glaucoma may be a "silent" disease, all those over age 35 should have a tonometry test periodically, as recommended by your eye doctor. Some people with special risk factors should have more frequent examinations. If you experience any severe eye pain that might signal acute glaucoma, go immediately to a hospital emergency room for treatment.

MACULAR DEGENERATION is the most common cause of legal blindness in the United States. It is a degenerative disease of the macula, tissue in the central portion of the retina, and most often strikes the elderly. Because the disorder usually develops very slowly and is painless, it can sneak up on a person who may not seek medical help until considerable vision has been lost. However, the diagnosis of macular degeneration must be made early to begin therapy and preserve maximal vision for as long as possible.

What are the symptoms?
When the macula is damaged or diseased, central vision begins to blur. You develop difficulty in reading small print, as well as seeing distant objects such as street signs. When both eyes are affected, reading and other activities requiring sharp vision eventually become impossible. However, because macular degeneration does not affect side vision, you may still be able to get around independently when you adjust to the condition.

How did I get it?
The cause of macular degeneration is unknown, although it may involve a hereditary predisposition. When the disease begins, small blood vessels may grow abnormally in the macular region between the retina and its supporting layer of tissue. The blood vessels may become narrowed and hardened, impairing the blood supply to the macula. If these vessels leak blood, the retinal cells that are responsible for central vision can be damaged. Almost invariably, both eyes are affected, either at the same time or sequentially.

How is it diagnosed?
Macular degeneration can be detected easily by your eye doctor as part of a regular checkup with a painless ophthalmoscope examination.

How is it treated?
Until recently, doctors could do little to help people with macular degeneration. However, in some cases, a laser beam can seal off newly formed

abnormal blood vessels. Such therapy can reduce or slow the pace of vision loss. However, to be successful, laser therapy must begin early in the course of the disease, preferably before symptoms appear.

> Self-Care: In the early stages of macular degeneration, magnifying glasses may be prescribed to help you read. Even if vision deteriorates markedly, special eyeglasses can help. If you completely lose your central vision, you can learn to function with your side vision, which is not affected by macular degeneration. However, you should contact your local association for the blind in order to get helpful counseling on everyday life with low vision.

MENIERE'S DISEASE is a disorder in the inner ear that causes severely uncomfortable attacks of vertigo, tinnitus, and hearing loss. It is more common in women than men and usually begins in midlife.

What are the symptoms?
Meniere's attacks usually begin with ringing in the ears and a sensation of fullness or pressure in one or both ears. Then severe vertigo, nausea, and vomiting occur. Attacks may also be accompanied by some hearing loss and migraine headaches. Attacks last from several hours to several days, and may recur weekly or monthly. You may be completely incapacitated during an attack.

How did I get it?
A rise in fluid in the labyrinth causes increased inner ear pressure and disrupts your sense of balance. Although doctors don't know what triggers the pressure buildup, it may be related to the degeneration of hair-like structures in the inner ear.

How is it diagnosed?
A complete examination is necessary to rule out other possible causes of your symptoms. Then an ear doctor performs a variety of hearing tests and ear evaluations. You may be asked to avoid drinking fluids or to take a diuretic for a period of time before a hearing test. In another examination, your ears are irrigated with water, and your subsequent eye movements are observed. In some cases, you may require electrocochleography, performed under general anesthesia, in which a probe is inserted through your eardrum to measure electrical activity.

How is it treated?
Your doctor may prescribe a low-salt diet and medications to reduce excess fluid in your body to help prevent attacks, as well as drugs to control vertigo and nausea when Meniere's hits. Because taking anything by mouth can be difficult or impossible during an attack, medications may be provided as a skin patch or suppository.

> Self-Care: Restricting your intake of fluid and salt may help reduce the frequency and severity of attacks. During attacks, you will be more comfortable staying in bed, as still as possible, in a darkened room.

OTOSCLEROSIS is a degeneration of the bones that conduct sound in the ear. It affects women more than men and can cause potentially permanent hearing loss. The composition of the ear bones changes from hard to spongy. The base of the stapes bone becomes fixed to the softened bone structure of the inner ear, preventing it from transmitting sound waves.

What are the symptoms?
Hearing loss develops gradually between the ages of 20 and 40, in the absence of any ear infections or other disorders that might cause the loss. It usually affects both ears.

How did I get it?
Otosclerosis is believed to be an inherited condition.

How is it diagnosed?
An ear doctor performs hearing tests to measure the degree of hearing loss and to assess whether the loss stems from conductive mechanical problems in your ears.

How is it treated?
At present, no medication seems to help otosclerosis. In some cases, one of two surgical procedures may be performed. In stapedectomy, the damaged stapes is removed and replaced with a metal prosthesis. In stapedotomy, a hole is made in the base of the stapes and a small prosthetic device is inserted. These procedures permit the vibration necessary for normal hearing. If you are not a candidate for these procedures, a hearing aid may help you hear better.

Self-Care: Be alert to signs of hearing loss throughout life. Take notice if friends or family complain that you turn the radio or TV on too loud or if you often do not understand what other people are saying. Such warning signs should prompt a visit to an ear doctor.

RETINAL DETACHMENT is partial separation of the retina from the back of the eye. Although it occurs most commonly in middle-aged and elderly people who are nearsighted, it can develop at any age. If not treated immediately, it can cause blindness.

What are the symptoms?
The most common warning signs are distortion of vision in one eye, blurring of vision in one eye, or seeing sudden light flashes or an increase in floaters, dark and irregularly shaped spots in your visual field. Floaters are most easily seen when looking at a clear sky or a pastel-painted wall.

How did I get it?
Retinal detachment may occur as a result of a blow to the head or an eye injury, but it may even result from a violent sneeze or for no apparent cause. Detachment is more common in people who are nearsighted and those with diabetes, hypertension, and sickle-cell anemia, as well as in boxers who suffer repeated head blows.

How is it diagnosed?
Your eye doctor can often diagnose retinal detachment by examining your eye with an ophthalmoscope. This may require an extensive evaluation using special lenses to discover retinal tears. In some cases, when it is impossible to see into the eye clearly, you may also need an ultrasound evaluation to determine the extent of the detachment.

How is it treated?
You must be hospitalized immediately and the extent of the retinal detachment assessed. In some instances, it is important to immobilize the head. Further therapy depends on the extent and nature of the detachment. Surgery is usually needed to drain fluid that may have accumulated behind the retina, as well as repair and reattach the retina. You will probably have to stay in the hospital about a week to make sure that healing progresses normally. You may be advised to avoid jarring exercise even after healing.

Self-Care: Because retinal detachment can cause blindness, get immediate medical care if you experience any sudden changes in vision.

If you can't reach your eye doctor right away, go to a hospital emergency room, preferably a hospital that specializes in eye problems.

STRABISMUS is a condition in which the eyes do not always move in parallel fashion. When one eye turns inward, the condition may be called crossed eyes. When one eye turns outward, the condition may be called wall-eyed. When the condition occurs in young children and is not properly treated, it may develop into amblyopia or lazy eye syndrome.

What are the symptoms?
One eye focuses on an object while the other is turned in another direction, either upwards, downwards, or to either side. You may also have double vision. Babies and young children with the problem frequently cover one eye or tilt their heads in an effort to see clearly.

How did I get it?
These disorders are caused by a dysfunction in the muscles that control eye movement. Babies normally gain full control over their eye muscles by about six months of age. In children, strabismus is most often due to an imbalance in the eye movement muscles. However, if left untreated, amblyopia may develop as the brain attempts to overcome the double vision by suppressing the messages sent by the weak eye. If this situation persists, the brain loses its ability to interpret information from the weak eye and its vision may be permanently lost. In adults, strabismus may be caused by simple loss of tone in the eye muscle or by some underlying muscular or nerve disorder, such as diabetes, stroke, multiple sclerosis, or muscular dystrophy.

How is it diagnosed?
Although the eye movement disorder is easily observed, your doctor will also do a complete physical examination to determine if any underlying disorder is causing the problem.

How is it treated?
If an underlying disease is found, its treatment can often alleviate the abnormal eye movements. If no such problem is found, you may be referred to an eye doctor for special glasses, a temporary eye patch over the strong eye, and training in eye exercises to strengthen the surrounding muscles. If these techniques fail, surgery may be performed to bring the eye muscles into better alignment.

Self-Care: Never assume that a youngster will grow out of abnormal eye movements. Any type of abnormal movements that persist beyond the first year of life should be called to an eye doctor's attention. If treatment is delayed until the school years, all vision in one eye may be lost. If vision training is prescribed, be sure to do your exercises at home as often as prescribed in order to regain normal muscle balance and control.

11

Skin and Hair Disorders

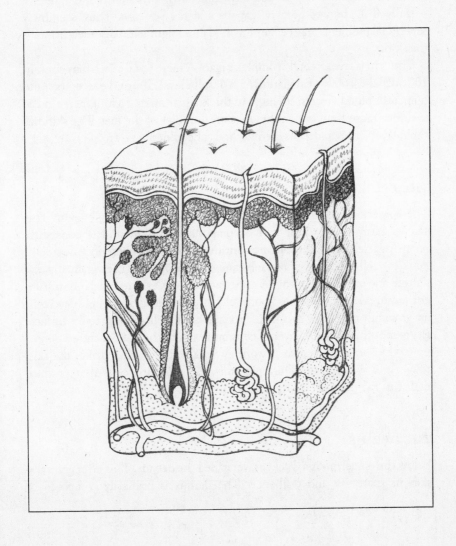

HOW THE SKIN AND HAIR WORK

The skin is one of the body's largest organs, weighing close to ten pounds in the average adult. The outer covering of our bodies, it holds organs and fluids within and protects us against invasion by germs and other hazards. The skin also helps regulate body temperature and maintain fluid balance in the body. It activates vitamin D upon exposure to the sun and is the body's center of touch sensation.

Although most skin disorders are minor, some can be quite serious. Skin problems may also be symptoms of more severe underlying illness. An abnormal complexion—the color, texture, and appearance of the skin—especially if it changes quickly, can be a sign of disease. Thus, seemingly superficial problems may be harbingers of more significant disorders beneath the skin.

The skin is an extremely complex organ. A mere square inch may contain 100 oil glands, 600 sweat glands, 65 hair follicles, 1,500 nerve receptors, and numerous blood vessels. It ranges in thickness from half a millimeter in the eyelid to more than two millimeters on the soles of the feet. The skin has three layers: the epidermis, dermis, and subcutaneous layer.

THE EPIDERMIS

The **epidermis** is the thin, semitransparent, outer covering of skin. This surface layer is the most active component of skin and is constantly renewing itself. Its inner cells are continually dividing to produce new cells. As these cells fill with a hard substance called **keratin,** they gradually die, flatten, and move up to form the upper surface of the skin, called the **stratum corneum.** As your body rubs against clothing or washcloths, these dead cells are gradually rubbed away, making room for new cells coming to the surface. Every month, an entire layer of cells moves from the base of the epidermis up to the surface, where it is worn away. Keratin is what makes the skin tough and waterproof. The epidermis also contains cells that produce **melanin,** the pigment that gives skin its color.

THE DERMIS

Below the epidermis is a thicker layer called the **dermis.** This layer gives the skin its elasticity and resilience. The dermis is primarily composed of

collagen, a fibrous protein that has been called the "glue" that holds the body together.

The upper dermis contains nerve receptors that send information about touch sensations to the brain. It also contains blood vessels that contract in cold weather to help conserve temperature in the core of the body and dilate in warm weather to get rid of body heat.

Deeper within the dermis are oil glands that help maintain skin moisture, sweat glands that produce perspiration to further aid in body cooling, muscle cells that produce shivering to help warm us when we are cold, and hair follicles. The lower level of the dermis is composed of connective fibers.

THE SUBCUTANEOUS LAYER

The lower or **subcutaneous** layer of skin is composed largely of fat, the amount of which varies throughout the body. The fat serves as an insulating layer, helps protect inner organs from injury, and is a source of reserve fuel for the body.

HAIR

Hair ranges from the small, fine hairs on the body that can barely be seen to the thicker, longer hairs found on the scalp and, in adults, under the arms and in the pubic area. Hair has important protective roles. Eyelashes help protect the eyes from foreign objects. Eyebrows help protect the eyes from sweat. Hair in the nose and ears filters out dust and other debris. Scalp hair provides cushioning against injury to the brain as well as insulation against cold.

Like the epidermis, the hair is composed of keratin. Hair is formed in the bulb of the hair follicle, where living cells continuously divide and push dead keratin cells to the surface. An erector muscle in each hair root responds to extreme cold or fear by contracting, causing the follicle to stiffen and the external hair to straighten—just as skin cells contract to cause the small bumps we call gooseflesh.

Hair grows cyclically; that is, any one hair may grow for months or years and then fall out. The follicle remains dormant for several months until it renews hair production. At any moment, each hair on the body may be in a different stage of this cycle. The result is that scalp hair generally grows about a half-inch each month.

The average person has about 100,000 hair follicles on the scalp and many more all over the body. Only the soles of the feet and palms of the hand have no hair follicles.

NAILS

Fingernails are produced by cells similar to those in the hair follicles. These cells are located under the cuticle at the base of each nail. Like the epidermis and hair, nails are composed of keratin.

SYMPTOMS AND SOLUTIONS

ITCHING

Itching skin can be an excruciating experience, and because it is difficult to avoid scratching, an "itch-scratch-itch" cycle can develop that may be difficult to halt.

> If you experience any persistent itching that cannot be explained by lifestyle causes discussed in this section, call your physician. Describe what is happening so that the doctor can decide whether you should be seen immediately.

Causes and Treatment of Itching

The most common cause of itching, without a rash or other skin lesion, is very dry skin. If you live in a dry climate or in a residence that is overheated, you tend to develop such dryness. Dry skin can be worsened—or caused—by frequent bathing or showering and the use of soap, all of which can strip skin of its natural oils. As we grow older, our skin produces less oil. If we continue daily baths or showers with plenty of soap, skin can become overly dry and itching can develop.

If you have itching in the absence of any rash or indication of other possible cause, consider buying a humidifier if your home is overheated. Also consider bathing less often. Wash with warm rather than hot water. Avoid deodorant soaps and others that may contain harsh chemicals. Choose a soap for dry skin. After bathing, pat your skin dry rather than rubbing it. Before you are totally dry, apply a light moisturizing lotion to your whole body.

If you develop itchy skin when you are wearing a new garment, or one that has just been washed in a new detergent, you may be having a mild reaction to the fabric or chemicals in the detergent. Wash the garment in a mild soap, and your itching is likely to disappear.

If neither dry skin nor irritation seems to be causing itching without a rash or other skin lesion, see your doctor for a complete checkup. Such itching also may arise from an underlying disease, such as a disorder of the blood, kidney, liver, or thyroid.

RASHES

Rashes can be caused by a wide range of problems, ranging from insect bites to serious diseases. The size, shape, and color of the rash, as well as whether or not it is hot to the touch or whether itching or pain is present, are all important factors in evaluating rashes.

If you develop **hives** (page 340), as well as a runny nose, wheezing, pale skin, and cold sweats, you may be having a life-threatening allergic or anaphylactic reaction.

- Call your doctor for instructions. Make it clear to whoever answers the doctor's phone that **this is an emergency.**
- If you can't reach your doctor immediately, go to a hospital emergency room by the fastest method—ambulance, car, or taxi. If possible, take someone with you. You may collapse on the way.
- Take nothing to eat or drink.
- Take no medication unless it was previously prescribed and is urgently needed or you are told to do so by your physician or emergency medical personnel.

Most rashes are far less severe. However, if you have any persistent rash that does not respond to self-care described in this section, call your physician. Describe what is happening so that the doctor can decide whether you should be seen immediately.

Causes and Treatment of Rashes

Rashes that occur in conjunction with fever usually signal an infectious disease (see Chapter 9).

Itchy rashes can be extraordinarily uncomfortable. **Hives** (page 340) are raised pink or red round lesions called wheals. They are hot and itchy and have flat tops. They range in size from a quarter of an inch to an inch and a half or longer. Because they are allergic skin disorders, taking an over-the-counter antihistamine can help speed hives away. If you have widespread or persistent hives, call your doctor.

Many itchy rashes are caused by fungal infections. If the eruption is between your toes, it is probably **athlete's foot** (page 336). Try over-the-counter topical antifungal agents—cream for dry eruptions or powder for wet ones. If you have no improvement within a week, call your doctor.

Other itchy fungal infections, also called **ringworm** (page 345), may arise elsewhere on the body as round, scaly lesions that are clear in the center. On the scalp, little bald patches reveal scaly skin. Toenails or fingernails may become yellow, thickened, and crumbly. See your doctor to confirm the diagnosis. Most such infections respond to topical antifungal agents. More severe infections may require oral drugs.

A persistent red, itchy rash that oozes and forms crusting lesions on the face and scalp of an infant may be **eczema** (page 339). In children and adults with eczema, the skin becomes brownish gray, dry, scaly, and thickened with symptoms more common in the elbow and behind-the-knee creases, face, neck, and upper chest. Itching is at its worst at night. Avoid over-the-counter creams and lotions because some may make your situation worse. Your doctor can prescribe medication to break the itch-scratch-itch cycle. Also learn to avoid the environmental factors—ranging from certain foods to wool clothing or temperature extremes—that are most likely to trigger your eruptions.

With **impetigo** (page 341), an itchy, red rash forms many small, itchy blisters. When the blisters break, pus may erupt and yellow crusts form. Impetigo is a bacterial skin infection that usually requires antibiotics for a cure. Never self-treat with an over-the-counter cortisone cream if you suspect impetigo. Until you can get to the doctor, cover the blisters with gauze and avoid infecting others.

If you have been exposed to **poison ivy, poison oak,** or **poison sumac** (page 343), you may develop a red, itchy rash that soon causes blisters that burst, oozing clear fluid, followed by crust formation and healing. Try to control the itching and swelling by applying an over-the-counter cortisone cream or calamine lotion. Call your doctor if the itching becomes unbearable; the rash becomes painful or oozes pus; the rash is extensive or near your mouth, eyes, or genitals; or you develop a fever, headache, weakness, or swelling anywhere on your body. You may need oral medication.

An unpleasant rash that tends to recur and may or may not itch is **psoriasis** (page 344). A red patch covered by silvery scales, it most commonly occurs on the knees, elbows, lower back, and scalp. Although psoriasis can't be cured and may recur, your doctor can prescribe medications and perhaps ultraviolet light treatments that can speed healing.

A painful, blister-like rash that also may or may not itch can be caused by **shingles** (page 349). The condition most commonly occurs on the chest, stomach, or back. Pain may occur beneath the rash, in the abdomen, or along the spinal cord. You also may experience appetite loss, stomach upset, fatigue, fever, and chills. Shingles is caused by a virus. Although it can't be cured and may recur, your doctor can prescribe painkillers and medication to alleviate symptoms more quickly. Capsaicin is a topical analgesic cream that may provide pain relief after the lesions have healed.

If you have flaking from your scalp, you call it dandruff. Your doctor calls it **seborrhea** (page 348). In its more severe form, the scalp and sometimes the face and other parts of the body are covered with a greasy crusting and red scaling rash that may cause mild itching or a burning sensation. Mild dandruff can be controlled by twice-weekly washings with a commercial antidandruff shampoo. More severe cases warrant a doctor's care.

The most common cause of a nonitchy facial rash is the **acne vulgaris** (page 334) that afflicts adolescents and young adults. It is usually limited to blackheads and whiteheads, known as superficial acne. Don't pick or squeeze them, wash twice daily with an antibacterial soap, and use antiseptic creams or lotions containing benzoyl peroxide to help dry the pimples. More severe acne causes painful eruptions that look like large red boils and may spread to the neck, shoulders, upper chest, and back. This type of acne warrants medical attention.

Boils (page 337) are abscessed skin infections that cause painful red lumps that come to a pus-filled head and eventually burst. Clusters of boils are called carbuncles. Again, don't squeeze. Applying warm compresses can ease discomfort until the boil bursts and healing occurs. If the boil lasts longer than ten days or is near your eyes, call your doctor.

OTHER SKIN ABNORMALITIES

Skin has many normal variations that do not warrant treatment, but some changes can signal more serious problems.

Causes and Treatment of Other Skin Abnormalities

Moles (page 342) are pigmented benign skin growths that vary in color from brown to black and may be flat or slightly raised. Most are harmless, but

> If you develop any sore that bleeds or does not heal, or notice a change in the size or color of a lump or mole, or observe any new growth on your skin that is not explained by lifestyle causes discussed in this section or not described as normal, you might have **skin cancer** (page 350). Call your physician. Describe what is happening so that the doctor can decide whether you should be seen immediately.

some may be at risk of turning into a dangerous form of skin cancer known as malignant melanoma. If moles become irritated, bleed, cause itching or pain, or change in shape, color, or size, see a doctor immediately because skin cancer may be a possibility.

Warts (page 351) are painless benign tumors that are usually totally harmless. They vary from flat to slightly raised rough-textured growths that may match the skin or range in color from yellow to tan to gray. Warts in the genital area are pink or red and may grow in cauliflower-like clusters. Don't use over-the-counter wart removers because they can damage surrounding skin. Most warts can be ignored. They often disappear on their own within a year or two. The exceptions are plantar warts on the sole of the foot, which can be painful, and genital warts. Both warrant a visit to your doctor and prompt removal.

If your hands are extremely sensitive to cold, and the skin over the fingers seems to be becoming hard, thick, and sausage-like, perhaps with small ulcers forming at the fingertips, you may have **scleroderma** (page 346). This is a potentially very serious connective tissue disorder. Such symptoms merit comprehensive physical examination.

If you develop a nonitchy rash that ranges from a mild blush to red scaliness to severe blistering on your face, across the bridge of the nose, and on either side, you might have **systemic lupus erythematosus** (page 116). The rash is more likely to occur after even brief sun exposure and may be accompanied by fatigue, joint pain, and mild fever. This is another potentially very serious connective tissue disorder. See your doctor promptly.

HAIR LOSS

It is normal to lose some hair every day when you comb or brush, because hair constantly renews itself. Hair loss only becomes a problem if it is excessive and leaves bald patches or overall increased thinness.

> If you experience any persistent hair loss that cannot be explained by lifestyle causes discussed in this section, call your physician. Describe what is happening so that the doctor can decide whether you should be seen immediately.

Causes and Treatment of Hair Loss

The most common cause of hair loss is called male pattern baldness—a hereditary pattern of receding at the front hairline or thinning of hair at the top of the head. Women may also experience a hereditary pattern of hair loss, although it is more likely to occur as overall thinning rather than in just one or two areas. Such hair loss is usually gradual.

Although many unproven remedies for such hair loss are on the market, only a prescription drug called minoxidil has been shown to help slow this type of balding and, in some cases, reverse it. Chances of success correlate with your age, the length of time hair has been falling out, and the size of the balding area. A dermatologist can evaluate your hair loss and help you decide whether to try this drug.

Among women, hair loss is more likely to be caused by mechanical damage, such as frequent use of hair dye, permanents or straighteners, curling irons, hot rollers, ponytails, or cornrows. For example, hair rollers create a lot of tension on the hair and loosen the roots, resulting in patches of baldness. The same problem can be caused by tight braiding or pulling the hair tightly in a ponytail, and is often seen in children. Overly vigorous teasing or brushing, or frequent combing of wet hair with a fine-toothed comb can also result in loss of hair luster and flexibility. Changing your hair grooming methods usually allows your hair to recuperate and return to normal growth. However, if you persist in causing such damage, with time, the hair will not regrow.

Female hair loss may be caused by hormonal changes. It is not uncommon for women to experience hair thinning a few months after giving birth; hair thickness will soon return to normal. Some women also experience hair loss after menopause.

If you have had a severe illness with a high fever, you may experience significant hair loss a few months later. Because the fever may have halted new hair growth temporarily, hairs caught in that cycle will not regrow at their normal pace. This is a temporary result of the illness. Hair growth should return to normal within a few months.

If you are being treated with chemotherapy for cancer, temporary hair loss is very common. Anticancer drugs are designed to kill rapidly dividing cells, which describes both malignant cells and those in hair follicles. Hair will regrow after therapy ends.

Sudden hair loss in circular patches, in the absence of any other signs of scalp problems, is likely to be alopecia areata and can occur in adults and children. The cause of this condition is not certain, but it is believed that hereditary factors and stress may be involved. Although the hair usually grows back within six months to a year, your doctor may prescribe topical steroids to halt the damage and speed regrowth.

Sudden hair loss in small patches that are itchy and reveal scaly skin probably indicates a form of **ringworm** (page 345) called tinea capitis. If topical antifungal ointments don't help, consult your doctor. You may need oral prescription medication.

Gradual hair thinning, especially in women, can be a sign of **systemic lupus erythematosus** (page 116). If you also experience exhausting fatigue, joint pain, a blush or rash on the center of your face, and/or low-grade fevers, see your doctor for diagnosis and treatment.

COMMON DISORDERS OF THE SKIN AND HAIR

ACNE VULGARIS, usually called acne, is a disorder that causes a variety of skin eruptions, including red bumps, whiteheads, and blackheads. The severity varies markedly from one person to another—from occasional pimples that disappear by the end of adolescence to severe lesions that leave pitted scars and continue into adulthood. Acne has long been the scourge of adolescence, although new medications are now available to treat and, in some cases, cure acne.

What are the symptoms?
In the first stage, the hair follicle is simply blocked with oil and dead skin cells, which produces a blackhead whose dark surface is caused by chemical change in the material in the pore. In the second stage, bacteria in the follicle multiply, and the resulting inflammation leads to pus-filled white-heads. Both of these stages are called superficial acne. For most teenagers, that's the extent of the problem, with pimples limited to the face. If the pimples are not squeezed, picked, or scratched, permanent scarring is unlikely. For others, a third stage called deep, inflammatory acne develops.

The skin lesions are larger and the inflammation is deeper, with bacteria causing significant infection and inflammation in the underlying skin layers. This type of acne occurs on the face, neck, shoulders, upper chest, and back and can cause scarring. For some, an even worse stage known as cystic acne develops in which infections join together beneath the skin surface in small canals and pockets of pus. This type of acne can be physically painful.

How did I get it?
Acne usually begins at puberty when the level of androgen, a male sex hormone, rises in both males and females. This hormone stimulates increased production of sebum, an oily substance that lubricates the skin. Males usually have worse acne than females because they have more androgen. Acne starts in the hair follicles, which contain glands that produce sebum. If sebum is overproduced and becomes trapped in the follicle, the stage is set for acne. Heredity seems to play a role in the development of severe acne. Fried or fatty foods and sweets don't bring on acne. Sebum is manufactured locally on the skin and occurs even in those on fat-free diets.

How is it diagnosed?
Doctors usually can diagnose acne simply based on observation of the characteristic lesions.

How is it treated?
Most acne responds well to self-care. If your acne is more than superficial or if you find the pimples very distressing, see a dermatologist. Depending on your age, gender, and the severity of your acne, the doctor may prescribe stronger lotions to help unplug pores and cause mild peeling of blocked-skin layers; oral or topical tetracycline, an antibiotic that kills the bacteria inflaming the follicles; oral estrogen to counteract the hormone androgen, a therapy for women only; or oral or topical tretinoin, a derivative of vitamin A commonly known as Retin-A.

Self-Care: Don't pick or squeeze the pimples. Wash the skin gently twice a day with a soap containing antibacterial agents. Don't use a complexion brush or anything rough that will irritate the skin. Antiseptic creams or lotions that contain benzoyl peroxide also can help dry up the pimples.

ATHLETE'S FOOT is a harmless but uncomfortable fungal infection that causes foot rash. It is called athlete's foot because the underlying fungus is most apt to flourish in skin softened by perspiration, especially on the feet, as is common among people who participate in active sports. It is also known as ringworm of the feet or by its medical name, tinea pedis.

What are the symptoms?
Athlete's foot causes an itchy rash between the toes and on the soles or sides of the feet. The rash may be dry and scaly or wet and blistery. If not treated, the disorder can lead to cracks in the skin and painful open sores between and at the base of all toes. It can also infect the nails, which become thickened and discolored. Athlete's foot can occur elsewhere on the body because of fungal transfer, a problem that is most apt to occur in women. If you nick yourself while shaving your legs and then transfer the fungus from foot to leg with a towel, it may grow on dead hair in living tissue under the skin. The result is Majocchi's granuloma, which looks like little pustules on the skin.

How did I get it?
Athlete's foot is caused by a fungus, a tiny plant that does not contain chlorophyll. The fungus takes up residence on your skin and is nourished by absorbing dead, protein-rich material from the top layer of the skin. Athlete's foot occurs more often in warm weather, when you are apt to perspire. However, it can occur at any time of the year in people who sweat a lot. The fungus is highly contagious. You catch athlete's foot from another person by using his or her damp towel to dry your feet or even by walking on a damp surface where the infected person has walked. Walking around a pool or in the shower area of your health club without wearing shoes or slippers is inviting infection.

How is it diagnosed?
Most doctor's can spot athlete's foot by the characteristic lesions, as you may be able to do if you've had it before. Rarely, microscopic examination of a skin scraping is necessary.

How is it treated?
Use a topical over-the-counter antifungal agent, such as tolnaftate, clotri-mazole, or miconazole. Choose a cream for a dry eruption or a powder for a wet one. Apply the medication at least once a day after you wash your feet and scrupulously dry them. Use the agent more often if your feet get damp

during the day. Once fungi take up residence on your body, they can be difficult to get rid of unless you practice strict sanitary and self-care procedures. If you're not sure you have athlete's foot, or if you have had no improvement after a week of self-treatment, call your doctor. A stronger antifungal agent can be prescribed for skin application. If the condition still doesn't heal, oral medication may be recommended.

> Self-Care: Scrupulous self-care can often prevent athlete's foot as well as help cure it. Fungi cannot penetrate the skin when it is intact and dry; they grow best in dark, moist environments, such as between damp toes. Keep your feet clean and dry at all times. Don't wear the same pair of shoes everyday. Allow shoes to air and dry between wearing. In humid weather, change socks often. Always wear some type of footwear in moist areas, such as around pools and public showers. If you are prone to athlete's foot, use an antifungal powder daily, as well as before and after every exercise session.

BOILS are abscessed skin infections that usually begin in hair follicles. Their medical name is furuncles. If the infection spreads through small tunnels beneath the skin, the condition is called carbuncles.

What are the symptoms?
A boil causes a painful red lump that may range in size from a quarter of an inch to an inch and a half. Within a week or so, a pus-filled head slowly forms and eventually bursts. A carbuncle may look like a cluster of boils or just like a bumpy red area that is painful. It, too, forms a cluster of pus-filled heads that burst and heal, albeit more slowly. Although boils can arise anywhere, they most often occur on the neck, face, breast, and buttocks.

How did I get it?
Most boils are caused by bacterial infections, usually due to staphylococcal bacteria. These germs are a constant in our environment, so boils are very common. You are more apt to get them if you practice poor hygiene, if you are under stress, or if you have some illness that lowers your resistance to infection.

How is it diagnosed?
If you have ever had a boil, you are likely to be able to recognize a recurrence. Carbuncles may be difficult to differentiate from severe cystic acne, and they warrant a doctor's examination.

How is it treated?

Most boils respond to the self-care described below. Call your doctor if a boil or carbuncle lasts longer than ten days or if it is near your eyes. Your doctor may lance and drain the boil. Rarely, an antibiotic may be prescribed.

> Self-Care: Never squeeze or lance the boil yourself because you may only spread the infection. Apply warm compresses to the boil for five or ten minutes several times a day to ease discomfort and speed the bursting and healing process. Wash your hands carefully after touching the boil.

CORNS and **CALLUSES** are thickenings of the epidermis, the outer layers of the skin.

What are the symptoms?

Corns often grow over bony areas, such as the toe joints, and appear as small, tender, raised bumps with hard centers. They are usually less than an inch in diameter. Calluses grow in areas that experience repeated pressure or irritation, such as the knees, hands, or soles of the feet. They appear as rough, thickened patches of skin.

How did I get it?

Corns and calluses represent the body's defensive action. They form to protect the skin from recurrent irritation or pressure. The most common cause of corns and calluses are poorly fitting shoes.

How is it diagnosed?

You can usually spot corns and calluses yourself. If you have any condition, such as diabetes, that could complicate the problem, you may have to consult a physician.

How is it treated?

Most corns and calluses respond to self-care. If you have a corn or callus that does not do so or that causes discomfort, or if you have diabetes or poor circulation, which increase the risk of infection, see your doctor. Depending on the extent of the problem, the doctor may inject the area with cortisone to relieve inflammation or prescribe topical ointment to peel off the upper layers of the corn or callus.

Self-Care: Do not try to cut off corns or calluses. You may cause serious skin damage and infection. Try to remove the source of pressure that caused the problem—buy properly fitting shoes. Soak thickened areas in warm water, rub them with a pumice stone to remove dry skin, and then massage with a moisturizer to help soften the remaining skin.

ECZEMA is the medical term for a persistent itchy rash that often begins in infancy and may recur throughout life. It is also called atopic dermatitis.

What are the symptoms?
Infantile eczema usually begins at about two months of age, when red, itching, oozing, and crusting lesions occur on the face and scalp. The rash may worsen after immunizations and during teething, but it disappears in almost half of all patients between the ages of two and four. Eczema may continue in childhood or develop for the first time. At this age, the areas most severely afflicted are the creases in the elbows and behind the knees, where skin becomes brownish gray, dry, scaly, and thickened. Again, the problem may disappear only to arise again in adolescence or adulthood with similar symptoms that may also occur on the face, neck, and upper chest. Itching usually is worst at night. Although eczema usually ends by the age of 30, it persists throughout life in some people. People with chronic eczema also are at greater risk of having severe reactions to injections of penicillin and other drugs and vaccines.

How did I get it?
Eczema tends to run in families, suggesting a hereditary predisposition. The rash is believed to be some type of allergic reaction, although the precise cause varies from one person to the next and may not always be identifiable. Eggs, milk, seafood, wheat, and other foods, as well as wool clothing, are often involved. Temperature extremes, high humidity, or stress may also trigger flares.

How is it diagnosed?
You may be referred to a dermatologist who can diagnose eczema based on your personal and family medical history and examination of the rash. Allergy tests may also be performed to try to identify substances that contribute to your problem.

How is it treated?
Treatment varies, depending on the areas affected and the degree of itching. Avoid over-the-counter medications unless recommended by your doctor;

some contain benzocaine, lanolin, or petroleum jelly, which can make your problem worse. Doctors attempt to alleviate the itching—in order to break the itch-scratch-itch cycle—because scratching only worsens the rash. In addition to self-care, your doctor may prescribe ointments containing coal tar, selenium sulfide, or cortisone to decrease inflammation, oral antihistamines to help reduce itching, and, in the worst cases, oral cortisone to reduce inflammation. If scratching has caused bacterial infection, you may need antibiotics.

> Self-Care: If you or your doctor can identify any substances or situations that tend to trigger outbreaks of eczema, try to avoid them. Because soap will tend to dry the rash areas, use soap substitutes that do not remove skin oils. Wash with lukewarm, not hot, water, and use oil-free moisturizers after showering. Avoid sudden environmental temperature changes, and try to minimize going out in extremely hot or cold weather. Avoid fuzzy, rough, and woolen fabrics. Avoid working around dust, industrial chemicals, fumes, sprays, and solvents—all of which tend to aggravate eczema. Try to avoid exposing yourself to people who have colds. Upper respiratory infections can lower your body's resistance and aggravate your skin rash. Beware of people who have cold sores or other forms of herpes, because the viruses that cause them can provoke very serious—even life-threatening—eruptions of eczema.

HIVES, also known as urticaria, are an allergic skin disorder. Although hives are usually a minor but irritating problem, they may occasionally be a harbinger of potentially fatal anaphylactic or severe allergic reactions.

What are the symptoms?
Hives are raised pink or red round lesions called wheals. They are hot to the touch and itchy and have flat tops, ranging in size from a quarter of an inch to an inch and a half or larger. In more severe cases, called angioedema, the hives are larger, link up with one another, and penetrate more deeply into the skin. Rarely, hives in the esophagus can obstruct breathing or may be the first sign of a life-threatening anaphylactic reaction, which may be signaled by wheezing, pale skin, cold sweats, and a runny nose.

How did I get it?
Hives are most often caused by food allergies, the most common offenders being shellfish, nuts, eggs, chocolate, and fruits. Some people may also break

out in hives in response to contact with cats or other animals, insect bites, certain drugs, or even exposure to cold, heat, or sunlight. Less commonly, hives may be the first sign of viral infections, like hepatitis or mononucleosis, or of other serious disorders, such as lupus, lymphoma, or hyperthyroidism.

How is it diagnosed?

A doctor can diagnose hives simply by looking at them, and you will probably be able to do the same if you have them more than once. If you have recurrent hives and are unable to discern the cause, your doctor may perform a variety of skin tests to identify substances to which you are allergic. If no allergies are identified and you have persistent hives, more extensive testing will be necessary to find a possible underlying cause.

How is it treated?

Hives will disappear on their own within a few hours or days. If the cause is not obvious and you are taking any medication, call your doctor to ask about possible discontinuation. To ease the itchy discomfort, you can take an over-the-counter antihistamine. If hives are widespread and severe, your doctor may prescribe oral prednisone. If you develop any symptoms of an anaphylactic reaction, go to a hospital emergency room immediately. You may need urgent medication, such as epinephrine.

> Self-Care: If you have frequent bouts of hives, keep a food diary to try to identify—and then avoid—the foods to which you are allergic. Also discuss with your doctor whether you should carry epinephrine with you at all times; such self-medication can be lifesaving in those at risk for anaphylactic reactions.

IMPETIGO is a common but painless skin infection that is highly contagious. Although mild and easily cured in most people, it occasionally causes serious kidney inflammation.

What are the symptoms?

Impetigo causes a red rash with many small, itchy blisters, some of which contain pus. When the blisters break, yellow crusts form. Some people have a slight fever with impetigo.

How did I get it?

Impetigo is caused by streptococcal or staphylococcal bacteria. It can be caught either by direct contact with an infected person or by sharing washcloths, razors, or other personal grooming materials. You are at greater risk of infection if your resistance has been weakened by illness or fatigue or if you practice poor hygiene.

How is it diagnosed?
Your doctor will take a sample of cells from the sores for laboratory examination to diagnose impetigo.

How is it treated?
If the infection has been diagnosed early and affects only a very small area, the use of a prescription antibiotic ointment may be sufficient. However, in most cases, you will need a course of oral antibiotics, such as penicillin, taken for 10 to 14 days. In addition, your doctor may also recommend use of a nonprescription ointment containing bacitracin or neomycin. Rarely, impetigo infections may lead to inflammation of the kidneys, a serious condition that can be life threatening if not treated promptly.

Self-Care: Never use an over-the-counter cortisone cream on any skin rash that might be impetigo. Wash the rashy areas with antiseptic soap and gauze or paper towels, not a washcloth. Break open the blisters and remove crusting areas to expose and cleanse the lesions. Cover the sores with gauze to keep from touching or scratching them. The infected person's bed linens and any clothing that may have touched the sores should be washed separately in the hottest possible water. The affected person and other household members should take a daily bath in water with an antibacterial solution and take other precautions against contagion as prescribed by your doctor.

MOLES are pigmented, benign skin growths also known as nevi. Virtually everyone has a few moles, and some people have hundreds. They are usually harmless. However, some physicians believe that certain moles may be at risk of turning into a dangerous form of skin cancer known as malignant melanoma.

What are the symptoms?
Moles vary in color, from brown to black. Some are flat but do not darken or increase in number when exposed to the sun as freckles do. Others may be slightly raised or markedly elevated. Their texture may be smooth or rough, and some may have hair growing out of them.

How did I get it?
Moles form when, for unknown reasons, pigment cells cluster. It is believed that excessive sun exposure can sometimes convert some moles to cancerous growths.

How is it diagnosed?
A dermatologist can usually diagnose harmless moles simply by observation. If there is any suspicion of cancer, the mole can be removed for laboratory examination.

How is it treated?
Most moles require no treatment. However, if you want to get rid of a mole for cosmetic reasons, or if it is located in a spot where it is constantly rubbed or irritated, it can be removed surgically or with a laser.

Self-Care: Do not irritate moles by scratching, rubbing, or picking. Call your doctor if you notice any change in the shape, color, or size of a mole; it bleeds or develops a discharge; or it causes any itching or pain.

POISON IVY, OAK, and **SUMAC** are plants that, despite their names, are not poisonous. However, about 70 percent of people whose skin comes into contact with any of these plants, or whose clothing or other items have touched the plants, develop severe rashes.

What are the symptoms?
The rash may develop as soon as a few hours after exposure or as long as one to two weeks later. In most people it occurs within a day or two after plant contact. A red, itchy rash develops that leads to the formation of multiple blisters. Within a week, the blisters burst, oozing clear fluid. Crusts then form and the rash dries and usually disappears within another week or two.

How did I get it?
These plants have substances that cause the immune system to develop an allergic reaction. Antibodies formed by the body lead to the release of other body chemicals that provoke the rash.

How is it diagnosed?
Your doctor can usually diagnose these rashes by observing them, especially if you report that you have recently been in an area where you may have brushed against the causative plant.

How is it treated?
Most infections respond to self-care. Call your doctor if the itching becomes unbearable; the rash becomes painful or oozes pus; the rash is extensive or near your mouth, eyes, or genitals; you develop a fever, headache, weakness, or swelling anywhere on your body. You may need oral antihistamines or cortisone or antibiotics to treat any secondary infection.

> Self-Care: Try to prevent this uncomfortable rash by avoiding contact with poison ivy, oak, and sumac. Wear long pants when walking in wooded areas. If contact was made with your clothes, don rubber gloves to remove them and wash them in hot water with a strong detergent. If you have skin contact, washing off the chemicals with soap and water within five minutes may be able to prevent a skin reaction. If you develop a rash after known exposure to these plants, try to control the itching and swelling by applying an over-the-counter cortisone cream or calamine lotion.

PSORIASIS is a skin disease that causes a potentially disfiguring rash. More than one out of every 100 Americans suffers from psoriasis. It is more common among whites than blacks. It is rarely found in infants or the elderly, but affects people in almost every other age group, most commonly between ages 10 and 40.

What are the symptoms?
The rash is a red, scaly patch, with the affected area covered by silvery scales. It may or may not itch. Psoriasis most commonly occurs on the knees, elbows, lower back, and scalp, although it can occur anywhere on the body. In some people, the nails are pitted and grooved by psoriasis. The condition often recurs at unpredictable intervals.

How did I get it?
The cause of psoriasis is unknown. Although it seems to run in families, it is not contagious. It may be worse in the winter and is often precipitated or aggravated by physical or emotional stress, upper respiratory infections, and strep throat.

How is it diagnosed?
Your doctor can usually spot psoriasis by the characteristic skin lesions.

How is it treated?
Psoriasis cannot be cured. However, many creams, ranging from lubricants to topical corticosteroids, can be prescribed to help remove the scales and reduce the redness. Special baths and shampoos may be recommended. Some powerful medications, with potentially serious side effects, may be taken orally, but they are used only for severe psoriasis. Your doctor also may prescribe a program of sunbathing or carefully controlled exposure to an ultraviolet lamp. People with psoriasis may be at risk for a form of arthritis that comes and goes as the rash does. This can become a disabling disease if not medically treated.

> Self-Care: Beware of over-the-counter medicines unless recommended by your physician. Some promise miraculous cures but provide only dismal disappointment. Many are a waste of money and can delay your getting to a physician for proper treatment.

RINGWORM is a general term used for several fungal infections of the skin, scalp, and nails. The name is a misnomer because no "worm" is involved and the rash may not be circular. The medical term for these superficial fungal infections is tinea. The most common ones are tinea corporis, the classical ringworm of body skin; tinea capitis, which erupts on the scalp; tinea ungulum, also called onychomycosis, that attacks the toe- and fingernails; and tinea pedis, more commonly known as **athlete's foot** (page 336).

What are the symptoms?
Itching is the most common symptom on the body and scalp. In tinea corporis, round, scaly lesions that are clear in the center appear on the body; the raised circle grows larger as the fungus depletes the central "food supply" and spreads out. It occurs most commonly on the trunk of the body or the arms. In tinea capitis, hair breaks off, revealing little bald patches of scaling skin on the itchy scalp. In tinea ungulum, the toe- or fingernails become yellow and thicken, then crumbly and discolored.

How did I get it?
The infectious organism is a dermatophyte, literally, a skin fungus. Like their mushroom cousins, fungi prefer dark, moist environments in which to grow. They are ubiquitous in our environment, so you can pick them up almost anywhere, including from pets, other humans, and soil. Fungal infections

are particularly common among people involved in sports, because sweating softens the skin, making it easier for fungi to invade. For the same reasons, fungal infections are more common in hot summer weather. Once fungi invade your skin, they nourish themselves by absorbing the dead, protein-rich material called keratin that composes the outer layer of skin.

How is it diagnosed?

Your doctor can usually diagnose ringworm simply by observing the characteristic rash. If there is any doubt, a painless skin scraping provides scales for laboratory examination. In other cases, especially if the rash is on the scalp, the doctor may use a Wood's lamp, which emits ultraviolet light that causes some fungal infections to fluoresce with diagnostic colors.

How is it treated?

Most fungal infections are easily treated with topical antifungal creams. Tolnaftate, clotrimazole, and miconazole are successful drugs available over the counter. Although improvement will begin quickly, complete cure of even simple ringworm may require therapy for as long as a month. If you don't improve within a week of using such a product, call your doctor. More severe fungal infections may require either stronger, prescription topical medications or oral drugs, as is often the case with ringworm of the scalp. Topical drugs tend not to work on the scalp because the fungus has taken up residence in the hair follicles. Ringworm of the nails may take months to resolve completely.

> Self-Care: To help heal the infection and prevent new ones, lessen the moisture from perspiration in body folds by applying an antifungal powder in hot weather and before exercise sessions. Especially use powder under the arms and between the toes. After sweating, shower and dry skin carefully, applying powder again. Wear cotton socks and underwear, rather than synthetics, to absorb perspiration. Do not use other people's towels, washcloths, and hairbrushes.

SCLERODERMA literally means "hard skin." Although skin symptoms are the most obvious, this is a connective tissue disorder in the rheumatic family of diseases and can cause damage throughout the body. Also known as progressive systemic sclerosis, it most commonly develops in women between the ages of 30 and 50. Problems may be relatively mild in some people. In others, the condition may be limited to the skin, joints, and digestive system for many years. However, severe scleroderma involving the heart and kidneys can be fatal.

What are the symptoms?
The disease varies widely in severity and how it progresses. The first and most prominent symptoms affect the hands, which become extremely sensitive to cold and may turn white or bluish upon exposure to cold, a condition known as Raynaud's phenomenon. In addition, skin over the fingers becomes hard and thick, the fingers feel numb, and small skin ulcers develop at the fingertips. Skin all over the body may harden and thicken, with facial skin becoming tight and losing its elasticity. Arthritis problems, including pain, stiffness, and swelling, may affect joints throughout the body. Also common are digestive symptoms, including difficulty in swallowing, indigestion, heartburn, feeling as if food is stuck in the chest, bloating after eating, and weight loss. Muscle aches, weakness, and fatigue may also occur. In the most severe cases, the heart, kidneys, and lungs are damaged.

How did I get it?
Scleroderma is believed to be an autoimmune disease in which the body turns against itself and destroys its own connective tissue as if it were an outside invader. Although a genetic predisposition may be inherited, what triggers the destructive course is unknown.

How is it diagnosed?
If scleroderma is suspected, you will probably be referred to a rheumatologist for extensive tests. Depending on what parts of your body are affected, these may include blood and urine tests, taking a sample of affected skin for laboratory examination, chest X-rays, and lung function tests.

How is it treated?
Scleroderma cannot be cured. Depending on your symptoms, you may be given drugs to dilate blood vessels, lower blood pressure, or alleviate heartburn. To slow progression of the disease, you may be given immunosuppressive drugs. Nonsteroidal anti-inflammatory drugs may be given to ease arthritis symptoms. You may also be referred to a physical therapist to learn simple exercises and other techniques to help maintain skin and joint flexibility and enhance circulation.

Self-Care: Try to avoid anything that will constrict your blood vessels, such as smoking and exposure to cold weather. If you have digestive problems, eat several small meals rather than three large ones. Chew carefully and drink plenty of fluids with your meal. Learn biofeedback techniques that can help enhance circulation in your hands and feet.

SEBORRHEA is the medical term for a range of skin problems characterized by excessive flaking or scaling of skin, most commonly on the scalp. In its mildest form, the disorder is known as dandruff. In its worst form, it is called seborrheic dermatitis.

What are the symptoms?
Dandruff is characterized by white flakes of dry skin shedding from the scalp. In seborrheic dermatitis, the entire scalp and sometimes the face and other parts of the body are covered with a greasy crusting and red scaling condition of the skin. In either form, seborrhea may also cause a mild itching or burning sensation.

How did I get it?
Although the underlying cause is unknown, the skin flaking is due to excessive turnover of the cells that form the outer layer of the skin. The skin constantly renews itself, with the top layers falling away. Normally, such dead cells are barely visible and, on the scalp, fall away during regular shampooing and brushing. However, in seborrhea, the cells age too rapidly and too many keratin cells are pushed to the surface—so they come off in large visible flakes. The condition may be aggravated by stress.

How is it diagnosed?
You can spot the light flakes of dandruff on your shoulders when you wear dark clothes. However, if you have anything more than mild dandruff, or if it does not respond to a few weeks of self-care, see your doctor. You may have seborrheic dermatitis or another condition with similar symptoms, such as psoriasis, eczema, or lupus.

How is it treated?
The severity of your seborrhea will determine treatment beyond the self-care measures discussed below. Your doctor also may prescribe scalp lotions to help loosen the scales. If itching and inflammation are part of your problem, a cortisone solution or cream may be prescribed for use several times a day. Once the inflammation is under control, you will probably need to use this cortisone treatment once a day for an extended period of time to keep the inflammation from coming back.

Self-Care: Mild dandruff can be controlled by twice-weekly washings with a commercial antidandruff shampoo. Brush your hair for about five minutes before shampooing to get rid of excess flakes. If your scalp is oily, choose a drying shampoo containing sulfur; after shampooing, use a rinse of one cup of lukewarm water containing the juice of one lemon. Then rinse with cool water. If your scalp is dry, choose a shampoo containing zinc pyrothione; before shampooing, massage a warm lanolin lotion or cream into your scalp and wrap your head in a hot, wet towel for 15 minutes. If your scalp is normal, more frequent brushing and daily shampoos may be sufficient to control your dandruff.

SHINGLES is the common name for a skin disorder that doctors call herpes zoster. The most noticeable indicator is a painful rash. Although anyone can get shingles at any age, it is more prevalent and more severe in older people.

What are the symptoms?
Shingles causes tingling skin sensations, pain, itching, and a blister-like rash. The rash most commonly occurs on the chest, stomach, or back, usually extending in a line and almost always on one side of the body only. Pain may be experienced beneath the rash, in the abdomen, or along the spinal cord. In addition, some people experience loss of appetite, stomach upset, fatigue, fever, and chills. Rarely, it may attack facial nerves and cause vision or hearing problems.

How did I get it?
Shingles is caused by the varicella virus, the same virus that causes chickenpox. It is believed that the virus remains dormant in the body after a childhood chickenpox infection. Why it reemerges years later to cause shingles in some people is unknown. It may be triggered by stress, aging, or some illness. The virus can attack nerve roots anywhere in the body, from head to toe, leading to a rash along the path of the involved nerve.

How is it diagnosed?
Early diagnosis can be difficult if only pain, tingling sensations, fever, and fatigue occur. However, once the blisters appear, your doctor usually can diagnose shingles by the characteristic lesions.

How is it treated?
Shingles cannot be cured and may recur. Usually, the condition disappears within a few weeks but, in some people, it may linger for months or years. The best odds for rapid healing come from early treatment. Depending on the severity of the attack, your doctor may prescribe soothing lotions to help dry up the blisters, steroid medications to shorten the period of inflammation, analgesics for severe pain, or antibiotics if secondary infection occurs. If you have a very severe attack, or if your immune system is weakened by cancer or other diseases, you may be given an antiviral drug to speed healing.

> Self-Care: Take aspirin or ibuprofen to reduce inflammation, and apply cool, wet compresses to ease discomfort. Get plenty of rest, and try to avoid stress.

SKIN CANCER is the most common of all cancers and often the most curable, if found and treated in time. Unfortunately, because skin cancer is so common, many people underestimate its potential seriousness. The most common type is basal cell cancer; although it can penetrate deep into the skin, it is highly curable if diagnosed and treated promptly. The second most common type is squamous cell cancer; it too is highly curable if found early but can be deadly if it spreads to other parts of the body. Far less common, but much more threatening, is malignant melanoma, which is apt to spread rapidly and be fatal within months if not diagnosed in its earliest stages.

What are the symptoms?
Skin cancer usually occurs on sun-exposed surfaces of the body, such as the face, neck, and arms. Be suspicious of any sore that bleeds or doesn't heal; a change in the size or color of a lump or mole; or any new growth on your skin. Basal cell cancer most often appears as small, rough lumps that are raised and have a waxy appearance. There may be a sore or ulcer present that seems not to heal over a period of time. Squamous cell cancer occurs not only on the skin but also on the lips, the lining of the mouth, and the tongue. Malignant melanoma may begin as a common birthmark or mole. If such a lesion starts to darken in color, itch, bleed, or enlarge, the change may signal melanoma.

How did I get it?
Most skin cancer is caused by too much exposure to the sun. However, industrial workers who are exposed to certain chemicals can have skin cancer, as can people who are overexposed to radiation. Squamous cell

cancer of the lower lip is also more common in pipe smokers and those with poor oral hygiene.

How is it diagnosed?
Your doctor may suspect cancer simply by observing the lesion. However, to confirm the diagnosis, a small piece of skin must be removed and studied under the microscope. If squamous cell cancer or melanoma is diagnosed, your doctor probably will recommend further tests to determine whether it has spread to other parts of your body.

How is it treated?
If the cancer was small and fully removed to take the biopsy sample, no further treatment may be needed. If it has penetrated the skin more deeply, surgical removal of the cancer is usually essential. Small cancers may be removed in your doctor's office, with local anesthesia, by freezing or laser destruction. Rarely, radiation may be used to kill the cancer cells. Very early basal cell cancers may be treated by applying a drug called 5-fluoracil to the skin. If skin cancer has spread to other parts of the body, chemotherapy may be required.

> Self-Care: Those who spend a lot of time outdoors should be very careful of sun exposure. Fair-skinned, fair-haired, blue-eyed people should take extra precautions. Everyone who is out in the sun should use sunscreen lotions rated 24 or higher. Also consider wearing a hat, long sleeves, and pants. Particularly avoid prolonged exposure between 11 A.M. and 2 P.M., when the sun is strongest. Deliberate tanning, with either natural or artificial sunlight, increases the risk of skin cancer and also prematurely ages the skin.

WARTS are benign (noncancerous) tumors that are painless and usually totally harmless. However, women who have had genital warts are at greater risk for cancer of the cervix and vulva and should have regular Pap tests.

What are the symptoms?

• *Common*, or *vulgar*, *warts*, the most frequently seen, are raised, rough-textured growths that start out skin-colored and eventually turn yellow to gray with age. They vary in size from a pinhead to a large mass and grow singly or in clusters. They often occur on fingers, hands, and soles of the feet.
• *Flat*, or *plane*, *warts* are smooth, flesh-colored or tan, slightly elevated

growths. They are usually less than a quarter-inch in size, appearing primarily on the face and hands.

• *Plantar warts* are similar to flat ones but appear on the soles of the feet; they may cause pain when walking.

• *Genital warts*, also called *condylomata*, are pink or red growths that range from isolated bumps, to elongated ridges, to cauliflower-like clusters. They may grow externally in the genital region or around the anus or inside the vagina or rectum. They may cause itching.

How did I get it?

Warts are caused by papilloma viruses that are spread by direct contact. The virus tends to enter the skin or mucous membrane through any small cut or abrasion. Genital warts are highly contagious and are transmitted during sexual relations. People who have allergies or suppressed immune systems are at greater risk of developing warts.

How is it diagnosed?

Doctors usually can differentiate warts from other growths simply by examination. Vaginal warts may be discovered only during a pelvic examination when a vinegar wash is applied. In some cases, particularly with genital warts, a sample of the wart may be taken for laboratory examination to make sure it is not some other type of growth.

How is it treated?

Treatment depends on the type of wart and its location. Doctors often urge that warts be left alone because they tend to disappear on their own within a year or two. If a wart appears on the face or otherwise disturbs you, or if a plantar wart becomes painful, removal is appropriate. A dermatologist may do so by using liquid nitrogen or an electric needle to destroy the wart or, in the case of plantar warts, by a multistep process using acid applications. Genital warts may be removed with applications of a chemical called podophyllin or by liquid nitrogen, lasers, or surgery. If you have multiple warts that proliferate, oral drugs may be prescribed. Unfortunately, warts often recur at the same location.

Self-Care: Never use over-the-counter wart removers. They may damage surrounding skin. Don't pick at warts, because you may then spread the virus—and the warts—to other parts of your body. If you have had genital warts, use a condom during sexual relations to avoid spreading the virus to your partner; certain types of the virus may cause squamous cell cancer of the cervix or penis.

Index

(Page numbers in **boldface** refer to main discussions of common disorders.)

WITHDRAWN